Globalizing Feminist Bioethics

Globalizing Feminist Bioethics

Crosscultural Perspectives

Rosemarie Tong

with
Gwen Anderson
Aida Santos

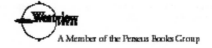

A Member of the Perseus Books Group

Copyright © 2000 by Westview Press, A Member of the Perseus Books Group

Published in 2000 in the United States of America by Westview Press, 5500 Central Avenue, Boulder, Colorado 80301-2877, and in the United Kingdom by Westview Press, 12 Hid's Copse Road, Cumnor Hill, Oxford OX2 9JJ

Find us on the World Wide Web at www.westviewpress.com

A CIP catalog record for this book is available from the Library of Congress
ISBN 0-8133-6615-1

The paper used in this publication meets the requirements of the American National Standard for Permanence of Paper for Printed Library Materials Z39.48-1984.

10   9   8   7   6   5   4   3   2   1

Contents

Part 3

Medical Research and Treatment

Tables and Figures

Acronyms

ACTG	AIDS Clinical Trials Group
BDPA	Beijing Declaration and Platform for Action
CEDAW	Convention on the Elimination of All Forms of Discrimation Against Women
CIOMS	Council for International Organizations of Medical Sciences
EMEA	European Agency for the Evaluation of Medicinal Products
FAB	International Network on Feminist Approaches to Bioethics
FDA	Federal Drug Administration
GDI	Gender-Related Development Index
GEM	Gender Empowerment Measure
HHRP	Health and Human Rights Project: Professional Accountability in South Africa
ICH	International Conference on Harmonisation
ICPD	International Conference on Population and Development
ICSI	intracytoplasmic sperm injection
IRRRAG	International Reproductive Rights Research Action Group
IVF	in vitro fertilization
MASA	Medical Association of South Africa
NIH	National Institutes of Health
NRT	new reproductive technology
RWS	Race Welfare Society
SADF	South African Defence Force
STD	sexually transmitted disease
TRC	Truth and Reconciliation Commission
UAGA	Uniform Anatomical Gift Act
UNAIDS	United Nations Program on HIV/AIDS
WPRO	WHO Regional Office for the Western Pacific

Acknowledgments

This anthology is the result of an exceptionally large team effort. If we have inadvertently neglected to praise or praise adequately a contributor, we beg her or his understanding. Among the individuals most responsible for this book's coming to press are Nancy M. Williams, Kristin Garris, and Paul S. M. Tong. Nancy, who will leave UNC–Charlotte next year to pursue a Ph.D. in philosophy, served as the co-coordinator of the book's entire writing team. Without her help, the project might have collapsed. Enormously talented, Nancy is also generous with her limited time. It was a pleasure to work with such a gifted young feminist philosopher, who will be helping develop feminist thought for many a year to come.

Much credit is also due to Kristin Garris, who brought her editorial skills to the project and sacrificed most of her weekends to further the book's progress. Similar kudos are due to Paul S. M. Tong, who managed to bring formatting unity to a set of documents that each seemed to speak a different language.

We also wish to thank our advisory board: Nikola Biller, Julien S. Murphy, Leslie Bender, and Cynthia Cassell. In addition, we wish to thank our respective institutions, particularly the University of North Carolina–Charlotte for extra secretarial support. We also wish to applaud Sarah Warner, Elizabeth Twitchell, Lori Hobkirk, and Chrisona Schmidt, our magnificent copy editor, for their patience, support, encouragement, and hard work on our behalf. Finally, we wish to thank the International Network on Feminist Approaches to Bioethics (FAB) for bringing the contributors of the book together—for inspiring them to speak to each other and to work together. In particular, we owe much to Anne Donchin and Becky Holmes, without whom FAB would not be the thriving, vibrant, meaningful organization it is.

Rosemarie Tong, principal editor
Gwen Anderson, coeditor
Aida Santos, coeditor

Introduction

ANNE DONCHIN

From its inception in 1992, the International Network on Feminist Approaches to Bioethics (FAB) has aimed to truly internationalize bioethics: to rectify the sweeping disregard of women's health care issues within mainstream bioethics literature and to build a nonhierarchical, nonelitist, geographically diverse grassroots movement with a collaborative structure that is open to all—academics and professionals, health care activists, and concerned groups in all fields. This anthology builds on a previous collection of essays inspired by the initial 1996 FAB conference.[1] The introduction to that collection includes a brief history of the network and its aims. As Laura Purdy and I edited that collection, we became aware of the need to encourage further work that addressed the global dimensions of feminist bioethics. So for the 1998 FAB conference in Japan we sought funding to assure representation of a broad cross-section of feminist theorists and activists. Through the generosity of the Ford Foundation we were able to secure a grant to fund the travel of fifteen participants from developing countries. Their presence considerably enriched cross-fertilization of feminist perspectives and facilitated further collaboration across geographical boundaries. Briefer versions of the essays by Ford recipients appeared in the May 1999 issue of FAB's newsletter.

The essays that are included as chapters in this volume transcend the usual dichotomies dividing the contemporary world into developed/developing economies and technological/nontechnological societies, addressing a broad array of concerns pertinent to projects in feminist bioethics and paving new ground at the intersection of the feminist and human rights movements. Several overriding themes predominate. Science, a number of contributors note, has become a collective international project, but the world community has yet to learn how to utilize scientific developments responsibly. Dominant Western technological practices tend increasingly to cross geographical boundaries and extend their ten-

1

tacles into developing economies, often appropriating morally dubious Western technological practices and diverting scarce resources from basic health care services. A number of authors stress the need to educate policymakers and local leaders about both harmful traditional practices such as clitoridectomy and modes of transmission of newly proliferating diseases such as AIDS. The principles stressed by Wan Jin-ling in her paper on AIDS and prostitution in mainland China feature prominently in the work of the anthology authors. She urges policymakers to institute reforms based on respect for the human dignity of all people, promotion of distributive justice across all groups, and education to increase all people's opportunities for freedom and well-being.

Part 1: Theoretical Perspectives

The chapters in Part 1 focus explicitly on the need to reconceptualize mainline bioethical theory to address the intersection of local and global concerns. Both Susan Sherwin and Rosemarie Tong point to tensions between specific cultural practices and features of our common humanity that override geographical, cultural, and racial difference, most conspicuously childbirth, illness, disability, and death. But, Sherwin warns, universal value commitments that have emerged out of particular historical and geographical locations, as well as an exclusive focus on global features of the human condition, can obscure the continuing operation of power relations. Dominant cultures, she cautions, tend to be oblivious to the reality of alternative moral systems, particularly those that privilege personal autonomy over group values. She proposes three ways of understanding the role of moral theories in bioethics that need not abstract from such particulars: as metaphors displacing foundationalism (which is, after all, an architectural metaphor); as frameworks that may appeal to different moral theories depending on the particular dimensions of the project we seek to illuminate; and as lenses that allow us to view a culture's practice in multiple ways and address problems that might not lend themselves to global solution. She favors the lens metaphor as the one that provides the best moral clarification of both local and global issues. Her reconceptualization is particularly evocative when read in conjunction with several other articles included here, such as Loretta Kopelman's discussion of ethical relativism and female circumcision.

In Chapter 3 Gwen Anderson, Rita Monsen, and Mary Rorty address the changing work of the nursing profession, particularly in light of the growing proliferation of genetic interventions, and argue for redirection of institutional policies. They enumerate several global forces that will increase future demand for genetic services. Two of these also feature prominently in other chapters in this collection that address expanding world population (Alexander) and the spiraling impact of Western medicine on developing economies (Diniz). At the intersection of these forces is a third factor: the expansion of global data collection facilities and increasing utilization of new genetic diagnostic tools. Drawing largely on the U.S. experience, in which nurses lack an institutionalized role as providers of genetic services, Anderson, Monsen, and Rorty argue for new transdisciplinary models of nursing-patient relationships that will speak to these issues. Their concerns about the need for reforms in genetic services intersect several other contributions included here, most notably Chapter 5, by Debora Diniz and Ana Cristina González Vélez on bioethics in Brazil, and Chapter 14, by Fernanda Carneiro and her colleagues calling for transformation of the relationship between geneticists and their clients.

Chapter 4, Leonardo de Castro's sensitive study of a central concept in Filipino bioethics, draws its examples from another area of health care services (organ transplant), yet her commitment to advancing concerned and caring social relationships overlaps values underlying the aims of Anderson and her collaborators. De Castro painstakingly explains how *kagandahang loob* (roughly translated, a deed motivated from within) functions in Filipino social relations. She draws analogies between this concept and Nel Nodding's moral orientation and contrasts this moral discourse to the dominant Western beneficence ethic. The concluding chapter in this section, Chapter 5, by Debora Diniz and Ana Cristina González Vélez, considers the influence of the principlist formulation of bioethical theory in the United States on the development of bioethics in Brazil and other "peripheral bioethics countries." They critique the practice of unreflectively importing theories and practices from countries in the center of medical developments to countries at the periphery, as though biomedical theory and its applications could be relocated to a different culture without modification. Feminist bioethics, they argue, provides the conceptual apparatus to unmask this error by exposing both the roots of the principlist bioethics framework in middle-class culture and the power imbalances among providers and patients, asymmetries that are likely to intensify in developing countries.

Part 2: Reproductive, Genetic, and Sexual Health

Though feminists have written prolifically on reproductive issues, both the burgeoning development of ever more exotic technologies and the disclosure of non-Western women's experiences (evident in this volume) motivate further interpretive analysis. In Chapter 6 Vangie Bergum and Mary Bendfeld challenge the supposed universality of the pregnancy experience by exploring the different ways in which cultures shape the subjective consciousness of pregnant women in accord with their world-views. Drawing on prior feminist scholarship, they show how expectant mothers are constructed as objects of the medical gaze in dualistic Western technological cultures. Nondualistic cultures, on the other hand, tend to regard pregnant women and their fetuses as an organic whole and give broader play to the felt dimensions of pregnancy. Bergum and Bendfeld argue, however, that neither worldview is adequate to resolve the dilemmas that surface when women consider pregnancy termination. The organic model reduces women to their functions, denies the intentionality of individuals' actions, and leads to characterizations of infertile women as defective. The technological model leads to self-objectification. The visual image of the fetus becomes more "real" than the felt experience. Thus neither model is able to capture the conditions leading a woman to decide to end her pregnancy. Bergum and Bendfeld's analysis is particularly insightful if read in conjunction with Chapter 9 by Naoko Miyaji on contraception in Japan and Chapter 10 by Jing-Bao Nie on abortion in the People's Republic of China.

In Chapter 7 Susan Sherwin addresses a broad array of reproductive interventions, both old and new, and critically scrutinizes the social contexts in which they have been introduced. She documents how technologies created to meet specific needs quickly tend to become normalized and are incorporated into routine medical practice. She calls for the adoption of a relational model of autonomy that recognizes the complexity of relations between persons and their culture. Such a conception is needed, she insists, both to make visible the ways social norms tend to condition individual preferences and to explain why the expression of an informed preference may not be an adequate measure of autonomous choice. In Chapter 8 Jurema Werneck and her collaborators within the black Brazilian feminist movement reiterate in a distinctive voice some of Sherwin's concerns about the capacity of new technologies to undermine women's autonomy. In less developed economies the means available to women to control their fertility are often less effective than those available in more developed economies. Under pressure by northern commercial interests, surgical sterilization (though technically illegal) is commonly performed, particularly on indigenous black women. Only upper-class women are offered the array of new reproductive technologies available to women in developed countries. The authors show that within the impersonal apparatus of this institutional world, people are rendered anonymous, are effectively deprived of their autonomy, and are forced to chose among "technologic market options." Within this cultural milieu the desire for a child is transformed into a demand for "child-merchandise." They call for a broader bioethics that addresses the reality of poor countries and the issues they face—child abandonment, lack of social support for mothers and children, high maternal mortality, and the burdens of poverty. They plead for courageous reflection among feminists in both North and South to reconfigure the desire for a child to encompass the needs of existing, often abandoned, children.

Turning to women's condition in Japan, in Chapter 9 Naoko Miyaji exposes the need for legal reforms to force men to share the burdens of unwanted pregnancy with women equally. In virtually all cultures, she argues, unwanted pregnancy perpetuates women's subordinate status. She argues that women who consent to sex while assuming that their partner is protecting them from pregnancy are subjected to a force similar to that experienced by rape victims. If men were made responsible for contraception, the incidence of unwanted pregnancy would be considerably lower. Drawing on major international documents, she proposes legal sanctions against men who fail to take adequate contraceptive measures. Her argument challenges traditional perceptions of contraception as predominantly a women's responsibility. Read in conjunction with Vangie Bergum and Mary Ann Bendfeld's discussion of the history of official Japanese resistance to oral contraception, Miyaji's proposal takes on added urgency. The Japanese government, they explain, deliberated for nine years before finally approving the use of the birth control pill in 1999. Governmental delay meant that many women had no choice but to opt for abortion, a practice prohibited to practicing Buddhists. A ritual called *mizuko kuyo* was developed to acknowledge women's continuing memory of their fetus and heal the broken connection. During my own stay in Japan I asked about the red scarves draped around many statues on the precincts of Buddhist temples. In halting English a guide told me that they had been placed there by women mourning their lost "little ones."

In Chapter 10 Jing-Bao Nie extends the discussion of abortion within the context of social policy in mainland China. Though many Westerners assume the "one child" policy leaves women the option of remaining childless, Nie points out that, paradoxically, bearing a *healthy* child remains the number one duty for women in Chinese society. The policy restricting the number of children does not free women from the social obligation to bear children altogether. Evident also in his discussion of women's subjective abortion experiences is the Chinese government's reliance on Western technological practices to enforce that policy. Nie's narratives of Chinese women's abortion experiences are reminiscent of Carol Gilligan's famous abortion study, which also testifies to the complexity and diversity of women's subjective responses within a seemingly homogeneous cultural context.

Chapter 11 by Mary Mahowald and Chapter 12 by William Alexander converge on issues surrounding the recent explosion of genetic knowl-

edge and resulting implications for technological development. Mahowald's discussion of the use of sex selection technologies across considerable cultural differences grapples with the central question raised
by Jing-Bao Nie: how to reconcile cultural norms with respect for the autonomy of individual citizens. Nie's chapter provides a test case for the
kind of egalitarian feminist standpoint Mahowald defends. William
Alexander's study of the disproportionate number of males in the population of some developing economies serves as a grim reminder, however, that although social practices favoring male offspring may be facilitated by technological innovation, they can be advanced just as readily
by such nontechnical measures as selectively withholding basic health
care and nutrition from girl children.

Unlike the systems of sex selection that frame Mahowald's and
Alexander's thinking, the social implications that will follow the development of human cloning technologies are still open to conjecture. In
Chapter 13 Julien Murphy applies an interesting historical phenomenon
that Sartre labeled "counterfinality" to speculation about the implications of cloning. This occurs when a human intervention produces results
contrary to the intended aim. Historic examples include deliberately
flooding farmland to maximize growth and production, which in China
actually resulted in deforestation of land, and intentionally hoarding
gold, which in Spain ultimately reduced its price by deflating monetary
values. So cloning would free gay men and women from dependence on
gamete donors but could unintentionally undermine freedom by reinforcing social prejudice against gays and bolstering deterministic clichés
about sexual orientation.

The study performed by Fernanda Carneiro and her colleagues on genetic counseling for breast cancer, described in Chapter 14, carries one
facet of Murphy's theme forward with great immediacy. Their focus on
the medical and social values embedded in genetic counseling as practiced in Brazil exposes the underside of a technology that purports to free
women to make autonomous decisions but, within specific social contexts, can actually intensify geneticists' dominance over them. In Chapter
15, in her discussion of moral relativism and female circumcision, Loretta
Kopelman extends the dialogue on the relevance of social context in evaluating interventions. She argues that conventionalist approaches to com-
bating genital mutilation (applying norms accepted within that culture)
do not accomplish what they set out to do. The practice of female genital
surgery, condemned by UNICEF, WHO, and AMA, among others, is
widely considered a form of child abuse. Her argument defends the
moral authority of intercultural judgments and raises searching questions about both the overlapping boundaries of cultures in today's global
economy and the limits of any specific culture's moral authority. Her cri-

tique of moral relativism extends and amplifies the primary concerns Mahowald raises in the context of the sex selection practices of diverse cultures.

Wang Jin-Ling presents astonishing data in Chapter 16 about the spread of HIV/AIDS in mainland China. The dominant route of transmission has been misrepresented (most cases are transmitted through blood supply and IV drug use). Yet policymakers continue to target the commercial sex trade, a blindness that the author attributes to cultural bias against women, who are stereotyped as seductresses preying on weak men. The moralizing official policy is ineffective, she argues. A more realistic policy is needed that stresses condom use (currently rarely employed), particularly in the commercial sex trade, rectifies gender inequities in AIDS prevention and control, reconceptualizes AIDS as an occupational disease, and provides education to commercial sex workers, who are often impoverished and illiterate.

Part 3: Medical Research and Treatment

The chapters in Part 3 offer feminist analyses of troubling moral quandaries in medical research. In Chapter 17 Nadine Taub tackles the knotty issue of including women in clinical drug trials. She argues that policies in both the United States and the European Union that bar women from participating in the early stages of drug development fail to give consumers the right to decide, instead imposing state-mandated authority. No such limitations are forced on men, she notes, though potential exposure to or ingestion of, say, carcinogens by men can also affect any future child. She urges including women in all phases of trials, as well as initiatives by international bodies to harmonize policies. The issue she confronts has direct application to the conduct of AZT drug trials on HIV-positive pregnant women in sub-Saharan Africa, which is Florencia Luna's topic in Chapter 18. Luna confronts head-on the conflict between universal and local research norms and problematizes the risk-benefit assessment employed by those who designed these trials. Had the women research subjects in these trials been granted the opportunity to assess risks and benefits, would they have come up with the same results as the "outsiders" who designed the study? She considers alternative policies for enhancing the social equality and self-determination of the women subjects and explores several decisionmaking processes that aspire to democratic norms. Assessing the strengths of human rights appeals to mandate uniform standards across cultures, she notes the enormous difficulties involved in implementing such standards. Lisa Eckenwiler, in Chapter 19, also focuses attention on the inadequacy of prevailing models of research design and the need for more adequate models that promote gender equality and democratize decisionmaking. She urges a participatory model that includes actual women who will be affected by the outcome of a trial in the design, review, and funding of clinical research.

In Chapter 20 Carol Quinn turns to the global implications of using data gleaned from flagrantly unethical experiments performed on inmates in Nazi death camps. She draws analogies between uses of Nazi data and data based on the Tuskegee syphilis studies and the Willowbrook hepatitis studies in the United States. Her essay adds an additional dimension to an issue at the locus of Eckenwiler's and Luna's chapters. She effectively shifts the terms of the mainline bioethics debate about legitimate uses of such data to the question of who should have the authority to make such decisions—researchers or victims. She urges adoption of the victim's standpoint and recommends giving victims control over the use of ill-gotten data, thereby restoring their lost dignity and aiding their healing. To ignore their perspective, she argues, is to continue to treat them as objects, which further intensifies the harms they have already suffered.

In Chapter 21 Kathleen Kurtz considers organ transplantation, a topical issue initially raised by Leonardo de Castro in her discussion of bioethical values in Filipino society. Kurtz, however, turns the discussion to allocation issues and their moral implications: questions of justice, fear of death, and the need for dialogue in determining policy—a theme that intersects Eckenwiler's discussion of clinical research policies.

Finally, in Chapter 22 Jeanelle de Gruchy and Laurel Baldwin-Ragaven relate the horrific tale of the violation of women's rights in apartheid South Africa and lay bare the collusion between South African physicians and apartheid patriarchy. They show how apartheid corrupted health services and the training of health professionals. Several examples illustrate how medical personnel actively subverted professional and human rights principles, using their power to develop and implement nonvoluntary sterilization programs. The struggle against such abuses will not end, they caution, until a culture of respect for human rights replaces the racist and sexist constructions of black women that medical professionals used to justify their practices. Their chapter picks up the strands of Carol Quinn's discussion in Chapter 20 insofar as abuses suffered by South Africans at the hands of medical authorities parallel experiments carried out by Nazi doctors in the World War II death camps. Both atrocities serve as continuing reminders of the flagrant abuses that are possible when medical power runs amuck and colludes with oppressive state power.

Many of the contributors included here offer novel strategies to interject women's standpoints into policymaking processes and transform bioethics and medical practice in ways that will heighten responsiveness to the situation of women and other marginalized groups. Several stress programmatic themes that feminist bioethicists need to work out more systematically in the future. Feminists in both developed and developing economies stress the need to transcend individualistic biases that so often pervade masculinist formulations of bioethics and the representation of women's perspectives conveyed within them. In feminist writing cultural differences often seem to relate to specific topical issues rather than underlying values. In affluent countries debates tend to cluster around issues at the cutting edge of technology, but in poorer countries "everyday" issues loom larger. And all point to the need to listen to one another across cultural boundaries, to fully respect the local knowledges that inform our perspectives, and to attend to the full complexity of our diverging and intersecting identities. As Barbara Nicholas so persuasively points out in the initial FAB volume, we need to continue to hear stories of transformative strategies that have worked—stories by women near the centers of power and by those at the margins.[2] Only through such continuing dialogue can we hope to interject feminist concerns into the dominant discourses and practices that define the norms of medicine and health care delivery services.

Notes

1. Anne Donchin and Laura Purdy, eds., *Embodying Bioethics: Recent Feminist Advances* (Lanham, Md.: Rowman & Littlefield, 1999).
2. Ibid., p. 249.

PART ONE

Theoretical Perspectives

1

Feminist Reflections on the Role of Theories in a Global Bioethics

SUSAN SHERWIN

From the beginning of their reflections, bioethicists have been uneasy in their relationship to moral theories. They have felt the attraction of comprehensive moral theories as a way of systematizing moral knowledge, providing their work with theoretical legitimacy and coherence and offering a logical methodology for investigating the hard cases they confront. On the other hand, most bioethicists have been uncomfortably aware of the fact that when faced with difficult cases, they are unlikely to be happy with the strategy of deducing answers from a single moral theory. Most find themselves reasoning in a fashion that is significantly more involved and complex than the relatively straightforward task of applying a single theory. For example, they are likely also to be occupied with deciding how to understand and categorize the problem before them lest they leap to a description with a prescribed solution that does not meet their intuitions (e.g., should physician-assisted suicide be classified as murder, mercy killing, suicide, or medical termination of suffering?).

There are other difficulties as well with the typical view of theories as the basis of moral reasoning. For example, when bioethicists try to invoke major moral theories, most find it difficult to fit the theories' criteria to the problems before them, a restriction that clearly limits their practical usefulness. Moreover, many bioethicists find that a single comprehensive moral theory is inadequate to capture all of their moral intuitions; in such cases, they may sometimes find themselves tempted by the attractions of alternative theoretical approaches for addressing different sorts of issues. However, theoretical disloyalty or inconsistency in theoretical perspective is not tolerable under standard views of the role of moral theories.

Another complication is many bioethicists' feeling responsible to consider the geographical and political scope of their positions. Many of the issues they explore arise in various forms around the world. This is not surprising, since all societies must deal with questions of how to handle childbirth, illness, disability, death, and dying in morally responsible ways. The difficulty is that local conditions can vary considerably. For example, there can be very great differences in the sets of expectations and opportunities that surround local discussions of particular bioethical issues, and the range of available practical options can be diverse (as happens when the rich have access to types of care unavailable to the poor). The question arises, then, of whether or not to seek common ethical answers to similar problems as they arise in culturally different contexts. Most moral theories would tell us that there is some underlying commonality in moral commitments that should transcend local variations, even though current conditions may determine how a theory applies in a particular society.

In general, feminist bioethicists have been especially dissatisfied with the centrality of traditional moral theories in bioethics. They note that the theories ignore rather than highlight and critique the ways in which oppression is woven into the various medical practices under review. By abstracting away from the details that are specific to particular patients (or research subjects, caregivers, policymakers, etc.), traditional moral theories obscure the ways in which power relations structure health care practices. Focusing on the generic human being (or generic patient, research subject, etc.), they have generally imagined that what is arrogantly believed to be the norm for all persons (white, educated, healthy males) is representative for all people in the same circumstances. This has allowed bioethicists to ignore the implications of gender, race, class, age, disability, sexuality, ethnicity, and other forms of difference associated with power in their analyses.[1]

Many feminist bioethicists have learned from their colleagues in feminist epistemology that knowledge claims, in ethics as in science, are inevitably situated in particular social and historical locations. That means that the moral beliefs each of us acquires and the moral analyses we bring to problems reflect the particular values, attitudes, and needs of our own historical position. Many feminists urge us to be careful in our use of the universal voice when addressing moral matters and to recognize that our commitment to the specific (universal) values we hold dear has emerged in a particular time and place. This awareness suggests that we need to learn to listen attentively to different voices and perspectives if we hope to understand where moral intuitions can legitimately be shared crossculturally and where they founder on differences in experience and cultural values. This recognition of the specificity of our particular moral views does not mean that we must adopt unconstrained moral relativism or moral nihilism, but it does require that we speak cautiously when we attempt to make universal claims and that we attend carefully to possible sources of difference.[2]

There is a tendency in any culture to judge alternative conceptual and value systems as incomprehensible and then to either dismiss them altogether from consideration or to "translate" them into something more familiar. Unless we make explicit efforts to hear and understand alternative perspectives, it is easy to assume that they are either misguided or reducible to one's own. Efforts to articulate a common basis of moral concern are especially vulnerable to inappropriate universalization when they reflect the moral values and priorities of the currently dominant global culture, since it is in the nature of dominant cultures to be ignorant of not only the reality but also the possibility of alternative (legitimate) moral systems. Thus, for example, it is important to be particularly wary of attempts to export uncritically the distinctly American value of privileging the autonomous individual above other moral concerns. Cultures that do not share Americans' enthusiasm for individualism (or, for that matter, Americans' understanding of individuals) have a difficult time expressing their alternative moral conceptions to those who assume that a moral perspective must begin with a belief in the fundamental importance of respect for the individual.

We need, then, to consider how we can understand the role of basic moral beliefs and theories in ways that leave space for respecting alternative moral positions and perspectives as legitimate guides to bioethical analysis. Rather than try to impose their own moral beliefs on other cultures, bioethicists would do well to consider the insights available to them if they examine different perspectives. I propose that we view alternative moral theories and positions as representing a collection of available guides to bioethical reasoning. To do this, we need to reconsider the role that is usually assigned to moral theory in bioethics. In the remainder of this chapter, I shall explore three different ways of understanding the role of moral theories in bioethics.

The Role of Metaphors

The most common way to think of moral theories in bioethics is to credit them with providing foundations for the more specific moral judgments of practical moral life. Many bioethicists speak of the need to appeal to well-developed foundations to ensure the legitimacy of their claims. The

implication is that if we can "ground" our bioethical views on a solid theoretical footing, we can establish the validity of our practical judgments.
Whenever we make this sort of reference to a theoretical foundation, we
are appealing to a familiar and evocative structural metaphor: just as the
foundations of buildings are meant to provide a strong, solid base for
whatever rests on them, so too theoretical ethical foundations should
provide the necessary support to justify the bioethical claims that rely on
them.

It is important to recognize the role of metaphor in this picture. Understanding that the foundational view of theories is metaphorical allows us
to understand both the virtues and the limitations associated with the
foundational conception. Moreover, it provides us with the conceptual
space to consider alternative, less familiar metaphors in its place. I shall
take advantage of that space to compare how two other metaphors—
frameworks and lenses—can provide different, and I think better, understandings of the place of moral theory within bioethics.

Before turning to the specific metaphor of foundations for ethics, let us
briefly consider the necessary role that metaphors play in bioethics.
Metaphors are pervasive throughout the domains encompassed by
bioethics—medicine, nursing, law, health policy, and ethics itself—as
they are in other areas of abstract thought. Probably the most familiar
and least controversial task of metaphors is their aesthetic role, for it is
clear that they can add color and interesting connections to discussions.
It is also the case that metaphors perform an important epistemological
function; this role is especially important in any task that involves abstract reasoning. In ethics, they provide us with access to moral understandings that may be unavailable through other means. They aid in the
understanding of complex ideas by transferring the relations that hold in
the domain of the metaphor to those that exist within the domain of the
field we are contemplating.[3] For example, we can speak of a sports team
as being "hot," "cold," or "heating up" to describe its recent record as
successful, poor, or improving. This understanding is possible because
the metaphor works by transferring the relations among temperature
ranges to the realm of sport. Similarly, when we speak of medicine as
waging a "war" against disease, we are suggesting that illness is similar
to an invasion of some alien force (or internal subversion). When our
goal is taken to be eradication of the harmful agent, we speak of strategies that involve the use of available "weapons" in the form of medical
interventions. We grant the physician the authority of a military com-
mander, and we often reduce the patient to her body, which is treated as
a battlefield.

Metaphors also play an important ethical role, for they determine our
understanding of the practices in question and, in doing so, they influ-

ence our evaluation of each. For instance, when we think of the subjects of medical care as "patients"—passive recipients of medical interventions—we evaluate medical practices differently than we do when we think of patients as active participants engaged in decisionmaking about their own health. Labeling them "consumers" or "clients" invokes quite different sorts of behavior and relationships than the term "patients" and creates other sorts of distortion in understanding the relation between physicians and those who consult them. These understandings determine the sorts of interactions we expect to find in medical encounters. When it comes time to morally evaluate those encounters, our analysis will be conducted according to what sorts of behavior seem to be appropriate to the relationships that the central metaphor has helped us to imagine. Hence, paternalism is a meaningful option to explore within the traditional patient metaphor, but it is quickly dismissed in the type of encounter suggested by the consumer metaphor. By the same token, we have no difficulty imagining the need for "caveat emptor" warnings in the consumer–provider framework, but such advice is disturbingly jarring in traditional doctor-patient relationships.

Metaphors have other important functions, as well. For one thing, they translate affective attitudes or emotions from one domain to another— one wages war against something that evokes feelings of dread and hostility, and one nurtures that toward which one feels protective. Moreover, the metaphors that are selected often affect our ability even to perceive the possibility of other approaches to a problem. When metaphors become so well entrenched that they seem natural and fully accurate descriptors, alternative ways of constructing the relations in question seem artificial and misleading, if they can be imagined at all. These limits on the ways of understanding a phenomenon limit the responses that will be considered reasonable. For example, the metaphor of the body as machine supports development of high-tech medical interventions in response to illness, but it makes spiritual responses seem irrelevant. Thus metaphors not only shape our understanding of central concepts but also frame the issues we recognize as morally significant or problematic; they also inform our sense of available solutions.

All metaphors function as models or analogies. As such, they emphasize similarities between the two realms in question while obscuring differences. That is, in the process of helping us to understand one set of relations in terms of another, metaphors highlight certain features of the domain to which they are applied and, inevitably, they hide or distort others. Thus, while facilitating one way of understanding a concept, situation, practice, or theory, the specific metaphors invoked may limit our ability to conceive of alternative ways of interpreting the subject matter and may divert our gaze from other possible strategies.

Theories As Foundations

Consider, then, the very familiar metaphor of "foundations" for bioethics. Foundationalism is a highly attractive way of understanding the nature of abstract thought in ethics. It encourages us to believe that all true moral claims can (at least in principle) be "grounded in" solid, undeniable truths. It also directs us to evaluate controversial claims by considering whether or not they are supported by plausible theoretical assumptions. But we should keep in mind that foundationalism is a metaphor whose task is to transfer the relations of concrete physical structures to abstract theoretical claims. The governing architectural metaphor suggests that there is a well-ordered structural relation among different types of ethical claims. Specifically, it directs us to search for "deep" or "core" principles that "lie underneath" all other ethical claims, while advising us to assume that nonfoundational ethical claims must be shown to be "resting on" or "supported by" the deeper foundational claims. The structural metaphor of foundationalism illuminates relationships among different "levels" of moral claims and directs us to "dig deeper" when seeking justification for "ungrounded" claims. By implying the existence of an ultimately firm, concrete basis for all true ethical assertions, and by demanding that we direct our attention to the theoretical "base" for each practical conclusion, foundationalism provides both a sense of security in the reliability of bioethical claims and an implicit methodology for dealing with controversy. Since metaphors transfer emotional attitudes as well as structural relations, it provides a sense of solidity and reliability to a domain that is notoriously unsettled and disturbingly ambiguous.

At the same time, the metaphor of foundationalism also has some problematic implications. For one thing, it discourages us from asking questions about moral matters that do not fit within the structure imagined. For example, if the bioethical system is seen to be "built on" propositions as the foundational units, then nonpropositional sorts of moral understanding are likely to be overlooked.[4] Similarly, if the system is organized around a set of basic duties, then questions involving other moral categories such as character or attitudes are usually excluded. And if the foundation is a single comprehensive moral principle (such as the principle of utility) or even a set of principles,[5] then considerations that do not fall under the scope of the principle(s) identified (e.g., nonconsequential features or virtues) may simply not be addressed. Categories that do not consist of the particular building materials available are seldom recognized as falling within the sphere of ethics at all.

The problem is even more significant if we try to consider the role of theories in bioethics from a global perspective. Here the task is to reconcile moral understandings from many diverse cultural perspectives into a single, ordered framework. If we believe the ideal is to identify a coherent, valid, transcultural foundational set of principles or virtues that can support all practical moral reasoning, we will face enormous difficulties in settling on the concepts and priorities that merit foundational status. The temptation is to try to reduce local moral systems to a single overarching transcultural one that rests on foundations that appear solid and incontrovertible from the perspective of recognized bioethics authorities. Moral observations, concerns, and insights that are incommensurable with the types of moral truths that can be derived from the chosen foundations will not fit within this model; they are likely, therefore, to be discarded as incomprehensible or simply false. Although the foundational metaphor has room for local variation in terms of how its edicts are actually carried out—just as real foundations can support buildings made of brick, stone, wood, or plastic—the specific practices supported must still fall within the terms specified by the governing moral theory. (Foundations determine the shape if not the texture of what rests on them.) Practices rooted in different conceptual schemes or different social understandings may be too readily excluded from the domain of the moral.

It seems, then, that the foundational metaphor is inclined to restrict our thinking in various troublesome ways. It limits our awareness of what sorts of features are ethically significant to those that fit within the dominant moral conception or theory. It encourages us to dismiss, rather than address, insights that may fall outside of its particular ontology and structure. It requires that crosscultural ethical discussions be reducible to some prior sorts of moral claims in which those with more power are likely to be able to set the terms of discussion and determine which concepts are comprehensible and which are not. It seems, then, that it may not be the best metaphor to rely on for guiding activity in the sphere of bioethics.

There are other reasons to resist the attractions of a foundational approach to bioethics. An important one is its inability to fit with current cognitive science views about the ways in which humans actually reason about practical ethical matters. Empirical evidence suggests that humans do not reason about moral matters in the way that foundational theory prescribes. Those of us brought up to believe that strictly logical reasoning is the proper (and only) model for deliberation can turn to cognitive science to appreciate the possibility of other approaches to moral (and other) types of reasoning. For example, prototype theory offers an alternative theory of moral deliberation that is better supported by the empirical evidence. Although prototype theory was originally designed to account for concept formation, Mark Johnson speculates on its usefulness for understanding the process of moral reasoning.[6] He cites abundant empirical evidence to suggest that ethical reflection begins with a set of core ethical beliefs that describe clear cases of morally objectionable or praiseworthy behavior that constitute the prototypes of ethical delibera- tion. When confronted with cases that do not fit neatly into any of the available prototypes, people typically struggle to expand their moral un- derstandings by using a variety of imaginative strategies to help them re- flect on the cases' similarities to and differences from the prototypes that constitute their settled moral intuitions.

Whether or not prototype theory ultimately turns out to provide the most accurate model of moral reasoning, it does free us of the need to re- main tied to the less convincing foundational model. Specifically, it re- lieves us from the need to accept foundationalism's central presumption that we reason about difficult moral cases by finding deep and timeless moral laws from which we can deduce the appropriate applications in complex new domains. Many bioethicists already resist this description of moral reasoning (the "top-down" version) and suggest that practical moral deliberation proceeds by induction, not deduction (the comple- mentary "bottom-up" alternative). But even "bottom-up" versions may be foundational if they assume that we use our practical moral intuitions to reason inductively to some abstract moral law that can then be applied deductively to support all relevant examples. Neither version seems to correspond with empirical evidence about how people actually proceed to address difficult moral problems, however.

Of course, just because we are inclined to reason in a certain way does not mean that it is the morally correct way to reason; nor does the fact that foundational strategies are difficult to apply prove that they are mis- taken. It is, however, sufficient grounds to give us pause in our commit- ment to foundationalism. At the least, it shifts the burden of proof to those who would argue that we should train ourselves to reason accord- ing to the deductive demands of foundationalism despite the conflicting reality of moral psychology. It also reveals the possibility of a different approach to moral deliberation—one that is not dependent on the logical structure of foundationalism. When we add the practical difficulty asso- ciated with applying foundational methodological prescriptions to the observation that there is no consensus as to what theoretical claims are certain enough to do the work of solid foundations, and to the recogni- tion that foundational views tend to exclude potentially important moral insights, we have good reason to consider alternative approaches.

Theories As Frameworks

Thus, I suggest, bioethicists would do better to move away from the rigidity implicit in the foundational metaphor for ethics, appealing in- stead to metaphors that support more imaginative approaches to ethical deliberation. To capture feminist and crosscultural interests in not prematurely excluding diverse perspectives, we should seek alternative metaphors that will encourage ideas of plurality and diversity in available ethical approaches. Consider, for example, the images associated with thinking of moral theories as providing frameworks for alternative approaches to practical ethical deliberations. This metaphor opens up spaces that can be filled in multiple ways, and it encourages us to appreciate the value of being receptive to different theoretical approaches.

Such openness accords well with the common practical experience of ambivalence that many bioethicists feel toward different theoretical perspectives. Most bioethicists are aware of the powerful critiques that have been developed against each type of theoretical approach that has been recommended for bioethics (Kantian, utilitarian, social contract theory, ethics of care, communitarian, principles-based, etc.). Nevertheless, many feel an undeniable attraction toward some of these theoretical positions; indeed most people would acknowledge that there seems to be value in many of the proposed theoretical perspectives. Thus, instead of trying to force bioethicists to choose a single, comprehensive theory to apply to all cases, I find it preferable to view different theoretical perspectives as providing alternative "frameworks" or "templates" for different sorts of approaches to problems.

This metaphor acknowledges that each theory has a definite appeal in a certain range of cases. Some problems seem to best fit the framework offered by consequentialist theories (e.g., those dealing with truth-telling issues); others fit more comfortably in frameworks offered by deontological theories (e.g., those dealing with the rights of subjects of clinical research trials); still others seem to evoke appeals to an ethics of care (e.g., those dealing with care of the dying). Often many theories will seem relevant to a particular dilemma, but they all frame the problem differently. The reason for this variation, I believe, is that each sort of theory helps clarify certain dimensions of the topic that may be inaccessible (or at least unlikely to be perceived) when other approaches are being used. Or, to put it another way, each provides distinct prototypes that we may want to call upon to help guide our thinking when we confront difficult problems.

This metaphor offers a radical reinterpretation of the nature of theories. It rejects traditional understandings of theories as absolute and comprehensive (i.e., as foundational) on the grounds that the foundational understanding is incompatible with the facts of moral psychology and the belief that no theory has proven to be adequate to embrace all morally relevant concerns. In other words, I am claiming that no moral theory can do the work normally expected of it: none provides reliable grounds for resolving all morally difficult problems through deductive application of its central principles. Nonetheless, each of the major moral theories provides important insights that can be enlisted in our efforts to address difficult moral issues. I am proposing, then, that moral theories be reconceived as providing partial and overlapping resources, not definitive, exhaustive truths. To make clear the more modest role I am suggesting, let us relabel these theoretical positions "moral perspectives" rather than the more ambitious "theories."

As in the case of metaphors, there is a "flip side" to the observation that each type of theory highlights certain aspects of a problem: each type of approach is also likely to obscure important dimensions that are easily visible within a competing framework. Consider how this works in a single complex area of bioethical thought: physician-assisted death. Kantian theory suggests the importance of keeping to universalizable principles when we enter such murky moral terrain. It insists on an uncompromisable duty to respect the autonomy and dignity of patients. In the current climate, where third-party payers are pressuring physicians to cut back on expensive treatment whenever possible, there is unquestionable appeal to the idea of relying on an absolute principle that keeps such powers out of the hands of individual doctors.

At the same time, reflecting on the effects that the different possible policies may have on the various parties involved—patients, families, physicians, other care providers, and future patients—does seem to be essential. Consequentialism's recognition of the importance of considering the likely consequences of different policy options also seems to be an essential part of a thorough analysis of the practice of physician-assisted suicide. The effects of different practices on the welfare levels of all affected surely have a place in a full ethical analysis of the subject.

Similarly, the perspective of an ethics of care enriches our analysis of this topic by directing us to try to understand how different policy options will affect the nature of the relationships involved. We must, for example, consider how a permissive policy of physician-assisted death will transform relationships between physicians and their seriously ill patients and how family members will respond to such options. Will the availability of this option facilitate or undermine trust? Will it necessitate improved communication or will it be fitted into current patterns of minimal exploration of patient values and concerns? Is it possible to develop a policy that is responsive to the particular needs of individual patients? Is there a way to develop a practice of physician-assisted death that promotes improved relationships between the very ill and those that care for them personally and professionally or is the very possibility of deliberately causing their death likely to increase anxiety? And who will assume the responsibilities associated with each policy option?

Those adopting a perspective of feminist ethics, as I understand it, will want to explore the questions raised by each of the leading theories and others besides. By insisting that bioethicists consider the role that specific policies and practices play in fostering or challenging existing patterns of oppression, a feminist bioethics framework would ask that we consider how a policy of physician-assisted death would affect those who are now oppressed.[7] It would direct us to ask, for instance, whether a policy that legalized and legitimized physician-assisted death increased the vulnerability of those who are most oppressed, since they are most likely to have their lives devalued and their interests neglected. Already receiving poor care, they face a high risk of premature death at the hands of physicians who are insensitive to their particular needs and interests. Feminist ethics would also direct us to ask, however, whether a policy that prohibited physician-assisted death could be supplemented by practices that reduce the disproportionate share of the burden of caring for the very ill that currently falls on members of oppressed groups.[8]

A global bioethics perspective, for its part, would direct us to inquire how to evaluate these various questions in very diverse cultural contexts. How attentive should a practice of this importance be to local conditions and values? Should a patient's right to seek an early end to suffering—or to be protected against an unchosen, premature death—depend on the society in which she finds herself? Such questions are particularly troublesome when we acknowledge that some citizens have very little respect and authority in their own communities.

Each of the leading moral theories has a contribution to make to the discussion. Each identifies different points as salient from its perspective, but each also makes it difficult to see the moral significance of factors that other positions treat as central. In many cases, all these diverse considerations seem to be morally significant. A thorough analysis of the topic of physician-assisted suicide, and of many others besides, cannot be done by limiting our focus to the issues that are of particular concern from a single theoretical perspective because whichever we choose is likely to obscure the importance of some morally important questions that are far more apparent from some other theoretical position. The framework metaphor grants legitimacy to each of the valuable perspectives.

I said earlier that all metaphors illuminate some features of the host domain at the expense of obscuring others. The difficulty with the framework metaphor is that it suggests walls and barriers that are not easily merged with one another. Where the image of frameworks implies the availability of alternative structural choices, it does not encourage us to combine or shift frameworks from within. Once we are committed to a framework, we seem to be unable to draw on the resources of any other, at least for the current issue. If we are working within a consequentialist frame, it is difficult to know where to "fit" deontological insights. Yet we often need to draw on insights from multiple theoretical perspectives as we struggle to determine the best way of thinking about the problem before us and the best way of responding to it. When we are confronted with moral problems that fall outside of our settled prototypes, we need to be able to draw on the resources of many different theoretical perspectives in our efforts to find the best way of addressing the problem before us.

Theories As Lenses

Since each major theoretical perspective helps to ensure that bioethicists discuss important moral questions that usually go unaddressed by those who use other theoretical approaches and since none exhausts all moral questions, we need a metaphor that allows us to combine as well as shift perspectives. I recommend that we think of the "competing" theoretical options as a set of lenses available for helping us understand the complex moral dimensions of bioethics. Lenses are readily switched when we want a different "view" of something; they may even be layered on top of one another. (I carry three different sets of eyeglasses with me so that I can see things at a distance, read fine print, and function in bright sunlight or at night.) Some lenses will provide clearer perceptions of particular problems than others, but we may still gain understanding by trying on different options (as, for example, we can benefit by studying a tree through both binoculars and a microscope—which instrument provides the "right" view will depend on our aims and needs at the time).

This metaphor provides us with a richer understanding of the value of exploring alternative cultural perspectives on issues, for it allows us to use diverse cultural positions as additional lenses. If, for example, we seek to understand the moral issues associated with adopting a concept of brain death to facilitate organ transplantation, it suggests the importance of trying to understand the resistance to this practice found among many Japanese and aboriginal people, as well as the enthusiasm for the practice that is common throughout the rest of the industrialized world. We may get a better appreciation of the issues involved if we look beyond the dominant Western view of the body as a machine with interchangeable, replaceable parts and consider the implications of adopting other ways of understanding the connection between persons and their vital organs. Just as adding a rose-colored tint can transform our appreciation of the world we see without affecting clarity, so too adopting (or at

least understanding) different cultural positions may change our attitudes toward different sorts of practices without requiring abandonment
of reason. It may highlight features (textures, perhaps) that look "flat"
from other angles.

The metaphor of lenses is particularly helpful in understanding the
ways in which feminist ethics can work with other moral perspectives
in approaching problems. As long as oppressive patterns structure social relations, all people bear responsibility for challenging and under-
mining the patterns that sustain oppression. Thus it is essential for
bioethicists to continually remind themselves of the moral injustice of
oppression and take care to ask how a particular practice or policy contributes to existing patterns of oppression; that is, they should think of
the feminist ethics lens as indispensible. Nonetheless, we must recognize that information about how a practice is likely to contribute to patterns of oppression will not, by itself, necessarily determine the moral
status of a practice; other moral factors are also likely to be relevant.
The lens of feminist ethics will seldom be sufficient, so we must also
keep other lenses handy.

The fact that multiple lenses are useful to bioethics does not mean that
all approaches are equally valid or that all proposed solutions are morally
acceptable. After all, not all lenses facilitate sight or understanding. Some
lenses obscure, invert, or distort everything and should therefore be discarded. And some cultural positions, such as those that thoroughly de-
mean and devalue certain types of people, should also be rejected out of
hand. If lenses can be seen to be badly flawed (cracked, say) or absent or
painted black, they need not even be tried. Similarly, moral positions that
fundamentally oppose deeply held moral convictions can be readily rejected. And just as some lenses will fit some people so poorly as to create
havoc, not sight, so too some cultural positions may be so incomprehensible as to be irrelevant to foreign users. And perhaps for some problems we
cannot all work with exactly the same lenses, given differences in our various kinds of unmediated vision (cultural frameworks). So too some moral
issues that bioethicists address do not admit of a common, global solution
but must be tailored to the specific cultures in which they arise.

Unfortunately, not all lenses will be compatible in all cases, for sometimes they lead us to conflicting conclusions. Different theoretical positions and different cultural perspectives will often take us in opposite directions. We cannot assume that adding lenses will always refine vision;
sometimes it will increase distortion (or perhaps lead to blindness, as for
example happens when differently polarized lenses are layered on one
another). In these cases, we are faced with the familiar difficulty of deciding which perspective(s) provides better moral guidance and which

should be abandoned for the moment. This is a task that the metaphor of lenses cannot resolve, but only explain.

Unlike the foundations metaphor, which promises to provide a definitive solution for every moral dilemma, we can anticipate an embarrassment of incompatible resolutions within the lenses metaphor. Nonetheless, it would be a mistake to return to the temptations of the foundations model, for, as we have seen, its solutions come at too high a price. The foundational metaphor would have us avoid such dilemmas by choosing up sides from the beginning; as a consequence, we are restrained from exploring morally important dimensions of the problems before us. The foundational metaphor may help us find a solution within the terms of a particular moral theory, but there are many reasons to doubt that it is a morally adequate one. The metaphor of lenses helps expand our moral vision and the price we must pay is that sometimes the light it lets in will be too bright (or too dim?) to see clearly by.

Such is the sad reality of moral life. The difficulty for bioethicists lies in learning which formulations are going to be the most morally instructive for a particular problem. None of these metaphors provides definitive advice as to which theoretical positions will be most valuable for specific issues, since even the foundation metaphor leaves us with the task of choosing the "right" foundations. Bioethicists are inevitably left with the difficult job of determining which considerations are morally important and how best to accommodate the multiple relevant factors in each particular problem area. The metaphor of lenses helps us appreciate that what appears to be a satisfactory resolution to a problem may well vary with the perspective we adopt. It challenges us not to settle too quickly for the most familiar and comfortable perspective but to seek out the best available lens(es) for each problem, even as it makes clear how difficult it is to know if we have been successful. (There is no standardized eye chart to judge by in ethics.)

Because the choice of ethical theory or perspective influences not only the answers we come up with but also the very problems we perceive, we cannot afford to restrict our vision from the full spectrum of moral problems before us. Doing bioethics well requires appeal to the insights provided by multiple theories. We should, therefore, resist depending on any single theoretical tool for addressing all of our problems. Rather, we should welcome the opportunities for expanded understanding that diverse theoretical voices bring to our deliberations. My contention is that the metaphor of lenses provides a more accurate and a more productive understanding of the role of theories in bioethics in a global context than do either foundations or frameworks. It has the added virtue of clarifying the vital role that feminist ethics should play in all bioethics deliberations, be they local or global.

Notes

The original version of this paper was presented at the Fourth World Congress of the International Association of Bioethics, Tokyo, Japan (November 1998). A shorter version of it appears in the selected proceedings of that conference in *Bioethics*. This version was developed at the Bellagio International Study and Conference Center, Bellagio, Italy.

1. For feminist discussion of these oversights, see, for example, (1) Helen Bequaert Holmes and Laura M. Purdy, eds., *Feminist Perspectives in Medical Ethics* (Bloomington: Indiana University Press, 1992); (2) Susan M. Wolf, ed., *Feminism and Bioethics: Beyond Reproduction* (New York: Oxford University Press, 1996); (3) Dorothy Roberts, "Reconstructing the Patient: Starting with Women of Color," in *Feminism and Bioethics*, pp. 116–143; (4) Rosemarie Tong, *Feminist Approaches to Bioethics: Theoretical Reflections and Practical Applications* (Boulder: Westview, 1997); (5) The Feminist Health Care Ethics Research Network, Susan Sherwin, coordinator, *The Politics of Women's Health: Exploring Agency and Autonomy* (Philadelphia: Temple University Press, 1998); (6) Susan M. Wolf, "Erasing Difference: Race, Ethnicity, and Gender in Bioethics," in Anne Donchin and Laura Purdy, eds. *Embodying Bioethics: Recent Feminist Advances* (Lanham, Md.: Rowman & Littlefield, 1999), pp. 65–81.

2. Susan Sherwin, *No Longer Patient: Feminist Ethics and Health Care* (Philadelphia: Temple University Press, 1992); Barbara Nicholas, "Strategies for Effective Transformations," in *Embodying Bioethics*, pp. 239–252.

3. George Lakoff and Mark Johnson, *Metaphors We Live By* (Chicago: University of Chicago Press, 1980); Eva Feder Kittay, *Metaphor: Its Cognitive Force and Linguistic Structure* (Oxford: Clarendon, 1987).

4. Susan Babbitt, *Impossible Dreams: Rationality, Integrity, and Moral Imagination* (Boulder: Westview, 1996).

5. Thomas L. Beauchamp and James F. Childress, *Principles of Biomedical Ethics*, 4th ed. (New York: Oxford University Press, 1994).

6. Mark Johnson, *Moral Imagination: Implications of Cognitive Science for Ethics* (Chicago: University of Chicago Press, 1993).

7. Sherwin, *No Longer Patient*.

8. Jocelyn Downie and Susan Sherwin, "A Feminist Exploration of Issues Around Assisted Death," *St. Louis Public Law Review* 15, no. 2 (1996): 303–330.

2

Is a Global Bioethics Possible As Well As Desirable?

A Millennial Feminist Response

ROSEMARIE TONG

Our world reminds us how different people are, but it also reminds us how similar people are. Because all human beings have bodies, minds, and spirits, all human beings are capable of feeling pain and experiencing suffering. This very simple yet profound truth invites health care theorists and activists to search for ways to improve people's health worldwide. A global bioethics—meaning a bioethics that takes into account the diversity of peoples and cultures in our world, as well as the fact that our planet and its resources provide the bases for all our lives—is desirable because "we can no longer examine medical options without considering ecological science and the larger problems of society on a global scale."[1] Technological and communications advances have made the world too small for any bioethics that is less than global. But do we have the conceptual tools to achieve such a bioethics, to create some sort of unity in and through our diversity? As I see it, feminist thought encompasses some of these tools. By examining power-focused feminist approaches to bioethics in particular, we can, I believe, learn how to identify and eliminate the factors that work against both the globalization of bioethics and the just distribution of health care services and goods worldwide.

Whereas care-focused feminist approaches to ethics and bioethics have as their main focus the rehabilitation of such culturally associated feminine values as compassion, empathy, sympathy, nurture, and kindness, power-focused feminist approaches to ethics and bioethics have as their first imperative the elimination or modification of any system, structure, or set of norms, including ethical rules, that contributes to human oppression, particularly women's oppression. Increasingly aware of how sexism, racism, ableism, heterosexism, ethnocentrism, and colonialism reinforce each other, as well as how the desires and needs of different groups of women are distinct, power-focused feminist bioethicists have wondered whether it is possible, let alone desirable, to say anything in *general* about women's health status or health care interests. For fear of being branded as absolutists or colonialists—insensitive to and disrespectful of people's diversity—many middle-class, Western, white feminist bioethicists have refused to make judgments about developing nations' systems, institutions, or practices that they would condemn as morally wrong and oppressive in their own nations. There is a problem with this well-intentioned reticence from a socially and economically privileged group of feminists, however. It threatens not only feminist politics and action but also any type of politics and action that require presumably good-willed and enlightened people to come together to forge *just* global policies—international policies that distribute freedom and well-being (in the form of goods and services) equally among all the individuals they affect. If feminists cannot agree on what is in women's best interests, on what sorts of policies promote gender justice, then how can we expect bioethicists from all over the world, bereft of a shared ideology, to develop policies that promote *international* human rights or *world* health or *global* anything?

The questions I just raised are neither new nor uniquely mine. My belief is that anyone who does not want to be either an oppressor or an oppressed person, but wants to work toward just policies at both the local and global levels, has asked them and has wondered how to mediate the differences that separate individuals and groups from one another. In the past, ethicists and bioethicists thought that the way to proceed was to appeal to our common human natures, to characteristics that are common to all people. In the United States, for example, civil rights advocates repeatedly proclaimed in the 1950s and 1960s that all "men" are created equal. Similarly, U.S. feminists in the 1970s and 1980s insisted on women's sameness, on women's sisterhood.[2]

But shifts in ethical and bioethical reasoning toward relativism, antifoundationalism, and postmodernism changed this way of seeing things, leading to a major transvaluation of values in which what had been good (the same) became bad, and what had been bad (difference) became good. Feminists, among others, initially affirmed the move in ethical deliberation from sameness to difference. They listened attentively to theorists like Elizabeth Spelman, for example, who urged them to resist the impulse to gloss over women's differences, as if there existed some sort of "Woman" into whom the autobiographical differences of all women could flow and dissolve.

In particular, power-focused feminist ethicists and bioethicists heeded Spelman when she pleaded with them not to make the mistake historian Kenneth Stampp made by asserting that "innately Negroes are, after all, only white men with black skins, nothing more, nothing else."[3] Why, asked Spelman, is it that *Negroes* are only white men with black skins? Why is it not instead that *Caucasians* are only black men with white skins? If a white man can imagine himself protesting his reduction to being only a black man with white skin, why does he have trouble imagining a black man protesting his reduction to being only a white man with black skin? Could it be that white people still think "white" is definitely the best way to be—the "gold standard" for all people? Fearing the presence of some *well-intentioned* "Kenneth Stampps" within their own ranks, power-focused feminist ethicists and bioethicists paid close attention to Spelman's warning:

> If, like Stampp, I believe that the woman in every woman is a woman just like me, and if I also assume that there is no difference between being white and being woman, then seeing another woman "as a woman" will involve seeing her as fundamentally like the woman I am. In other words, the womanness underneath the Black woman's skin is a white woman's, and deep down inside the Latino woman is an Anglo woman waiting to burst through a cultural shroud.[4]

If power-focused feminist ethicists and bioethicists really value equality, implied Spelman, then they cannot claim all women are "just like us."

The realization of power-focused feminists that the ideal of sameness can operate as a tool of human oppression—of moral absolutism and colonialism—initially led to many improvements in feminist thought and action. However, an overemphasis on the ideal of difference gradually has resulted in feminists' increasing inability to formulate policies aimed at expanding women's freedom and well-being in a just manner. In the name of respect for difference, power-focused feminists fail to confront some social injustices for fear of "imposing" their moral views on a culture different than their own. As a result, desperate health care needs of many women are not being met as often or as well as they should be met.

This frustrating state of affairs stymies the formulation of just global health care policies. Uma Narayan is a feminist of Indian background who came to the United States as a graduate student in her mid-twenties and has lived and worked there for over a dozen years. She illustrates these misunderstandings of cultural differences well. In her book, *Dislo-*

cating Cultures: Identities, Traditions, and Third World Feminisms, Narayan explains the ways in which Westerners ask her to play roles: emissary, mirror, and authentic insider.[5] According to Narayan, well-intentioned Westerners, but particularly well-intentioned Western feminists, try to view everything through the lenses of an anthropological perspective with two imperatives: (1) "It is important for mainstream Westerners to take an interest in Other cultures" and (2) "It is important that this interest not involve moral criticism of Other cultures by mainstream Westerners."[6] The first of these imperatives is based on a sincere desire to be less parochial and to expand one's limited intellectual horizons. It is also rooted in the growing realization that ignorance about other cultures is "increasingly impractical and imprudent in a world where an increasingly global economy reinforces all sorts of complex interdependencies between nations in various parts of the world."[7] The second of these imperatives is based on thoughtful Westerners' growing realization that Western theorists are largely responsible for unfavorable representations of the so-called Other as uncivilized, primitive, barbaric, or animalistic, and also for using such conceptual ammunition to defend its colonial policies, that is, its economic exploitation and political domination of the Third World. Western feminists in particular wish "to avoid contributing to a history of negative stereotypes about Third-World communities and practices."[8] Narayan believes that it is precisely this wish that is behind Western feminists' insistence that she be (1) an emissary of India's cultural riches, (2) a mirror in which the West can view itself as "big" and "bad" and the East as somehow "small" and "good," and (3) an authentic insider who is entitled to condemn oppressive features of Indian society that Western feminists also clearly see as harmful to women but dare not condemn out of a desire to respect cultural diversity.

Although Narayan is proud of many of India's cultural riches, it bothers her when Western feminists fail to see that the "riches" of other cultures are often "the cultural products of privileged sections of a society, whose social positions not only gave them privileged access to the domains of cultural achievement, but also gave them the power to constitute these achievements as 'definitive,' 'emblematic,' and 'monumental' aspects"[9] of their culture overall. Non-Western cultures can be just as guilty of marginalizing some of their members as Western cultures can be. What puzzles and concerns Narayan is the fact that the same Western feminists who readily condemn the past and present segregationist policies of the United States seem loath to condemn India's traditional caste system, for example. For fear of being branded as colonial absolutists bent on violating the cultural integrity of India, Western feminists often employ a sophomoric cultural diversity lens instead of their powerful feminist lens. Narayan stresses that she does not want Western feminists to "respect" her culture unreflectively but to show that what was and is wrong about U.S. segregation is essentially the same as what is wrong about the Indian caste system.

As uncomfortable as Narayan is with the role of emissary, the role of mirror is, in her estimation, a more tedious one which demands that she listen to seemingly endless lists of mea culpas by her Western feminist friends. Narayan notes that Western feminists, in conversations about Third World development, show a desire to blame the West, and only the West, for developing nations' economic and political problems, as if developing nations had no problems of their own making. Essentially, Westerners view persons in developing nations as mirrors in which they see those persons not as they really are but as they would have them be: "Poor Passive Victims of Western Imperialism, Western Capitalism and Western Political machinations" or innocent children incapable of committing adult sins.[10]

Of all the roles she is asked to play, however, Narayan claims that the role of authentic insider is the most taxing one. Often Narayan's Western feminist friends have appointed her *the* spokesperson for the "Third World position" on a wide range of practices, as if she were some sort of encyclopedia or as if the "Third World" really had a singular position on anything. Even worse, says Narayan, her Western feminist friends have expressed disappointment in her when her views deviated from the view they considered the "authentic" Third World feminist position. For example, on several occasions, when Narayan offered her analysis of *sati* (a widow's self-immolation on her husband's funeral pyre), female genital mutilation, or sex-selective abortion, she was met with the following criticism: "Your analysis of this issue is 'the analysis of a Westernized feminist. What are the views of the women who actually undergo, or face the prospect of undergoing, these practices?'"[11]

As someone who has, on more occasions than I wish to admit, asked people—but particularly feminists in developing nations—to play the roles of emissary, mirror, and authentic insider, I have become painfully aware that the roles I have asked the Other to play have left me playing the awful roles of capitalist hustler, imperialist oppressor, and nonjudgmental outsider. This role playing must stop. Whether we label ourselves feminists or humanists or nothing in particular, we bioethicists must find the conceptual tools we need to chisel a measure of unity within our diversity so that we may shape a global bioethics strong enough to generate just public policies.

Within what is called multicultural and global feminism I believe there are several of these needed conceptual tools, ones that any bioethicist—nonfeminist or feminist—can use to achieve the kind of democratic consensus that leads to the formulation of just health care policies. Essentially, multicultural and global feminists desire to affirm their differences from each other as basic to their self-identity. Therefore, multicultural and global feminists initially rejected approaches such as Robin Morgan's attempt—in her book *Sisterhood Is Global*—to reaffirm women's universal sisterhood.[12] Among other feminists, Chandra Talpade Mohanty criticized Morgan for claiming that women share "a common condition"[13] best described "as the suffering inflicted by a universal 'patriarchal mentality,' women's opposition to male power and androcentrism, and the experience of rape, battery, labor, and childbirth."[14] Mohanty took particular exception to Morgan's claim that if women asked themselves "*sincere* questions about [their] differences,"[15] they would discover that their ultimate goals are the same, namely, to constitute themselves *as selves*. For Morgan, white women and women of color, women in developed countries and developing countries, are united in their quest for "self identity," "self-realization," "self-image," and "the right to be oneself."[16] As Mohanty saw it, Morgan's ideas about all women's need for "selfhood" was nothing more than a "middle-class, psychologized notion"[17] conceived to gloss over the uncomfortable fact that most women of color in developed countries and most women in developing countries have little if any time to think about their "selves," let alone to develop them. They are, said Mohanty, usually too focused on surviving, on getting enough food, clothing, and shelter for themselves and their families, to worry about self-fulfillment.

Although I think Mohanty is right to emphasize women's differences, I think she may have become so enamored with the *idea* of difference that she is no longer able to recognize the *reality* of sameness. In a recent *Hypatia* article, Susan Okin reminds "First World" feminist *theoreticians* that feminist *activists*, particularly those in the "Third World," are finding that women have a lot in common after all.[18] Okin stresses that at several global meetings, women attending from countries throughout the world acknowledged "that women everywhere are greatly affected by laws and customs having to do with sexuality, marriages, divorce, child custody, and family life as a whole." They "are much more likely to be rendered sexually vulnerable than men and boys," and their "work tends to be valued considerably less highly than men and men's work."[19] Women in developed countries, implies Okin, should work with women in developing countries to achieve for *all* women the kind of freedom and well-being most women in developed countries already have. To do so is not an exercise in cultural imperialism but a simple response to a call for assistance.

Okin's case for cooperation between "First World" and "Third World" women is a cogent one that invites all bioethicists to engage in some form of what Alison Jaggar terms "feminist practical dialogue."[20] As Jaggar describes it, feminist practical dialogue typically begins not with the articulation of general moral rules or principles but with the creation of opportunities for participants to speak about their own moral experiences. These bits of personal narrative are then molded together through a process of collective reflection, the goal of which is to transform the tendency of individual women to think about their past situations and actions as merely "personal." Feminist practical dialogue debunks this notion by giving individual women the opportunity to hear that their personal experiences of gender oppression are anything but "personal." On the contrary, they are "political." They are a product of the large social systems and structures that maintain patterns of male domination and female subordination among us.

Jaggar cautions that feminist practical dialogue is not easy and has little in common with gossip or coffee house meetings. It takes more than goodwill. It takes effort, skill, and the practice of such virtues as responsibility, self-discipline, sensitivity, respect, and trust. It also assumes that "understanding between diverse people becomes possible only when those involved are for each other as specific individuals."[21] In this connection, Jaggar notes an article in which María Lugones and Elizabeth Spelman propose that neither self-interest nor duty but friendship is the only appropriate motive for Anglo and Hispanic women, for example, to come together to iron out their differences. Lugones specifically writes that a "non-imperialist feminism requires that . . . you [Anglo feminists] follow us into our world out of friendship."[22] Once there on the turf of the Others, the task for Anglo and Hispanic women is to find ways of interacting that are respectful of each other's cultural differences and yet courageous enough to articulate the gender-oppressive implications of these differences.

The most striking difference between feminist and nonfeminist versions of practical discourse is, in Jaggar's estimation, the nurturing nature of the former. She points out that speaking is not as important as listening in feminist practical dialogue. In other words, the goal of each woman is not to be thinking—while others are speaking—about how she will refute or interrupt them when they pause to take a breath. The goal is not to make sure that her own point of view is heard or prevails but, instead, to listen attentively to others' opinions in the hope of working with them to forge a consensus position on the issue being discussed.

As a realist, Jaggar cautions that feminist practical dialogue, like any theory, has its limitations in practical application. It sometimes fails to bring about the consensus it so urgently seeks. The goal of consensus may also open the dialogue process to abuse by those who would "screen" participants for agreement on a particular moral issue so that consensus is likely from the start. Furthermore, the ideals on which feminist practical discourse are based—for example, equal respect and consideration for persons—may be compromised by cultural limitations. Some women, especially those from non-Western cultures, may find feminist practical discourse alien if it violates their conventions of discourse regarding, for instance, self-disclosure, eye contact, forms of address, and direct disagreement. Other women may be unable to participate in feminist practical discourse because the very means of discourse are unavailable to them. In other words, their inability to engage in dialogue may result from speaking a language other than that of the discourse group, from physical challenges, from mental illness, or from a history of abuse that renders them unable to trust and communicate with others.[23] Nevertheless, provided that those who participate in feminist discourse continually remind one another of its limitations, this method of conversation, in Jaggar's view, holds out at least the hope of true consensus—a coming together of diverse minds.

A recent example of feminist dialogue is the collection of essays edited by Rosalind Petchesky and Karen Judd, *Negotiating Reproductive Rights*. These essays, written by members of the IRRRAG (International Reproductive Rights Research Action Group), reveal that women from diverse countries can achieve consensus on issues affecting women throughout the world. For example, one study described in the book takes into account the different political powers, religious majorities, and cultural contexts of seven different countries but still comes to some conclusions about the ways in which women think similarly about their reproductive rights. To be specific, low-income urban women in Brazil, Egypt, Malaysia, Mexico, Nigeria, Philippines, and the United States all tended to employ "motherhood" as their primary justification for their sense of reproductive entitlement: "since they (not husbands or partners) suffer the greatest burdens, pains and responsibilities of pregnancy, childbearing and childrearing, they therefore have earned the right to make decisions in these arenas."[24] Although it is vital to acknowledge that political, religious, and cultural contexts make the situations of women different around the world, it is also vital to acknowledge that the biological characteristics of females make *some* situations of women similar around the world. Petchesky and Judd's collection makes both of these acknowledgments, striving to emphasize similarities without erasing noticeable differences among women.

As important as the right kind of *dialogue* is, what is most important is the right kind of *action*—the kind of action that aims to eliminate the gap between the world's haves and have-nots. In other words, we bioethicists, nonfeminist as well as feminist, have to get serious about *distributive justice*, about eliminating the gaps between those who have too many health care goods and services and those who have too few. As long as these gaps exist, our health care goods and services will be used in morally inappropriate ways.

Clearly, bioethicists, beginning with feminist bioethicists, need to focus on our traditional goal—to make the world of health care one that structures and organizes itself so as to serve men and women (as well as races, classes, and, yes, nations) equally. If human beings have anything in common, it is our carnality and mortality. We all experience pain, suffering, and death. Because we are all equal in this way, it is the task of health care to serve each of us as if we were the paradigm case of treatment for everyone. Feminist bioethicists should be among the leaders in the movement to make health care attentive to people's *differences* so that it can help people become the *same*, that is, equally autonomous and equally the recipients of beneficent clinical practices and just health care policies.

Beginning with an inquiry into the status of women in health care and medicine, and specifically an investigation into those biomedical systems, structures, and policies that subordinate women to men, feminist bioethicists should aim to build health care and medical practices that contribute not only to gender liberation but also to race, class, and human liberation. The work of feminist bioethicists has begun, but it cannot succeed unless all bioethicists become what Aristotle termed partners in virtue and friends in action, that is, people who share meaningful goals and tasks in common. In recognizing each other's shared frailty and morality, we will perhaps be inspired to care enough about each other to produce globally just health care policies aimed at eliminating the patterns of domination and subordination, of arrogance and servility, that have characterized human relationships for too long.

Global bioethics is a possibility, provided we agree to see each other not through the eyes of justice blindfolded and holding a sword and scales, but through the open eyes of the Greek goddess Nemesis—she of the "third eye"—continually looking for wrongdoers, for oppressors.[25] We need to confront oppression with all our senses, with our emotions as well as with our reason. And we need to confront it whether it occurs in a developed or a developing nation. Unless we bioethicists learn to examine our own and each other's health care systems in the way Nemesis would, we will find ourselves the instruments of local and global injustice—a very unhealthy state of affairs that I, and I suspect you also, wish to avoid at all costs.

Notes

1. Van Rensselaer Potter, *Global Bioethics: Building on the Leopold Legacy* (East Lansing: Michigan State University Press, 1988), p. 2.

2. Alice Echols, "The New Feminism of Yin and Yang," in Ann Snitow, Christine Stansell, and Sharon Thompson, eds., _Powers of Desire: The Politics of Sexuality_ (New York: Monthly Review Press, 1983).

3. Elizabeth V. Spelman, _Inessential Woman: Problems of Exclusion in Feminism Thought_ (Boston: Beacon, 1988), p. 12.

4. Ibid., p. 13.

5. Uma Narayan, _Dislocating Cultures: Identities, Traditions, and Third-World Feminisms_ (New York: Routledge, 1997), p. 121.

6. Ibid., p. 125.

7. Ibid.

8. Ibid., p. 127.

9. Ibid., p. 128.

10. Ibid., p. 140.

11. Ibid., p. 146.

12. Robin Morgan, ed., _Sisterhood Is Global: The International Women's Movement Anthology_ (Garden City, N.Y.: Anchor, 1984).

13. Morgan, "Introduction: Planetary Feminism," in _Sisterhood_, p. 4.

14. Chandra Talpate Mohanty, "Feminist Encounters: Locating the Politics of Experience," in Michelle Barrett and Anne Philips, eds., _Destabilizing Theory: Contemporary Feminist Debates_ (Stanford: Stanford University Press, 1992), pp. 78–79.

15. Morgan, "Planetary Feminism," p. 36.

16. Ibid., p. 36.

17. Mohanty, "Feminist Encounters," p. 83.

18. Susan Moller Okin, "Feminism, Women's Human Rights, and Cultural Differences," _Hypatia_ 13, no. 2 (1998): 42.

19. Ibid., p. 45.

20. Alison M. Jaggar, "Toward a Feminist Conception of Moral Reasoning," in James Sterba, ed., _Moral and Social Justice_ (Lanham, Md.: Rowman & Littlefield, 1995), p. 115.

21. Ibid., pp. 131–132 (emphasis added).

22. Maria Lugones and Elizabeth Spelman, "Have We Got a Theory for You! Feminist Theory, Cultural Imperialism, and the Demand for 'The Woman's Voice,'" in Janet A. Kourany, James P. Sterba, and Rosemarie Tong, eds., _Feminist Philosophies_ (Englewood Cliffs, N.J.: Prentice-Hall, 1992), p. 363.

23. Jaggar, "Feminist Conception of Moral Reasoning," pp. 132–135.

24. Rosalind Petchesky and Karen Judd, eds., _Negotiating Reproductive Rights: Women's Perspectives Across Countries and Cultures_ (London: Zed, 1998), p. 362.

25. Mary Daly, _Pure Lust: Elemental Feminist Philosophy_ (Boston: Beacon, 1978), pp. 278–280.

3

Feminism and Genetic Nursing: Globalizing Transdisciplinary Teams

GWEN W. ANDERSON
RITA BLACK MONSEN
MARY VARNEY RORTY

"As society moves forward from a highly specialized, individualized, and competitive model of healthcare delivery,"[1] it is important to critique existing models of practice in order to construct new models that are more collaborative, interactive, multi-skilled, and non-hierarchical.

Feminist thought in the last few decades has both drawn on and contributed to a variety of critical social and intellectual movements. Thus it has been a rich source of insights and strategies for groups seeking to alter traditional hierarchies and oppressions.[2] Here we borrow some successful strategies from feminism to focus on a serious problem that the nursing profession currently faces—how to deliver morally appropriate genetic services globally as well as locally. Paramount among these feminist strategies are egalitarian views that seek to break down not only hierarchical social and economic structures but also hierarchical ideational and conceptual structures. Drawing our inspiration from feminist egalitarianism broadly interpreted, we propose a transdisciplinary model for disseminating genetic health care services that will enable nurses in a variety of disciplines to focus on their common challenge: improving health and adapting to new economic, political, technological, and social realities around the globe.

Three Global Forces

The recent explosion in genetics research and the proliferation of technologies associated with genetic medicine are already having a noticeable impact on delivery of health care and can be expected to have even
greater influence in the future. Among the global forces that will increase
demand for genetic services in the future are (1) the increasing world
population, (2) the increasing impact of Western attitudes toward applied technology on traditional societies, and (3) the increasing global desire to benefit from the fruits of the Human Genome Project.

The common thread tying these three forces together is their individual and synergistic potential to irreversibly alter civilization by changing
cultural patterns of procreation and societal definitions of what it means
to be human. We believe that it is imperative for health care professionals, particularly nurses, to collaborate in order to provide genetic services
in a manner that promotes trust, enhances quality of life, and prevents
unintended exploitation.[3]

The Increasing World Population

The world population—2.9 billion in 1960 and 5.8 billion in 1999—is projected to be 8 billion by 2015.[4] Introducing technologies associated with
genetics into the already problematic issue of population growth complicates a volatile issue. Who should reproduce, and what individuals or
groups should be reproduced? The outcome of individual pregnancies
can be more precisely predicted on the basis of various tests, some of
them genetic, which can determine the genetic makeup of future children. This may reduce the suffering associated with the birth of genetically anomalous progeny or limit the transmission of some genetically
linked diseases. Genetically determinable differences, however, have the
potential of becoming the basis for genetically driven discriminations (as
sex-selection abortion in cultures with a strong preference for male children has shown). Since the line between a debilitating genotype and a
merely undesirable phenotype is hard to draw, already disadvantaged
populations, ranging from people with minor genetic disabilities to
members of various minority groups, may fear genetics as another possible source of discrimination and control.

The Increasing Impact of Western Applied
Technology on Traditional Societies

Because social attitudes, legal remedies, and moral standards typically
lag behind scientific and technological developments, it is vital that sci-

entists and technologists consider how their new products might affect the people who use them, negatively as well as positively. A technology designed for a limited purpose can be applied beyond its original intent (e.g., contemporary uses of growth hormone to "enhance" normal growth instead of just compensating for inadequate growth), or its very availability can alter general expectations of what is possible or desirable. Therefore, the developers of new technologies cannot simply assume that they will be used in the beneficent ways they were intended to be used; rather, they must consider how their creations might be misused and alert the public to this risk.

Criticisms of how genetic information is presented to the public, initially brought to bear during the 1970s with the introduction of prenatal and sickle cell screening programs, continue to resurface.[5] Sickle cell screening in particular created wide public distrust because it was used to disqualify African Americans from economic advancement, many of whom were merely carriers and were not themselves affected by this genetic condition. Skepticism is raised when a priori assumptions dictate in advance what can be included or excluded in a particular definition of what is a preventable mutation, what is a known scientific fact, what is real as compared to what is ideal, and what merits allocation of scarce public resources. By selecting the "facts," the expert predetermines the "frame" through which the public will view a new technology.[6] How genetic technology is packaged for public consumption is especially significant, since this emerging technology threatens to reconceive human beings as nothing more then biologically determined organisms. Because scientists and technicians who specialize in genetics use methods that objectify, quantify, splice, and clone DNA, their worldview and its inherent assumptions could be dehumanizing. It is far too easy to overlook the fact that technology is not neutral. It is a way of thinking[7] that forgets aspects of being human that go beyond pure rationality,[8] thereby transforming our fundamental conception of what it means to be human.[9]

The Increasing Global Desire to Benefit from the Fruits of the Human Genome Project

Many people regard the enormous challenge of identifying the entire human genome sequence by the year 2003 as the key for unlocking human capacity to cure disease. As the human genetic map unfolds, it is clear that the promise of using genetic science to improve human health lies in the hands of biotechnology and pharmaceutical corporations that will translate genomics into therapeutics. Discoveries from large-scale sequencing projects of human DNA stimulate research and development that promotes prospecting for new drugs that target and repair DNA, trigger tissue regeneration, produce viral vaccines, and make effective gene transfer mechanisms that have both the potential to change human DNA permanently and the ability to simultaneously explore thousands of genes for deleterious mutations. As these new tools are brought to market, societies around the world must place their trust in health care professionals who will make use of these new genetic diagnostic and treatment capabilities. One of the most immediately problematic issues is the very practical one of cost versus benefit, and who will pay for which benefits. Scientific and technological expertise, as well as access to its (often expensive) products, varies considerably around the world. Only wealthy countries or the most wealthy individuals can expect to reap the benefits of recent scientific and technological advances. For economic reasons, the majority of the world's population will be deprived of any benefit from advances in genetic knowledge, despite the fact that many of these advances will have been made as a result of relatively risky research on them. The task that lies ahead, therefore, is to find a way of using genetic technology that spreads genetic benefits and risks equitably across the entire human population.[10]

Nursing, Genetics, and Nursing's Minimal Involvement in Genetics

Given the global genetic forces at work in the world today, it is clear that there is going to be an increasing demand for applications of human genetics. Because of the historical and continuing involvement of nurses in the provision of patient care and its role in the mediation of new medical diagnostics and therapeutics, the nursing profession will need to respond to increasing patient demand for genetic services and research. Unfortunately, nursing lags behind the disciplines of medicine and genetic counseling in terms of its readiness to utilize and disseminate genetic information about genetically mediated diseases, genetic diagnostics, genetic therapies, and genetic research nationally and internationally. Yet at the same time, because of its location in the forefront of health care delivery, and because of its traditional focus on the whole patient in the context of family and community, nursing, the largest profession, is ideally situated to broker this new knowledge. However, nurses must first gain adequate knowledge, training, or national certification in genetics to legitimate their position in the delivery of genetic services or genetic research. With proper knowledge nurses can help create models for delivering genetic services in a patient-centered, humanistic manner.

Few renowned nursing leaders nationally or internationally have given thought to exploring or defining what and how nurses might contribute to the delivery of genetic health care and research in a global society. To adequately address society's expectations of professional nursing, leaders in the discipline must develop a strategic plan to develop formal links to disciplines in different societies and genetic communities around the world. Collaboration with other disciplines in these communities will foster dissemination of genetic knowledge into nursing practice as well as dissemination of nursing knowledge and practices into the delivery of genetic services and research. As part of this dialectical process, nurses will need to articulate their role as advocates for patients, families, and communities in the context of partnerships with educators, other clinicians, researchers, policymakers, and professional organizations in local and global genetic communities.

where is this now?

From a feminist perspective, there are two major factors that help explain the discipline of nursing's minimal involvement in genetic research and its applications in clinical settings: (1) the subordination of nursing to medicine and (2) conflicting epistemologies present in nursing and medicine. Feminism contributes to changing the status quo for nurses by sensitizing nurses to the importance of disparities of power in institutional settings, by challenging nurses to develop humanistic models for understanding the impact of genetics on families and populations, and by reminding nurses of the importance of context in applying genetics in different cultures. Publicly acknowledging the historical context that has shaped nursing makes it possible for nurses to increase their understanding of the potential barriers that stand in the way of developing new dialogues among nursing leaders and between nursing and other disciplines, and to use this understanding to forge new avenues for integrating genetics into practice, education, and research.

Subordination of Nursing to Medicine

During the 1960s and 1970s, the introduction of new medical technologies began to transform the face of medicine. As the profession responsible for bedside care, nursing assumed increasing responsibility for machines at the bedside, from ventilators and dialyzers to the increasingly sophisticated monitors that fill contemporary ICUs. Nurses embraced machine technology in an effort to make their practice more scientific, to improve the reliability of their observation of human functioning, and to strengthen the nurse–physician relationship. However, "transfer of technology from medicine to nursing reinforced the subordination of nursing to medicine and impeded the development of nursing as a valued province of knowledge and practice."[11] Despite its history, nursing has been and continues to be thought of as medicine's subsidiary rather than a separate and unique discipline by a majority of physicians around the world.[12] At the end of the twentieth century biomedical science is the champion of cause-and-effect theories of human disease and curative practices based on empirical science.

Success from basic and applied science continues to reward medicine with the top positions in the medical hierarchy, rewarding physicians in particular with "a vastly inflated status within the hospital."[13] True to Darwinian form, the most powerful are presumed to be the most fit. Nationally and internationally, medicine not only survives but also gathers authoritative power, control, and economic privilege within all health care and research settings, whereas the discipline of nursing is eclipsed as a "soft" complement to the "hardness" and rigor of science. In this social structure, nurses are viewed as physicians' helpers.[14] As handmaidens, nurses were once trained to do services that promoted medical goals, and they were "primarily accountable to physicians for patient care."[15] In modern and not-so-modern societies around the globe, they are still obliged to obey physicians' orders rather than think critically about their practice or openly advocate for the welfare of patients and families. To a large degree nurses' identities and roles are controlled overtly and covertly by the authoritative and "expert" power of medicine. Economically and intellectually, nursing education, nurse-conducted research, and holistic nursing practices are systematically oppressed within a physician-dominated, directed, and oriented model of medicine that has been adopted as the only bona fide model for all health care systems. Nevertheless, nurse academics in particular have courageously pursued humanistic and holistic practices and ways of respecting and communicating with patients that are contrary to the medical model (and perhaps heretical).[16] They have sought to integrate into nursing practice multiple ways of knowing and being human—the empirical, aesthetic, personal, ethical,[17] and moral.[18]

Conflicting Epistemologies in Nursing and Medicine

The epistemological and ontological presuppositions of nursing differ in many respects from those of modern medicine.[19] Discussions in nursing raise important questions about what counts as knowledge, how knowledge is obtained, and the ways it is applied in human contexts, questions to which many of the conclusions of feminism have great relevance. Likewise, feminists have urged acknowledgment of a variety of sources of information that are required to deal sensitively and comprehensively with human beings—sources such as the ethical, aesthetic, and subjective understandings that are often neglected by an empirically driven scientific objectivism and medical rationalism.[20] For nurses who believe in holistic practice, a philosophy of science that holds rationalism and objectivism preeminent in "medical services" is problematic because it creates "a false universalism that silences the voices of all those other than the dominant group by presuming that it can speak for all."[21]

As a practice, the art of nursing is founded on traditions of caring, nurturing, healing, listening, intuiting, presencing, and understanding holistically instead of curing disease and prolonging human life, practices dominant in medicine.[22] Nurses believe that all people deserve to be treated in a manner that recognizes their equality and strives to promote their human potential, integrity, dignity, social reciprocity, spirituality, and wholeness.[23] These beliefs enable nurses to create respectful, genuinely caring, and interconnected relationships with the patients and the families who are the recipients of their health care. Feminist writings that espouse an ethics of care—a relational ethics—have found practical applications in nursing, where caring is conceptualized as a basic human trait, a moral imperative, a therapeutic intervention, and an essential attribute of the nurse-patient interpersonal relationship.[24]

Competing Models of Practice

This history of alliance in clinical practice but divergence in philosophy and theory between medicine and nursing, which we have recounted, points to substantial reasons why the involvement of nursing in the global delivery of genetic health care is crucial. Nursing's views of epistemology and ontology, so similar in many ways to some feminist approaches, may very well prevent leaders in nursing everywhere from buying into the principles and practices inherent in the philosophy of atomism, reductivism,[25] biological determinism,[26] and scientism[27] that underlie the science of medical genetics and some of its applications in health care services and research. Nurses think that there is something fundamentally wrong with these principles and practices as the preeminent paradigm in health care services and health care research, including genetic technology transfer. They wonder, "Is it not possible to practice in an environment where humanists and natural scientists collaborate and respect each other's different perspectives so that patients and families can benefit from both old and new philosophies of science?"

In the following section of our analysis we respond that, yes, it is possible for nurses and everyone to practice in just such an environment, provided that all health care professionals, beginning perhaps with nurses, learn how to think in a transdisciplinary manner. If it is important for nursing to become more involved in the utilization and dissemination of genetic information, genetic diagnostics and therapies, it is equally important that the profession think seriously about how that involvement should be structured. Borrowing some ideas from contemporary feminist analyses that focus on the effect of power distributions in institutional structures, we recommend a transdisciplinary model that values professional diversity and allows all participants to collaborate for the benefit of the individuals and populations they cumulatively service. As we see it, this transdisciplinary model not only represents an improvement over multidisciplinary and interdisciplinary models of delivering health care but also provides nurses with a feminist structure for genetic nursing.

A Multidisciplinary Model of Practice

Members of an interprofessional team work in parallel or sequentially toward preestablished goals. Each person works from within his or her own disciplinary philosophy. Team members have a clearly specified role function and their participation is bounded by their disciplinary expertise.[28] The power, authority, and responsibility for a final decision about a plan of care lies with one discipline and often with only one person on the team. This occurs because team members are not considered equal in terms of their expertise, status, or function on the team. Usually the physician is the identifiable leader to whom other team members provide information. The physician utilizes this information to prescribe an appropriate medical intervention that other team members are charged to carry out. Services can be fragmented, and there may be discrepancies between team members about which interventions are most appropriate or how to carry them out. Lack of attention to relationship building among team members and a lack of understanding about what each team member has to offer can result in disputes over ownership of certain domains of service. This results in focusing on the integrity of professional practices and traditions rather than on the well-being of patients. To the degree that patients are "turfed" among a group of disharmonious team members, they tend to be viewed as parts of persons rather than as whole persons.[29] Competition for dominance, control, superiority, and extreme individualism threatens and inhibits team members from fully participating in decisionmaking, a state of affairs that deprives patients of the kind of holistic care they might have received otherwise.

An Interdisciplinary Model of Practice

Philosophically, the interdisciplinary model supposedly represents an improvement over the multidisciplinary model. It actively promotes collaborations across disciplines by gathering three or more practitioners into an interdependent working relationship.[30] Team members are likely to have some idea about the role functions, knowledge base, and general overall framework and approach used by other team members. As a result, program planning is more collaborative than in the multidisciplinary model. However, because each discipline implements the collaborative plan of care or program on its own, so to speak, the interdisciplinary model still tends to promote "hierarchical relationships."[31] In other words, in theory team members are supposed to be consulting with one another routinely, whereas in practice team members generally fail to consult each other and implement individual care plans unilaterally "without understanding the impact of their actions on other team members."[32] They thereby lose the full potential for innovative and creative problem solving in the clinical setting. In other words, the interdisciplinary model provides coordinated but not integrated family-oriented services.[33] Services remain fragmented because continuity of care is not systematically reinforced, nor is cohesiveness within the team valued as an everyday therapeutic strategy that serves the best interest of the patient and family.

A Transdisciplinary Model of Practice

In contrast to the multidisciplinary and the interdisciplinary model, in which occupational power, status, and professional recognition are key issues, the transdisciplinary model considers each member of the team an equal partner.[34] The unique professional abilities, personal qualities, values, cultural traditions, personal emotions, knowledge, special training, and life experiences of each team member are acknowledged and viewed as an attribute for the team's functioning. These attributes are thought to enrich the team process and enhance patient outcomes. In addition, the transdisciplinary model encourages team members to "transcend their separate conceptual, theoretical, and methodological orientations in order to develop a shared approach to . . . building a common conceptual framework."[35] The resulting *shared* philosophical perspective is then used as a conceptual reference point to provide a justification for the team's insistence on providing patients and their families a truly integrated set of services. Because team members pool their knowledge and learn from each other, boundaries between disciplines are loosened, overlaps in services are recognized and incorporated into care plans, and patients and families actually receive the kind of comprehensive and meaningful health care they desire.[36]

From what has been said about it so far, it is clear that the transdisciplinary model requires a change in how all health care services, but particularly ones related to genetics, are delivered, researched, and conceptualized. In both multidisciplinary and interdisciplinary models, medicine retains expert power, authoritative control, and economic privilege. In such a social/cultural environment other practitioners are all too often considered physician helpers or "handmaidens" whose purpose it is to further the curative powers of medical genetics.[37] A transdisciplinary model challenges this tradition by calling for a new way of thinking about the composition of team members and about team leadership (the best team leader will change as the context or stage of health care delivery changes). In addition, a transdisciplinary model invites each discipline to view patients as whole people living within multiple communities[38] and to provide them its special services as excellently as possible.[39]

Achieving a Transdisciplinary Model in Genetics

Throughout the course of their educational training and professional socialization clinicians need to be introduced to the transdisciplinary approach, particularly in those areas of medicine (e.g., genetics) that affect some of the most basic aspects of human personhood. Only when a transdisciplinary model is valued by every professional can it be used to achieve equality among professions and foster partnerships with the public during the discourse of daily practice. Once students become clinicians, they resist transdisciplinary team practices due to perceived barriers such as unequal workloads, insufficient time, disciplinary-specific jargon, and lack of willingness to teach each other decisionmaking and judgment skills as part of the process of role release.[40]

A transdisciplinary educational model must foster understanding and respect for differences and similarities in the role function of each professional involved in patient care. Valuing each other's differences and similarities fosters sharing and encourages the transferal of information, skills, and decisionmaking responsibilities across disciplines. Making the boundaries that divide disciplines transparent and permeable promotes cross-pollination of ideas, the building of new frameworks that establish a shared common social mission, and more variety in the goals to be achieved. Most importantly, however, a transdisciplinary educational model understands patients and family members as part of the "team." Precisely because they are not professionals, patients and family members bring to the decisionmaking process unique perspectives that might otherwise be neglected, ignored, or trivialized.[41]

Final Remarks

If the current promising possibilities for human genetics are to be realized in a positive way, greater involvement by nursing is inevitable and

[handwritten margin note: This is why they have different training.]

desirable. The humanistic perspective that the profession of nursing embodies, different in many respects from the techno-scientific philosophy that medicine promotes, offers an important resource for individuals, families, and communities in different cultures whose lives will be increasingly influenced by genetic technology.[42] But in order to use their resources in transdisciplinary teams, nurses must incorporate genetics into the perspective of *nursing* knowledge—as a dimension of teaching and practicing excellent nursing care—rather than allow nursing values to be subordinated to traditional medical values. In order to do this effectively, the discipline of nursing needs to include genetic content in its disciplinary knowledge base and generate genetic nursing research to provide evidence of the effects of its practice. The challenge that must be met is to find ways to train future generations of genetic nurses so they can clearly articulate their unique disciplinary paradigm. They must be taught how to contribute their nursing perspective to future developments in genetic services around the world, a shift that "parallels the process of enabling and empowering, which produces competence and hope."[43]

Integrating the efforts of practitioners, researchers, and theorists within nursing itself will contribute to this process, as practicing nurses better understand how to use genetic medicine to better meet the needs of a global community. Nurses must recognize their obligation to fulfill their social mandate by more effectively asserting their roles as patient advocates, coordinators, educators, and leaders. Within transdisciplinary teams, "the promising outlook for nursing is realization of the opportunity for advanced practice roles. . . . One discipline alone cannot serve the complex needs of clients with chronic, disabling, or developmental disorders. We must synchronize our paradigm shift as a team."[44] Relinquishing the image of nurses as "medicine's" handmaidens will enable nurses around the world to move to more complex, productive, and collaborative modes of being.

Patients, families, and communities expect scientists and practitioners in all disciplines to deliver services that ultimately mitigate their suffering and improve their quality of daily life without stripping them of their human dignity or wholeness. The ethical challenge we all face is to recognize and begin to deal with the fact that westernized approaches to science, technology, and geneticized health care should not be unreflectively transferred into populations with different cultural, religious, and historical traditions; this is done at the risk of doing serious damage to the cultures and people involved. Likewise, no single type or source of knowledge will be adequate to help the public come to terms with the idea that ethnicity (family and genetic heritage) and the global environment influence human health and illness.

The voices of all disciplines must be given an equal chance to contribute and to promote genetic information and genetic therapeutics as
human goods. Together, nurses, physicians, and other health care professionals are responsible for delivering genetic information and services
equitably. Otherwise they run the risk of alienating the public, who
might perceive advances in genetics as tools that benefit only those in society who are already privileged. Genetic health care must be delivered
within an environment of collaboration across clinical specialties, disciplines, and cultures. Collaboration will improve patient services by expe-
diting a compassionate and comprehensive response to patients and families who, despite some reservations, are looking to the new genetic
technologies for some healing balm.

Notes

Gwen Anderson and Rita Monsen wish to thank Nancy Diekelmann, who created an opening to critique nursing's involvement in genetics within a scholarly
community of postmodern nurse philosophers who were not afraid to question
their values, beliefs, and assumptions about nursing and medicine.

1. Cecilia Rokusek, "An Introduction to the Concept of Interdisciplinary Practice," in Bruce A. Thyer and Nancy P. Kropf, eds., *Developmental Disabilities: A Hand-
book for Interdisciplinary Practice* (Cambridge, Mass.: Brookline, 1996), pp. 4–12.
2. Nancy Tuana and Rosemarie Tong, eds., *Feminism and Philosophy: Essential
Readings in Theory, Reinterpretation, and Application* (Boulder: Westview, 1995).
3. L. Norsen, J. Opladen, and J. Quinn, "Practice Model: Collaborative Practice," *Critical Care Nursing Clinics of North America* 7, no. 1 (1995): 43–52; H. J. Ornstein, "Collaborative Practice Between Ontario Nurses and Physicians: Is It Possible?" *Canadian Journal of Nursing Administration* 3, no. 4 (1990): 10–14.
4. Data from the United Nations: on-line http://www.facingthefuture.org/
trends.html Accessed October 1999.
5. Abby Lippman and Benjamin S. Wilfond, "Twice-Told Tales: Stories About
Genetic Disorders," *American Journal of Human Genetics* Suppl. 1 (1992): 936–937; T.
Marteau, "Framing of Information: Its Influence Upon Decisions of Doctors and
Patients," *British Journal of Social Psychology* 28, no. 1 (1989): 89–94; Nancy Press
and C. H. Browner, "Collective Fictions: Similarities in Reasons for Accepting Maternal Serum Alpha-fetoprotein Screening Among Women of Diverse Ethnic and
Social Class Backgrounds," *Fetal Diagnosis and Therapy* Suppl. 1 (1993): 97–106.
6. Norman Fost, "Ethical Issues in Genetics," *Medical Genetics* 39, no. 1 (1992):
79–89; Nancy Press and C. H. Browner, "Risk, Autonomy, and Responsibility: Informed Consent for Prenatal Testing," *Hasting Center Report* 25, no. 3 (1995): S9–S12.
7. Kenneth Ketner Laine, "An Implicit World View in Technology and Its Consequences for Contemporary Life," *Nursing Outlook* 44, no. 6 (1996): 280–283.
8. Charles Taylor, *The Ethics of Authenticity,* 7th ed. (Cambridge: Harvard University Press, 1997).

9. Martin Heidegger, "The Phenomenological Method of Investigation in Being and Time," in D. F. Krell, ed., *Basic Writings: From Being and Time to the Task of Thinking* (New York: Harper & Row, 1977), pp. 72–89.

10. Alexander Capron, "Which Ills to Bear? Reevaluating the 'Threat' of Modern Genetics," *Emory Law* 39 (1990): 666–696; Press and Browner, "Collective Fictions," pp. 97–106; Colleen Scanlon, "Genetic Advances: Policy and Perils," in Felissa Lashley, ed., *The Genetics Revolution: Implications for Nursing* (Washington, D.C.: American Academy of Nursing, 1997), pp. 33–37.

11. M. Sandelowski, "(Ir) Reconcilable Differences? The Debate Concerning Nursing and Technology," *Image: Journal of Nursing Scholarship* 29, no. 2 (1997): 169–174.

12. S. Reverby, *Ordered to Care: The Dilemma of American Nursing, 1850–1945* (New York: Cambridge University Press, 1987); Daniel P. Chambliss, *Beyond Caring: Hospitals, Nurses, and the Social Organization of Ethics* (Chicago: University of Chicago Press, 1995), pp. 120–149; Martin Benjamin and Joy Curtis, *Ethics in Nursing* (New York: Oxford University Press, 1992).

13. Sandra Harding, "Value-Laden Technologies and the Politics of Nursing," in Stuary Spicker and Sally Gadow, eds., *Nursing: Images and Ideals* (New York: Springer, 1980), p. 60.

14. Ornstein, "Collaborative Practice"; Reverby, "Ordered to Care."

15. Mila Aroskar, "Envisioning Nursing As a Moral Community," *Nursing Outlook* 43, no. 3 (1995): 134–138.

16. K. Martin, "Coordinating Multidisciplinary, Collaborative Research: A Formula for Success," *Clinical Nurse Specialist* 8, no. 1 (1994): 18–22.

17. Barbara Carper, "Fundamental Patterns of Knowing in Nursing," *Advances in Nursing Science* 1, no. 1 (1978): 13–23.

18. Gwen Anderson, "Creating Moral Space in Prenatal Genetic Services," *Qualitative Health Research: An International and Interdisciplinary Journal* 8, no. 2 (1998): 168–187.

19. David Allen, Patricia Benner, and Nancy Diekelmann, "Three Paradigms for Research: Methodological Implications," in Peggy Chinn, ed., *Nursing Research Methodology: Issues and Implications* (Rockville, Md.: Aspen, 1986), pp. 23–38; K. Schumacher and Susan Gortner, "(Mis)conceptions and Reconceptions About Traditional Science," *Advances in Nursing Science* 14, no. 4 (1992): 1–11; Mary C. Silva, Jean M. Sorrell, and Carolyn D. Sorrell, "From Carper's Patterns of Knowing to Ways of Being: An Ontological Philosophical Shift in Nursing," *Advances in Nursing Science* 18, no. 1 (1995): 1–13.

20. Mary Ann Belenky et al., *Women's Ways of Knowing: The Development of Self, Voice, and Mind* (New York: Basic, 1986).

21. Georgia Warnke, "Feminism and Hermeneutics," *Hypatia* 8, no. 1 (1993): 81–98.

22. Ibid.

23. Patricia D. Barry, *Psychosocial Nursing Care of Physically Ill Patients and Their Families* (Hartford, Conn.: Lippincott, 1996), pp. 54–77.

24. Janice Morse et al., "Concepts of Caring and Caring As a Concept," *Advances in Nursing Science* 13, no. 1 (1990): 1–14; Petra Bowden, *Caring: Gender Sensitive Ethics* (New York: Routledge, 1997); Carol Gilligan, *In a Different Voice: Psy-*

chological Theory and Women's Development (Cambridge: Harvard University Press, 1982); Nel Noddings, "An Ethic of Caring," in Noddings, ed., *Caring: A Feminist Approach to Ethics and Moral Education* (Berkeley: University of California Press, 1984), pp. 79–103.

25. Taylor, *Ethics of Authenticity.*

26. Barbara Katz-Rothman, *Genetic Maps and Human Imaginations: The Limits of Science in Understanding Who We Are* (New York: Norton, 1999).

27. Hwa Yol Jung, "The Geneology of Technological Rationality in the Human Sciences," *Research in Philosophy and Technology* 9, no. 3 (1989): 59–82.

28. Patricia Rosenfield, "The Potential of Transdisciplinary Research for Sustaining and Extending Linkages Between the Health and Social Sciences," *Social Science and Medicine* 35, no. 11 (1992): 1343–1357.

29. Fred P. Orelove and Dick Sobsey, *Educating Children with Multiple Disabilities: A Transdisciplinary Approach* (Baltimore: Brookes, 1996).

30. Rokusek, "Concept of Interdisciplinary Practice."

31. Rosenfield, "Transdisciplinary Research," pp. 1343–1357.

32. Gwen Anderson, "Commentary: Prenatal Genetic Services Signals a Much Deeper Problem in Healthcare Delivery," *Nursing Ethics: An International Journal for Healthcare Professionals* 6, no. 3 (1999): 255–257.

33. Kara B. Jaffe and Patricia A. Walsh, "The Development of the Specialty Rehabilitation Home Care Team: Supporting the Creative Thought," *Holistic Nursing Practice* 7, no. 4 (1993): 36–41.

34. R. Kenen, "Genetic Counseling: The Development of a New Interdisciplinary Occupational Field," *Social Science and Medicine* 18, no. 7 (1984): 541–549.

35. Rosenfield, "Transdisciplinary Research," pp. 1343–1357.

36. N. Ferrer and T. Navarra, "Issues in Collaborative Practice: Professional Boundaries: Clarifying Roles and Goals," *Cancer Practice* 2, no. 4 (1994): 3111–3112.

37. Ornstein, "Collaborative Practice," pp. 10–14.

38. Rokusek, "Concept of Interdisciplinary Practice," pp. 4–12.

39. Jean Watson, "NLN Perspective: President's Message: From Disciplinary Specific to 'Inter' to 'Multi' to 'Transdisciplinary' Healthcare Education and Practice," *Nursing and Healthcare: Perspectives on Community* 17, no. 2 (1996): 90–91.

40. S. Ryan-Vincek, L. Tuesday-Heathfield, and S. Lamorey, "From Theory to Practice: A Pilot Study of Team Members' Perspectives on Transdiciplinary Service Dellivery," *Infant-Toddler Intervention: The Transdisciplinary Journal* 5, no. 2 (1995): 153–176.

41. Dorothy Hutchinson, "The Transdisciplinary Approach," in Judith B. Curry and Kathryn Peppe, eds., *Mental Retardation: Nursing Approaches to Care* (St. Louis, Mo.: Mosby, 1978), pp. 65–74.

42. Susan Sherwin, "Feminist and Medical Ethics: Two Different Approaches to Contextual Ethics," in Helen Holmes and Laura Purdy, eds., *Feminist Perspectives in Medical Ethics* (Indianapolis: Indiana University Press, 1992), pp. 17–31.

43. Shirley Hoeman, "A Research-based Transdisciplinary Team Model for Infants with Special Needs and Their Families," *Holistic Nursing Practice* 7, no. 4 (1993): 63–72.

44. Ibid., p. 71.

4

Kagandahang Loob: A Filipino Concept of Feminine Bioethics

LEONARDO D. DE CASTRO

The concept of *kagandahang loob* is central to ordinary Filipino ethical thinking. In this chapter I show how *kagandahang loob* can provide a perspective for understanding issues of bioethics. In the process, it also establishes the affinity of the concept to feminine ethics.

The feminine characterization of *kagandahang loob* is found in a number of features that have been mentioned in various accounts of feminine approaches to ethics, including (1) the recognition of "self-imposed" obligations arising spontaneously from the acceptance of a need to care, (2) an emphasis on the enhancement of relationships, (3) a high valuation of emotions and attitudes, and (4) stress on what may be considered a virtue of character. The features have been mentioned—separately or in combination—in various works highlighting the gendered profile of ethics discourse.

First, I will examine the literal meanings of the words that make up the term *kagandahang loob*, showing that its core meaning is located in the intentional aspects of human actions. Subsequently, I will examine both the uses of *kagandahang loob* in ordinary ethical discourse and the uses of related terms in feminine ethical discourse.

In Filipino ethics the concept of *kagandahang loob* is expressed routinely and in multiple ways. For general purposes, a good deed is ordinarily referred to as a *kagandahang loob*. Doing something good for somebody else is *pagmamagandang loob*. A good person is somebody who possesses something called *magandang kalooban*, a term that has the same root as *kagandahang loob*. In being helpful to others, someone is *nagmamagandang loob*.

51

The opposite of *kagandahang loob* is *kasamaang loob*, which may refer either to evil deeds or to evil intentions that attend human actions. Somebody who feels bad about being wronged has a *sama ng loob*. Those who perpetrate evil are *masasamang loob*.

Transcending the Physical

The word *kagandahan* has its root in *ganda*, which means beauty. On the other hand, *loob* means inside. Hence, *kagandahang loob* may be translated literally as beauty within. The words inside and within both suggest spatial relations. The effect of this spatial qualification is to put the focus on a person's emotions and motivation for acting. For it is the motivation that lies within, as opposed to the physical components of actions, which are exposed and directly observable.

A parallel rendering of the meanings of the two critical words *ganda* and *loob* supports this understanding of *kagandahang loob*. Although *ganda* is mainly used in Filipino in the expression of aesthetic judgment, it is also used as an expression of positive ethical judgments. The adjective *maganda* is used to qualify not only works of art or aesthetic experiences but also human actions. Additionally, *loob* may be taken to mean will. The *loob* or *kalooban* consists of one's inner feelings toward something or somebody else. Hence, *kagandahang loob* means goodwill. In a sense, it is the willing of something good for others and thus the manifestation of a caring attitude.

This emphasis on the internal aspects of human action notwithstanding, *kagandahang loob* transcends the physical. There is even a sense in which it transcends traditional physical-mental or corporeal-spiritual dichotomies, since within the context of the pertinent ethical discourse, it is important that the beauty within be manifested externally. *Kagandahang loob* is meant to be "shown" to others. It is part of the meaning of *loob*—of what lies within—that it must be ventilated. The *kalooban* lies inside but it must not be kept inside. In a way, it is "what-lies-within-that-lives-without." It can only be manifested and perceived externally. It is a good whose value is evident to the *kagandahang loob* community, something that is essential for that type of community and its members to flourish.

Manifesting *Kagandahang Loob*

To show *kagandahang loob* is to open up one's inside to another. It is to show the other that one means well. And one shows that one means well by performing actions meant to benefit others.

It is only through actions beneficial to others that *kagandahang loob* can be manifested externally. People perceive manifestations of the *kalooban*, rather than the *kalooban* itself directly. But externalization is only half of the story. The use of the word *loob*—instead of other Filipino words such as *kilos* or *gawa*, which stand for physical actions—indicates the significance given to the intentional component of human behavior in this discourse. What needs to be underscored is the integration of intention or will with the physical component of actions. Making ethical judgments of physical acts without regard for the emotions and motives of the person acting would be inappropriate.

In the context of *kagandahang loob*, what is most important about beneficial actions is that they be characterized by positive feelings toward the intended beneficiaries. It is not sufficient that they bear benefits, whether actually or potentially. In the reckoning of moral worth, the actual benefits may not even be necessary at all. It is the *kagandahang loob* attending the deed that carries the greatest weight.

In effect, to exhibit *kagandahang loob* is not just to allow others to notice it but to convey it to them: There must be an effort to make somebody the recipient of it. There must be a relationship with another. To convey *kagandahang loob* is to give part of oneself for the benefit of others. Through this conveyance, one expresses genuine concern and signals a caring relationship.

Of what, then, does *kagandahang loob* consist? How is it manifested?

Kusang Loob

A very important requirement for the conveyance—and flourishing—of *kagandahang loob* is the moral agent's exercise of *kusang loob* (free will). *Kusang loob* may be exercised only if the agent (1) is not acting under external compulsion, (2) is motivated by positive feelings (e.g. charity, tolerance, clemency, love, or empathy) toward the beneficiary, and (3) is not motivated by the promise of payment or reward. These conditions are evident in the use of *kusang loob* in ordinary discourse. Taken together, they stress personal spontaneity as opposed to socially imposed obligations. They emphasize the need for congruence between the motivation for acting and the agent's individual desires.

For an act to have moral worth, it is essential that the agent proceed without external compulsion. The desire to benefit others must arise as an unsolicited initiative. The *loob* must express itself freely. Genuine *kusang loob* flows spontaneously and without the agent having to be coached or intimidated. One may be able to bring benefits to others by complying with public expectations, but that would not amount to *kusang loob*. For if the beneficial acts are motivated by a desire merely to comply with public expectations, the motivation may come into conflict with the agent's personal preferences. If so, the spontaneity requirement cannot be met.

As an expression of concern for others, *kagandahang loob* is driven by positive feelings for the beneficiaries of the agent's actions. There must be a caring attitude. This means that the agent must be motivated toward the prospective beneficiary by positive emotions. These emotions bind the moral agent to the beneficiary of the *kagandahang loob* in a caring relationship.

Interestingly, Nel Noddings, a feminist philosopher in the United States, does much to capture the "committed" quality of care present in *kagandahang loob* when she writes:

> If I do either of these things without reflection upon what I might do in behalf of the cared-for, then I do not care. Caring requires me to respond to the original impulse with an act of commitment: I commit myself either to overt action on behalf of the cared-for (I pick up my crying infant) or I commit myself to thinking about what I might do.[1]

Equally helpful for a full appreciation of *kagandahang loob* is Noddings's explanation of "the impulse to act on behalf of the present other." She writes:

> Indeed, I am claiming that the impulse to act in behalf of the present other is itself innate. It lies latent in each one of us, awaiting gradual development in a succession of caring relations. I am suggesting that our inclination toward and interest in morality derives from caring. In caring, we accept the natural impulse to act on behalf of the present other. We are engrossed in the other. We have received him and feel his pain or happiness, but we are not compelled by this impulse. We have a choice; we may accept what we feel, or we may reject it. If we have a strong desire to be moral, we will not reject it, and this strong desire to be moral is derived, reflectively, from the more fundamental and natural desire to be and to remain related.[2]

This passage could very easily serve as an elaboration of important aspects of *kagandahang loob*. The notion that we are "not compelled" by the impulse to receive the other and feel the other's pain or happiness reflects the spontaneity condition for *kusang loob*. This condition is also evident in the reference to the "more fundamental and natural desire to be and to remain related."[3]

Actions done in anticipation of reward or personal gain are not done out of *kusang loob*. There can be no *kagandahang loob* if actions are tainted with selfish desire: "A deed lacks nobility if it is motivated by self-interest and not by a sincere desire to help."[4] Hence, actions calculated to derive public recognition or material reward do not have the purity that is essential to *kagandahang loob* even if they are truly beneficial to others. Within this context, intended beneficiaries may reject beneficial acts when such acts are ill motivated, or when they do not arise from a caring attitude.

The performance of a duty is not attended by *kagandahang loob* if there is no positive emotional involvement on the part of the agent. An agent who is motivated purely by a sense of duty does not act out of *kusang loob*. Instead, such an agent responds to what is perceived (though not in Immanuel Kant's view, perhaps) as an external call—an obligation imposed from without.

Kagandahang Loob and Beneficence

The three conditions identified as necessary for *kusang loob* are so important that if they cannot be complied with in the performance of a beneficial act, it might be better for that act not to be done at all. As a Filipino saying goes: *Kung nagbibigay mat mahirap sa loob/Ang pinakakain ay di mabubusog*. (Alms given without *kagandahang loob* will not be valuable to the recipient.) A corollary point is that the mere expression of *kagandahang loob* could be more valuable than the benefits derived as a consequence of the act. Another Filipino proverb declares: *Uray awan ti maypasango ti bisita, no laket nalawag ti rupa nga umawat caniada*. (It is not what is served to the guests but the *kagandahang loob* that counts.)

Thus the idea of pure beneficence provides a contrast that serves to bring out an important test of *kagandahang loob*. To be sure, there is an aspect of beneficence that is presumed in the concept under consideration. It is the beneficial intent that provides the most useful clue in distinguishing *kagandahang loob* from its opposite, *kasamaang loob*. Nevertheless, *kagandahang loob* cannot be understood merely in terms of this beneficial component. Again, this is a view that has a counterpart in Noddings's account of caring:

> I may or may not act overtly in behalf of the cared-for. I may abstain from action if I believe that anything I might do would tend to work against the best interests of the cared-for. But the test of my caring is not wholly in how things turn out; the primary test lies in an examination of what I considered, how fully I received the other, and whether the free pursuit of his projects is partly a result of the completion of my caring in him.[5]

The nature of this test can be illustrated as we look at some implications of *kagandahang loob* for practical decisions.

Organ Donation As Gift Giving

From the viewpoint that *kagandahang loob* offers, organ donation can naturally be seen as gift giving. As the literal giving of oneself, even if only in part, organ donation fits the *kagandahang loob* model. Hence it is instructive to examine various aspects of organ donation in terms of the components of *kagandahang loob*.

Organ donation involves giving part of one's physical self as a gift to an intended beneficiary. However, it is important not to get fixated on the physical component of the gift. For the significance of the action of literally giving a part of oneself to someone else lies in its being a manifestation of the beauty within one's self. The essence of the action lies in what the physical gift manifests, rather than in the physical gift itself. The beneficence model cannot go all the way in describing what takes place in the donation. If we view organ donation as nothing more than an act of beneficence, we cannot transcend the material exchange that takes place.

In relation to this, one senses the shortcomings of a Philippine organ transplant law that allows the removal of organs from the bodies of brain-dead patients whose relatives cannot be located within forty-eight hours. Under this law, hospital administrators may give the required authorization. It is obvious that the main consideration is to provide benefits to prospective recipients by making more organs available for transplant. However, the law does not make room for the flourishing of *kagandahang loob*. On the contrary, it provokes a negative emotion—*sama ng loob*—by tolerating (if not encouraging) a practice that puts beneficence at the forefront and takes emotions and motivation out of the decision equation. In effect, the law seeks to make an organ donor out of someone who may not have wanted to make any such donation in the first place.

When well-known doctors at a leading hospital retrieved and transplanted organs from a brain-dead patient without consulting the patient's family, they witnessed an extreme reaction of *sama ng loob* on the part of the family. The surprised relatives took the hospital and doctors to court over what blazing headlines in many newspapers reported as a "transplant murder." Although the defendants were eventually acquitted because of the protection given by the law, the case alarmed the public so much that medical authorities now worry about a major reduction in the number of Filipinos willing to serve as organ donors. Thus, because *kagandahang loob* was ignored, an action initially intended by some people to be of great benefit to someone in particular became of great harm to the nation in general.

What needs to be stressed is that *kagandahang loob* does not result automatically from attempts to benefit others. When organ "donors" are brain-dead and are not represented by family (i.e., by those who have the necessary familiarity with their *kalooban* and are in a position to speak in their behalf rather than in behalf of prospective beneficiaries), they clearly are not in a position to express *kagandahang loob*. A donation made under such circumstances does not meet the requirement for *kusang loob*.

In such situations, the spontaneity that characterizes unsolicited initiatives is missing. The "donor"—the source of the "gift"—does not actually do the giving. Somebody else performs the gift-giving function. The law undeniably invests the hospital administrator with legal authority. However, beyond the provisions of the law, the nonrelative is not perceived generally as speaking for the brain-dead person. The hospital administrator does not enjoy popular recognition as a moral surrogate. What effectively happens in such a situation is that the legally authorized person takes something from the "dead" person to give away, without the latter actually giving it. Thus there is no genuine donation or gift giving, and no authentic caring relationship to bind the donor to the organ recipient.

When beneficence completely takes over the ethical discourse to the exclusion of *kagandahang loob*, we are taken out of the personal world of feeling and caring, and into the territory of "traditional moral epistemology," which stresses that moral wisdom is to be found in being dispassionate:

> To make considered, sound moral judgments, we are told to abstract from our emotions, feelings, and sentiments. Emotions are not part of the equipment needed to discern moral answers; indeed, only trouble can come of their intrusion into deliberations about what to do, for they "cloud" our judgment and "bias" our reasoning. To be objective is to be detached; to be clear-sighted is to achieve distance; to be careful in deliberation is to be cool and calm. Further, the tradition tends to discount the idea that experiencing appropriate emotion is an integral part of being moral. Moral theory tends to focus exclusively on questions about what actions are obligated or prohibited, or perhaps on what intention or motive one should have in acting, not on what emotional stance a moral agent should be feeling.[6]

The emergence of recent legislation seeking to classify medical malpractice as a criminal act may be seen as a consequence of the general public's lack of appreciation for the Philippine organ transplant law. It reflects an attitude of suspicion toward the ideal of pure beneficence. In a context of *kagandahang loob*, the public expects greater respect for *kusang loob*. Filipinos seem to have learned their lesson and have decided to exercise greater vigilance in using the test of *kagandahang loob* to understand other issues of bioethics.

Kagandahang Loob and *Utang Na Loob* (Debt of Goodwill)

The concept of *kagandahang loob* cannot be defined solely in terms of a one-way caring relationship between someone who cares and someone who is cared for. Even if the one caring in the context of *kagandahang loob* must be presumed not to expect anything in return for the caring behavior, it does not necessarily follow that the beneficiary owes the benefactor nothing. Having been the recipient of *kagandahang loob*, the beneficiary incurs an *utang na loob*, or debt of goodwill (debt of gratitude).[7] This debt is something that the beneficiary ought to repay. However, the terms of repayment and the nature of the "ought" must both be understood from the perspective of *kagandahang loob* rather than from the perspective of contractual debt, where the terms are clearly spelled out in a formal agreement.

Some writers have argued that human beings have an obligation to participate as subjects in research designed to benefit the human population in general. They reason that because the knowledge derived from biomedical research is prospectively useful to all, everyone must share in the task of generating such knowledge by serving as research subjects.[8] This type of obligation is supported by H. L. A. Hart's principle of "mutuality of restrictions":

> When a number of persons conduct any joint enterprise according to rules and restrict their liberty those who have submitted to these restrictions when required have a right to similar submission from those who have benefited by their submission.[9]

However, the idea of an obligation to serve as a research subject is problematic. Even if it can be granted that such an obligation exists in general with respect to participation in medical research, it would still have to be separately proven that that obligation is enforceable with respect to each specific subject. Moreover, it must be established that serving as a research subject is the only correct way of "submitting to restrictions" in order to fulfill the obligation.

A specific difficulty lies in the idea of enforcement. If the obligation to serve as a research subject were truly correlated with the corresponding right of former research subjects to demand participation by others, enforcement would have to be done by legal authorities. This means having to rely on the government to make participation mandatory. In practical terms, mechanisms would be required that allocate and prioritize individual obligations to participate.

What comes to mind is the practice of calling up military reserves in time of war. But this comparison makes the idea of enforcing obligations to participate in medical research seem absurd. For one thing, we cannot easily identify an "extreme danger" to national security that can justify compelling citizens to participate in medical research against their will. Moreover, even when the state has to deal with a war situation, the first recourse should be to ask for volunteers rather than conscript reservists right away.

How, then, does one overcome the contradiction that exists between the idea of enforcement and the idea of voluntary participation in medical research? Since the middle of the twentieth century, much emphasis has been placed on the requirement that human participation in medical research be grounded on voluntary and informed consent. But can consent be regarded as voluntary when the participation is perceived as obligatory?

The combination of *kagandahang loob* and *utang na loob* may provide a way to answer this question in the affirmative. One may view the fulfillment of such an obligation as repayment of a debt of goodwill. The point is that beneficial actions of previous (or even future) volunteers may be construed as *kagandahang loob* that creates a debt of goodwill on the part of beneficiaries, provided that the requirements of *kusang loob* are complied with.

The key lies in the notion of "ought" embedded in these concepts. In order to explain this "ought" in the context of *kagandahang loob*, I borrow from Noddings's explanation of the ethical "must":

> I am obliged, then, to accept the initial I must when it occurs and even to fetch it out of recalcitrant slumber when it fails to awake spontaneously. The source of my obligation is the value I place on the relatedness of caring. This value itself arises as a product of actual caring and being cared-for and my reflection on the goodness of these concrete caring situations. . . . I have identified the source of our obligation and have said that we are obligated to accept, and even to call forth, the feeling I must. . . . it seems that I am obligated to maintain an attitude and, thus, to meet the other as one-caring and, at the same time, to increase my own virtue as one-caring.[10]

If the source of one's obligation is the value that one places on the relatedness of caring, then that obligation is something that is self-imposed. It does not require external compulsion. It does not have to comply with external authority.

From the perspective of *kagandahang loob*, one may appreciate the need to serve as research subject without having to be coached or coerced. This appreciation comes as a result of one's voluntary acceptance of indebtedness—*utang na loob*—to those who have contributed to medical knowledge by their own participation in earlier medical research. A person's awareness of being one with the rest of the human community in general is also an important factor in cultivating this sense of obligation. This awareness is emphasized when one is cognizant of a more specific relatedness—to a sick brother, a suffering neighbor, or a dying friend. If so, it would probably be more effective in generating the sense of *utang na loob*, thereby establishing the existence of an obligation. From this perspective, one's decision to participate in medical research could be reached not by appealing to deductive reasoning premised on universal ethical principles but by spontaneously responding with *kagandahang loob* to the recognition of *utang na loob*. It is not the mere calculation of benefits and risks that leads to the conclusion that participation would be morally worthwhile. The motivating factor is the fulfillment that the moral agent attains through the flourishing of *kagandahang loob*.

On the whole, then, one can argue that there is an obligation to serve as subjects in medical research. It is an obligation that does not follow necessarily from any rights that former participants have to require others to render similar service. Instead, it comes as an obligation to oneself, as part of an obligation to be self-fulfilled.

Kagandahang Loob As a Feminine Concept of Bioethics

In this chapter I endeavored to show points of contact that establish the affinity of *kagandahang loob* ethics to feminine ethics. I did not intend to show that the former can be subsumed under the latter. It would be self-defeating to seek to understand *kagandahang loob* ethics completely as a variant or subclass of feminine thought. Just as seeking to understand feminine ethics entirely in terms of "mainstream" ethical parameters would do it an injustice, so trying to find the significance of *kagandahang loob* wholly in its alignment with feminine ethics would be misleading.

The point has been to spell out a conceptual framework using a language expressive of a people's own experiences, concerns, traditions, perceived problems, dreams, hopes, and aspirations. After the features that indicate the affinity of *kagandahang loob* ethics to feminine approaches have been noted, the task ahead is to identify and appreciate the characteristics that differentiate the former perspective from the latter. These characteristics could well constitute the glue that binds a community under the umbrella of *kagandahang loob* and provides them with the inspiration to care for one another and adopt the caring attitude as an obligation; these characteristics, so far in the history of humankind, could well be ones that have been expressed more by women than by men.

Notes

This chapter is based on material earlier published in "Kagandahang Loob: Love in Philippine Bioethics," *Eubios Journal of Asian and International Bioethics* 9 (March 1999).

1. Nel Noddings, *Caring: A Feminine Approach to Ethics and Moral Education* (Berkeley: University of California Press, 1984), p. 81.

2. Ibid., p. 83.

3. Ibid.

4. Emilio Jacinto, quoted in Ed Aurelio C. Reyes, "Moral and Ethical Codes of the Katipunan," *Sunday Chronicle*, November 3, 1996, sec. 2., p. 16.

5. Noddings, *Caring*, p. 81.

6. Margaret Olivia Little, "Why a Feminist Approach to Bioethics?" *Kennedy Institute of Ethics Journal* 6, no. 1 (1996): 12.

7. "Debt of goodwill" is more accurate than "debt of gratitude" when referring to what the beneficiary owes the benefactor, since the former term clearly identifies the "goodwill" as the object of debt.

8. W. McDermott, "Opening Comments to Colloquium: The Changing Mores of Biomedical Research," *Annals of Internal Medicine* 67 (1967): 39–42.

9. "Are There Any Natural Rights?" *Philosophical Review* 64 (April 1955): 183.

10. Noddings, *Caring*, p. 84.

5

Feminist Bioethics:
The Emergence of the Oppressed

DEBORA DINIZ
ANA CRISTINA GONZÁLEZ VÉLEZ

The first two decades in the emergence and consolidation of bioethics were marked by the predominance of the principlist theory,[1] originally developed by Tom Beauchamp and James Childress in their *Principles of Biomedical Ethics*.[2] The principlist theory offered bioethicists four principles—autonomy, justice, beneficence, and nonmaleficence—for the purposes of resolving moral dilemmas. To the extent that bioethicists relied on these principles in their work, they became a veritable ethical "checklist."[3]

The principlist theory had a tremendous impact not only in central bioethics countries such as the United States but also in peripheral bioethics countries such as Brazil.[4] As we use the term, a "peripheral" bioethics country is one in which bioethics emerged relatively late and relies on bioethical theories imported from central bioethics countries in which bioethics first appeared.[5] Brazilian bioethics, the peripheral bioethics with which we are most familiar, has relied heavily on North American but especially U.S. bioethics. Beauchamp and Childress's principlism has had enormous influence in Brazil. Indeed, the majority of Brazilian bioethicists still refer to principlism as the only bioethical theory. As we see it, the persistent influence of the principlist theory in peripheral bioethics countries is largely the consequence of its seductive instrumentalism. One of the principlist theory's greatest merits is its ability to organize moral dilemmas and offer solutions to them in a way that a wide public uninitiated in bioethical studies finds comprehensible. The four principles have become a kind of magic formula that all too many bioethicists merely invoke whenever they need to resolve a moral dilemma. Unreflective use of principlism has resulted in a gross reductionism that has obscured some of its deepest and most demanding contributions to bioethical thought. An understanding of *Principles of Biomedical Ethics* demands more than simply reciting its four major principles.[6] Unfortunately, many "principlists" in Brazil have never really read the *Principles of Biomedical Ethics* from start to finish, relying instead on secondary references to the work. Limited by their thin knowledge of Beauchamp and Childress's book (which by the way has yet to be translated into either Portuguese or Spanish), all too many Brazilian bioethicists chant the "Georgetown mantra" without fully understanding it.

Although theories that diverged from the principlist theory—such as Singer and Kuhse's utilitarianism and Pellegrino's theory of virtues—existed from the start, these theories did not immediately enter into a critical dialogue with either principlism or, as we demonstrate further on, bioethics as a discipline. Only in the late 1980s and early 1990s did challenges to the theory of principlism in particular and the discipline of bioethics in general flower into a set of theories powerful enough to seriously challenge Beauchamp and Childress's paradigm, among them feminist bioethics.[7]

Not coincidentally, critiques of principlism were accompanied by a reexamination of the assumptions of bioethics as a discipline. Feminist bioethics formally arose in the 1990s, with the publication of the first books that interrelated feminism and bioethics.[8] Earlier, in the 1980s, a number of scattered studies on the topic were published, the debate focusing heavily on so-called feminine ethics,[9] articulated most notably in Carol Gilligan's book, *In a Different Voice: Psychological Theory and Women's Development*.[10] For feminist bioethicists as well as feminist ethicists, Gilligan's "feminine" ethics had tremendous repercussions. With daring originality, Gilligan developed the idea of a feminine ethics rooted in care (hence "ethics of care"), contrasting it with a masculine ethics guided by justice (hence "ethics of justice"). Gilligan's categories of care and justice as determinants of the ethical patterns of women and men, respectively, implied that feminine and masculine gender roles resulted in different ethical trajectories. The logical consequence of Gilligan's argument was that moral discourse should contemplate diversity (in her analysis, gender differences).

Gilligan enabled feminist ethicists and bioethicists to reflect on how gender identity and behavior roles affect moral behavior. But she did more than this. She inspired a wide variety of nonfeminist as well as feminist thinkers to acknowledge moral differences based on differences of class, race, ethnicity, and so on.[11] In the years since the publication of *In a*

Different Voice, however, Gilligan's theory of gender-differentiated ethics has been reassessed by feminist writers who have signaled its weaknesses as well as its strengths.[12] For example, in *Caring: Nurses, Women, and Ethics*,[13] Helga Kuhse argues that an "ethics of care," improperly formulated, leads to "essentialism," the assumption that gender differences in moral behavior are biologically determined.[14] As Kuhse sees it, viewing an "ethics of care" as a feminine ethics reinforces women's traditional roles, especially in woman-dominated professions such as nursing. Kuhse claims that the "ethics of care" requires nurses to be "good women," that is, self-sacrificial, obedient persons who dutifully and passively follow the instructions of physicians (mostly men). Insofar as female nurses and male physicians assume these gender roles, a moral division of work based on female subordination and male domination is created. Such a state of affairs in the realm of health care undermines the voluntary giving of care by both men and women.[15] As Tong puts it, "Genuine or fully authentic caring cannot occur under patriarchal conditions, that is, conditions characterized by male domination and female subordination. Only under conditions of sexual equality and freedom can women care for men without men in any way diminishing, disempowering, and/or disregarding them."[16]

Keeping Kuhse's criticism of the ethics of care in mind, it is not surprising that traditional bioethicists have embraced the ethics of care as a "good" one—especially for women. What they have not embraced, however, is the kind of power-focused feminist bioethics that seeks to identify and eliminate those principles, systems, and structures that contribute to women's oppression. Susan Wolf, among others, attributes the resistance of traditional bioethics to power-focused feminist thought to what she perceives as its vested interest in maintaining the status quo in both the practical and theoretical world.

Wolf challenges the supposed universality of the treasured principles of traditional bioethics, highlights the limits of its individualistic ideology, particularly its veneration of the principle of autonomy as the highest of values, and reveals how the structure of traditional bioethics preserves the interests of the socially advantaged, thereby constituting a "bioethics for the privileged."[17] Finally, she testifies to its insularity—its lack of engagement with cutting-edge thought within the academy such as feminist thought, critical race theory, and postmodernism.[18] In her estimation and ours, feminist bioethics clearly demands nothing less than the transformation of the deep structure of traditional bioethics—its very nature.

Given that post-Gilligan, feminist bioethics is particularly critical of the kind of universal or generalizable ethics that constitutes traditional bioethics, it has found common ground with other nonabsolutistic bioethical theories. However, this is not to claim that feminist bioethicists and their allies espouse relativism. Rather, they hold moral pluralism as a reference and value.[19] Unlike traditional bioethicists (and ethicists), feminist bioethicists do not insist that all people are the same and must share exactly the same moral views. On the contrary, recognizing just how different people are, and how their gender, race, ethnicity, and class, for example, shape (or mishape) their divergent moral views, feminist bioethicists seek to understand and mediate between people when their moral views conflict.[20] In the course of serving as moral mediators, however, feminist bioethicists do not accept as equally worthy and valuable the moral views of each individual or each society.

Refusing to recognize the relativist principle of "everything and anything goes," feminist bioethicists refuse to honor culturally based moral differences just because they express a given culture's current ethical beliefs. As Susan Sherwin notes, it is important for feminist bioethicists to distinguish between respecting moral differences and accepting all of them as equally good.[21] There is, she says, a difference between nonfeminist moral relativism and feminist moral relativism. Sherwin claims that nonfeminist moral relativism "takes communities as given, and says that what is moral is whatever we find accepted as moral within a particular community."[22] In contrast, feminist moral relativism does not accept as moral the practices of all communities, but only those communities that treat all of its members with equal respect and consideration. It refuses to recognize as moral "practices that exploit and entrench power differentials" among the groups that make up a society.[23] In other words, feminist moral relativism is a limited kind of relativism, according to Sherwin. It "remains absolutist on the question of the moral wrong of oppression"[24] and criticizes any practice that is the result of "oppressive power differentials," even when the majority of a community accepts the practices as morally permissible.

Analyzing the organization and the development of critical processes is an urgent task for bioethics. If feminist bioethicists want to serve women and men equally, they must recognize that men and women are, at present, not equal and then develop bioethical principles capable of illuminating and ultimately eliminating the causes and consequences of male domination and female subordination. For this reason, Sherwin stresses that critical to all her writings "are the understandings that women are oppressed, that this oppression is pervasive in all aspects of social life, and that political action (that is, collective action on a broad scale) is necessary to understand and eliminate that oppression from our world."[25]

Like Sherwin, we do not think that there is anything inherently wrong with the four major principles of traditional bioethics (autonomy, benefi-

cence, nonmaleficence, and justice). It is just that we, like Sherwin, think
these principles can be interpreted in perverse ways that serve to maintain the dominant order and the interests of those whom Wolf appropriately termed "privileged."[26] According to Wolf, if the principle of autonomy—treasured by feminist as well as nonfeminist bioethicists—does
not take into account differences in power based on people's gender,
race, and class, it will inevitably be used as a weapon against the vulnerable people it claims to protect. The same line of reasoning applies to the
principles of beneficence, nonmaleficence, and justice. Improperly interpreted, they will serve only to downgrade already less powerful people
to imperiled ones. Thus we believe, with Sherwin, Wolf, and other like-
minded feminist bioethicists, that the primary task of feminist bioethics
is to serve the interests of the oppressed rather than the privileged. Our
first and foremost goal must be to question any health care principle,
practice, or policy that contributes to the kind of inequalities between individuals that result in the creation and maintenance of unjust societies.

An interesting theoretical proposal for subverting the moral order in
the world of health care is found in one of Kuhse's books, *Caring: Nurses,
Women, and Ethics.*[27] Kuhse uses the process of decisionmaking related to
the end of life as a case study. Although discussions about disagreements
related to euthanasia or assisted suicide have traditionally revolved
around the figures of the doctor and patient,[28] Kuhse proposes the formal
entrance of a third figure in such discussions: the nurse. As Kuhse sees it,
in situations of moral conflict regarding the end of life, the competent patient's will ought to be sovereign. However, she contends when the patient is incompetent or largely incompetent, the nurse's ethical decision
should be respected even more than the doctor's. Starting with the assumption that the one who possesses technical knowledge does not by
definition possess the best ethical solution, Kuhse identifies the nurse as
an appropriate agent for legitimizing decisions regarding death, since the
nurse generally establishes a closer link with the patient than does the
doctor. Comments Kuhse:

> My own view would be that ultimately, at least in the area of terminal care,
> final decision-making authority should be vested in nurses. While this
> would not exclude shared decision-making, that is, the consultation of doc-
> tors by nurses, the final responsibility would be the nurse's. . . . While doc-
> tors would function as technical advisers and would, if so requested, pro-
> vide technical services, they would hold no formal decision-making
> authority.[29]

In bestowing the nurse with an active and responsible role in ethical
decisionmaking at the bedside, Kuhse expresses a position that is pro-

foundly disturbing for nurses as well as doctors, namely, the ethical independence of the nurse from the doctor. Kuhse challenges nurses to "view themselves as rebels fighting against an unjust hierarchical order who must have the courage to take the lead in restructuring the doctor-nurse relationship."[30]

Kuhse's model of rebellion can be extended to other relationships of dependence, such as that between the bioethics of the center and of the periphery.[31] The relationship between U.S. bioethics and Brazilian bioethics is a case in point. Brazilian bioethics is closely linked to the practice of medicine in all its aspects, from the choice of appropriate topics for inquiry to control over the academic and professional trajectory of its researchers.[32] Brazilian medicine, typical of the medicine of the periphery, imports medical theories and practices from countries at the center of medicine. This tradition of importing techniques is well accepted by the country's health care professionals, with Brazilian doctors feeling more comfortable when their medical practices closely match the medical practices of U.S. and Canadian physicians, for example. This kind of unreflective importation from central countries is even more problematic when morals, rather than techniques, are in question. As we have already suggested, a prime example of this kind of unreflective importation is the unquestioned adoption and thus improper use—and abuse—of Beauchamp and Childress's theory. In other words, all too many Brazilian bioethicists assume not only that all medical practices are transcultural but also that all bioethical theories are transcultural, regardless of their often local philosophical and moral inspiration, as in the case of the principlist theory, which is deeply rooted in U.S. (white, educated, middle-class) culture.[33] The result of the acritical introduction and application of U.S. principlism in Brazil is that Brazilian reality is forced to fit into a framework that best explains U.S. reality. And, as in the doctor-nurse conflict described by Kuhse, any possibility of change in this relationship of dependency can only come from the oppressed, in this case, Brazilian bioethicists.[34]

Brazilian bioethicists must claim the particularity of *Brazilian* reality as their own, being as attentive as possible to the differences that separate Brazilian reality from U.S. reality. They must create a unique bioethics for Brazil, which continually interprets and reinterprets principles such as autonomy, beneficence, nonmaleficence, and justice through the lenses of local wisdom. Brazilian bioethicists need to view U.S. bioethics as a beginning and not an ending point. They must use the insights of feminist bioethics as well as other revolutionary approaches to bioethics to gain the strength they need to stop viewing Brazilian bioethics as peripheral and U.S. bioethics, for example, as central.

Although we have consistently referred to feminist bioethics in the singular throughout this article, we recognize that feminist bioethics, as well as traditional bioethics, are not monolithic. On the contrary, there are a variety of strong feminist theories in bioethics. What unites them, however, is their concern with difference and their focus on unequal relations. Feminist bioethics is defined by the search for changes in social relations that are characterized by human domination and subordination and which, therefore, hinder the exercise of freedom. In her search to protect and legitimize the freedom of choice, feminist philosopher Victoria Camps, for example, substituted Kant's concept of a "categorical imperative" with the notion of a "heretical imperative."[35] The "heretical imperative," according to Camps, points out the failure of the Enlightenment project to construct a universal (bio)ethics based on reason and rejects the possibility of accepting a singular ethical spokesperson for all humanity; it takes delight in not believing that the status quo is inviolable and permanent, risking rejection by the establishment. Understood as part of an audacious project to rescue what has traditionally been left aside—the oppressed—feminist bioethics is about more than the ways health care has disserved women's interests and favored men's.[36] It is, as we see it, part of a revolutionary movement in Brazilian health care, a movement that hopes to provide equal health care for all Brazilian citizens irrespective of their class, race, and culture. For this reason alone, we recommend that all Brazilian bioethicists become feminist bioethicists.

Notes

This chapter is drawn from an article presented at the International Network Feminist Approaches in Bioethics, held in Tsukuba, Japan, October 31-November 3, 1998. The comments of Marcelo Medeiros and Ondina Pereira were essential to the initial article. For the final version of this chapter, we are grateful for the comments of Gwen Anderson, Helga Kuhse, and Rosemarie Tong.

1. Some authors have already noted the conceptual imprecision of referring to Beauchamp and Chidress's theory as "the" principlist theory, given that many other theories in moral philosophy are based on principles. Bernard Gert, Charles Culver, and Danner Clouser, *"Principlism" in Bioethics: A Return to Fundamentals* (New York: Oxford University Press, 1997), pp. 71–92; Renée Fox, "The Entry of U.S. Bioethics into the 1990s: A Sociological Analysis," in Ronald Dubose and Laurence O'Connel, eds., *A Matter of Principles? Ferment in U.S. Bioethics* (Pennsylvania: Trinity Press International, 1994), pp. 21–71. Nevertheless, we will refer to Beauchamp and Childress's theory as the principlist theory simply because it is better known than any other version of principlism in bioethics. (James Childress, "Principles-Oriented Bioethics: An Analysis and Assessment from Within," in *A Matter of Principles*, pp. 72-100.

2. Tom Beauchamp and James Childress, *Principles of Biomedical Ethics*, 4th ed. (Oxford: Oxford University Press, 1994).

3. Gert, Culver, and Clouser, "*Principlism,*" pp. 71–92. Danner Clouser and Bernard Gert, "A Critique of Principlism," *Journal of Medicine and Philosophy* 15, no. 2 (1990): 230–242.

4. For a definition of central and peripheral bioethics, see Volnei Garrafa, Debora Diniz, and Dirce Guilhem, "The Bioethical Language: Its Dialects and Idialects," *Reports in Public Health* 15, Suppl. 1 (1999): 35–42.

5. This idea was originally brought up by Roberto Cardoso de Oliveira when analyzing Brazilian anthropology. For other studies in which Cardoso de Oliveira's concept is developed, see "Peripheral Anthropologies Versus Central Anthropologies," in *O Trabalho do Antropólogo* (Brasília: Paralelo 15, 1998); "In Support of a Peripheral Etnography," in *Sobre o Pensamento Antropológico* (Rio de Janeiro: Tempo Brasileiro, 1988).

6. In the Brazilian case, for instance, the largest number of professionals working within bioethics come from the health care industry. Because they are unfamiliar with humanistic disciplines, they have real difficulty with theoretical language and philosophical abstraction.

7. The major authors who correlated feminism and bioethics, especially those analyzed in this article, avoid the concept "feminist bioethics." Like Tong, for example, who uses the expression "feminist approaches to bioethics," the majority of bioethicists oscillate between recognition of a new field—feminist *bioethics*—and the already legitimized field of feminist *ethics* (Rosemarie Tong, *Feminist Approaches to Bioethics* [Boulder: Westview, 1997]). With the likely intention of avoiding epistemological discussions about the adequacy of the concept, the most common reference is "feminist ethics." See, for example, Susan Sherwin, "Feminism and Bioethics," in Susan Wolf, ed., *Feminism and Bioethics: Beyond Reproduction* (Oxford: Oxford University Press, 1996), pp. 47–66. For the purposes of this article, however, we opt for the use of the term "feminist bioethics" because we believe that recent publications of feminist-inspired bioethicists (or "feminist bioethicists") contain a solid and well-argued theoretical body that justifies its use. In addition, we will use the concept in the singular because we believe that there is something in common among the various feminist theories which is, as Wolf notes, the study of power, hierarchy, and gender inequality.

8. Tong considers what feminist (bio)ethicists felt was a certain initial comfort with the principlist theory; Rosemarie Tong, "Feminist Approaches to Bioethics," in *Feminism and Bioethics*, pp. 67–94.

9. For a satisfactory distinguishing of "feminist" and "feminine" ethics, see Susan Sherwin, *No Longer Patient: Feminist Ethics and Health Care* (Philadelphia: Temple University Press, 1992); and Rosemarie Tong, "Feminist Approaches to Bioethics," pp. 67–94.

10. Carol Gilligan, *In a Different Voice: Psychological Theory and Women's Development* (Cambridge: Harvard University Press, 1982); Nel Noddings, *Caring: A Feminine Approach to Ethics and Moral Education* (Berkeley: University of California Press, 1984).

11. The legacy left by the author has also resonated in other nonfeminist bioethical theories rooted in the recognition of differences among peoples, cultures, and societies, that is, theories consistent with the highest postmodernist value, which is the polissemy or, more correctly, the disenso. The polissemy and

disenso values are part of a philosophical heritage left by the theorists of suspicion in the postmodern age. Philosophy after Friedrich Nietzsche's work did not succeed in establishing the existence of truth or the universality of moral standards. Therefore the concepts of diversity, polissemy, and disenso are used in this article as part of this heritage. Living in the aftermath of the breakdown of the Enlightenment project—the anguish left by the lack of a single Truth for humanity—we are forced to deal with the resulting conflict and tragedy as constitutive facts of moral life and of humanity. About these topics, see Richard Rorty, *Contingency, Irony, and Solidarity* (Cambridge: Cambridge University Press, 1988); and Clément Rosset, *Le Principe de Cruauté* (Paris: Les Editions de Minuit, 1988).

12. See, for example, Rosemarie Tong, "Feminist Approaches to Bioethics," pp. 67–94; and Tong, *Feminist Approaches to Bioethics*; Susan Sherwin, "Feminism and Bioethics," in *Feminism and Bioethics*, pp. 47–66; Laura Purdy, *Reproducing Persons: Issues in Feminist Bioethics* (Ithaca, N.Y.: Cornell University Press, 1996); and Susan Wolf, "Introduction: Gender and Feminism in Bioethics," in *Feminism and Bioethics*.

13. Helga Kuhse, *Caring: Nurses, Women, and Ethics* (Oxford: Blackwell, 1997).

14. The essentialist nature of *In a Different Voice* was not due to a biological naturalization of ethical behavior but to its social counterpart, a naturalization of the social roles of men and women.

15. Referring to the consequences of the moral-professional socialization of nurses based on an "ethics of care," Kuhse writes, "It may show no more than that these nurses have been socialized, corrupted if you like, into accepting a subservient role—a role that is, of course, incompatible with professionalism" (*Caring*, p. 218).

16. Rosemarie Tong, *Feminine and Feminist Ethics* (Belmont, Calif.: Wadworth, 1993), p. 103.

17. According to Susan Wolf, "The safeguards and principles we have developed in bioethics do not seem to apply equally to all. We have developed a bioethics primarily for the person with access to health care and with a doctor likely to listen to, understand, and respect that person. It is a bioethics for the privileged." See "Gender and Feminism in Bioethics," p. 18.

18. Tong, *Feminine and Feminist Ethics*, p. 103.

19. Within the idea of pacific moral pluralism, we believe bioethics should make better use of philosopher Richard Rorty's ideas about moral diversion. In Brazil, for instance, between bioethics and moral philosophy, there is an interesting phenomenon. On one side, bioethics is revolutionary because of its recognition of such values as freedom, autonomy, and moral pluralism—undoubtedly modern values. On the other side, bioethics is simultaneously conservative insofar as it remains beholden to such traditional philosophical theories as Platonism, Aristotelianism, and Kantism. Among Brazilian bioethicists there is very little awareness and acceptance of philosophical theories different from the conventional ones.

20. "What Differences Make a Difference?" was the topic of a major study known as the Pluralistic Project coordinated by the Hasting Center, begun four

years ago. See Eric Parens, "What Differences Make a Difference?" *Cambridge Quarterly of Health Care Ethics* 7, no. 1–6 (1998): 1.

21. A classic example frequently cited by feminist bioethicists that suggests the imposition of limits on cultural difference is that of female genital mutilation, a ritual suffered by women in Africa and elsewhere. Sherwin, *No Longer Patient*, p. 61.

22. Ibid.

23. Ibid., pp. 68–75.

24. For a fuller understanding of Sherwin's thesis, it is worth applying the ethical model to two situations of moral-cultural conflict: Whereas the genital mutilation of women would be considered unethical, the rejection of blood transfusions by adult Jehovah's Witnesses would be considered ethical. Of these two practices, only female genital mutation bolsters inequality between men and women.

25. Sherwin, *No Longer Patient*, p. 32.

26. Wolf, "Gender and Feminism in Bioethics," p. 18.

27. Kuhse, *Caring*.

28. It can be counterargued that in many situations of moral conflict, the doctor as well as the patient answers to social forces such as class attitudes, religious beliefs, family pressures, and so on, turning a conflict that seemingly occurs between two moral subjects into a conflict, in some measure, between collectivities. However, we believe that these social forces are "embodied" in the figures of the doctor and patient, allowing conflicts to be analyzed from that joint perspective. In Brazil, the doctor-nurse relationship is still characterized by an intense subservience of the nurse to the doctor in personal as well as technical matters. Such dependency begins in the education period but extends throughout the professional life of the nurse. In Brazil, just as in other parts of the world, the majority of nurses are women, whereas the majority of doctors are men. There is some resistance to this state of affairs by feminist bioethicist nurses, but their numbers are few. They aim to raise nurses' consciousness about the importance of coming to their own moral conclusions and counterpositioning them, if necessary, against the moral conclusions of physicians. Unfortunately, most Brazilian nurses are not ready to become revolutionaries, preferring not to take any risks that might jeopardize their jobs.

29. Kuhse, *Caring*, p. 217.

30. Ibid., p. 216.

31. Volnei Garrafa, Debora Diniz, and Dirce Guilhem, "The Bioethical Language," pp. 35–42.

32. Another example of how medicine and bioethics find themselves associated in the Brazilian context is the case of the country's most important scientific journal on bioethics *(Bioética)*. It is organized and sponsored by the Federal Council of Medicine (Conselho Federal de Medicina).

33. The idea of a transcultural and ahistorical ethics has been gradually challenged by other philosophical projects in ethics, which point to the relevance of cultural and moral differences among people. Good indicators of this are the proceedings from the fifth international meeting of the International Association of

Bioethics, where several researchers pointed out their new theoretical frameworks.

34. This idea that the principle agent of change is the oppressed is linked to the theory of standpoint, according to which the position of the oppressed is privileged in the critical analysis of power relations. See Wolf, "Gender and Feminism in Bioethics."

35. Victoria Camps, *La Imaginación Etica* (Barcelona: Seix Barral, 1983), p. 77.

36. Tong, "Feminist Approaches to Bioethics," pp. 67–94.

PART TWO

Reproductive, Genetic, and Sexual Health

6

Shifts of Attention

The Experience of Pregnancy
in Dualist and Nondualist Cultures

VANGIE BERGUM
MARY ANN BENDFELD

[The] absence of any adequate theory of maternity is sufficiently serious in itself. But the problem is exacerbated by recent scientific developments.[1]

Only by producing a model of motherhood that takes into account both its biological and psychological aspects will we be able to understand the natural maternity of women as well as technological (re-)production by scientific means . . . What is necessary is to reflect on maternity, to be aware of it so as to be able to use its creative and expressive potential.[2]

John Macmurray has claimed that the adoption of a dualistic perspective, such as exists in the Western world, "must either assimilate the material to the mental, or absorb the mental in the material" but that neither option produces an adequate understanding of human experience.[3] This is nowhere more evident than in the framing of a woman's experience of pregnancy in either of these two ways—what has been called the "organic" and "technological" worldviews—which misrepresents that experience. Such misrepresentations are revealed most vividly in the discussions of pregnancy termination. Visualization technologies have become an important part of health care in North America and are widely used for pregnant women, so much so that the sense of sight is privileged in the experience of pregnancy for many women over that of their "feeling" body. However, in other cultures, such as Japan, which have not adopted the dualistic perspective of mind and body,[4] women find it easier to integrate bodily experience and the ensuing emotions that arise out of that experience, even though they have adopted the technological devices used by North American women. As a result, they deal with the ambiguity of pregnancy and the termination of pregnancy differently than many North American women do. This would suggest that it is not primarily the technology itself that is at fault but the manner in which we prioritize and interpret the products of these visualization technologies.

John Macmurray's "form of the personal" constructs a paradigm that differs from the technological and organic worldviews through which we will examine the experience of pregnancy.[5] The response of Japanese women to the termination of pregnancy as recounted by Bardwell Smith suggests that in rejecting a dualistic perspective of mind and body, they have adopted a concept of a "personal" body such as Macmurray would advocate.[6] Macmurray urges us to shift our attention back to the "feeling" body, emphasizing the primacy of "feeling" over vision, as this is where our immediate awareness of the other begins. In this chapter, we take up Silvia Finzi's challenge and "reflect on maternity," attempting to understand some of the physical and psychological processes that a pregnant woman undergoes, and the potential that the examination of such processes holds for enhancing our ethical understanding.

The Pregnant Body

Barbara Duden noted that in the eighteenth century the experience of the pregnant woman determined how her pregnancy was conceptualized. The fact that "quickening" occurred established the existence of a (potential) child. "This was a time when women quickened; it was taken for granted that women have this experience, make it public, and thereby establish the fact of pregnancy."[7] Recognizing the phenomenon of quickening rooted the knowledge of her condition in the physical experience of the mother herself, not the physician who attended her. Duden says that quickening has been eliminated by science and has been lost from common use: "Quickening is at best a feeble reminder of what a woman already 'knows' because she, too, is able to look at her own inner body with medical optics that create scientific facts."[8] Susan Squier advances the argument that the visualization technologies, which claim to re-present experience, supersede the *immediate* experience (i.e., the physical feeling) of the mother and, in the process, construct her as "object" of the "medical gaze" rather than acknowledge her subjectivity.[9] As object, she can be regarded as a mere "vessel" for the fetus. The objectification of her experience, in its turn, forms the moral environment within which she forms her ethical questions and searches for their answers.

Technology, or the technological worldview, tends to privilege "sight" over "feeling," a notion that deeply troubled John Macmurray. He contends that "tactual perception is our only means of having a direct and immediate awareness of the Other as existent."[10] Knowledge has been construed on the model of vision, but vision has no immediate causal effect—visual perception is symbolic rather than immediate. We look at an object and form a representation of it in our mind, and thoughts or emotions are then stimulated by that representation. However, these thoughts or emotions are the result of processes of the imagination operating at a "distance" from the object. These responses differ in important ways from the *immediate* "feeling" or awareness that coming into contact with the object would arouse. Vision is always mediated by (and therefore, Squier would argue, constructed by) concepts we already hold—in this case, concepts that contributed to and are thus encouraged by modern technology. Modern technology relies on a dualism of mind and body that encourages an emphasis on the visual. In contrast, Macmurray argues that the primacy of "touch" over "vision" rests in the fact that "the core of tactual perception is resistance."[11] It is this resistance that makes us aware of the distinction between self and Other, but only because we must be aware of *both* at the same time. Knowledge itself depends on the *awareness* of this distinction—an awareness of an "I" that comes into contact with something that is "Not I." The "Other," he contends, "is discovered in tactual perception, both as the resistance to and support of action."[12] Contact makes me aware of the Other and the limitation it places on my movement. Although contact alone does not give me full knowledge of the Other, it stimulates a search for such knowledge and thus provides the ground for further action. Additionally, even though we perceive ourselves as individual or separate, physical contact can only be made in a shared space within a common boundary. Therefore, every action an individual makes is affected by or affects another individual as his or her action occurs within this communal space, forcing a connection between them.[13]

Vangie Bergum noted in her research that pregnant mothers are often amazed by the *simultaneous* awareness of connectedness to, yet separation from, their child to be, as that phenomenon evidences itself in their pregnancy. Late in pregnancy, women describe the fetus as having a life of its own:

> It [the fetus] definitely has a life of its own. I had been reading on my side and then I turned on my back and the baby didn't like that position and then it started moving. It had these deliberate movements. I knew that somebody else was in there. It was a "somebody" who could decide when it wants to do something, a deliberate turning over and pushing and getting more space. It was definitely someone separate.[14]

The awareness of the Other stimulated by "feeling" the Other shifts one's attention from self to Other, and back again. This activity has important implications for conceiving a theory of maternity, as feeling shapes our thoughts differently than vision does, a topic we will return to later in more detail. In preparation for that discussion we will turn to Robbie Davis-Floyd's essay "The Technocratic Body and the Organic Body," in which she describes women's experience of pregnancy and birth customs as "integrated systems [technocratic or organic] of knowledge and praxis."[15]

The Technocratic Versus Organic Body

Davis-Floyd analyzed women's differing conceptualizations of their relationships to their fetuses—whether they preferred to emphasize the physicality of their body and their ensuing feeling of the fetus (organic) or the technologically mediated conception of the fetus (technocratic). Davis-Floyd notes that the "technocratic extreme is dominant in most American hospitals and . . . this technocratic paradigm metaphorizes the female body as a defective machine unable to produce a healthy baby without technological assistance."[16] Alternatively, she characterizes the "organic" model as one that "interprets the female body as an organic system, and birth as an ecological process that can only be harmed by dissection and intervention."[17] The technocratic model is based on a material conception of the world that blurs the distinction between animate and inanimate objects. It is threatening because it detaches from the human that which is integral to being human, such as our specific modes of perception, reasoning processes, and the capability of intentional action, which we then judge as ethical or not. On this view, the individuality of the mother, as a mother, is overlooked in favor of her sameness to all gestating women and the biological matter they share. The mother as individual, as subject, is negated.

Surprisingly, then, the research of Davis-Floyd shows that the mothers who wholeheartedly adopted the technological paradigm viewed themselves as "future-shapers"—persons who creatively constructed their world according to their own desires. However, they could do this only by adopting the belief that their self was their mind, not their body. Davis-Floyd adds that this group of women conceived of their body merely as "a vehicle, a tool for the self." As a corollary of that they "tended to see the pregnant body as a vessel, a container for the fetus (who is a being separate from the mother) and to interpret its growth and birth as occurring through a mechanical process in which the mother [was] not actively involved."[18] They relied for knowledge of their fetus on technological means (i.e., ultrasound photographs) and electronic amplification of the fetal heart rate, not from individual acknowledgment and interpretation of their own bodily feelings and the movements of the fetus within.

In contrast, the group that adopted the "organic" model of the birth process did not separate the body and mind but rather experienced "the body as the self, or as part of the self . . . stress[ed] in belief and behavior the body's organic interconnectedness, as opposed to its mechanicity, and . . . view[ed] the female body as normal, attractive, and healthy."[19] The organic model, or holistic model, as Davis-Floyd calls it, views "*mother and baby [as] essentially One—that is, they form part of an integrated system that can only be harmed by dissection into its individual parts.* Much more than a passive host, or 'vessel,' *the mother sees herself as actively growing the baby*" (emphasis added).[20] Accordingly, these women held that their individual "inner knowing" or "bodily knowing" was as reliable as the information they received from technological tests. They did not view their uterus as a "vessel" but as a part of a whole that constituted the emotional, physical, and spiritual aspects of themselves. This had important consequences for the manner in which they conceptualized their pregnancy, and we will attempt to understand why this was so by looking at how "seeing" another entity or "feeling" it influences our apprehension of it.

The Primacy of Feeling

As noted earlier, Macmurray argued for the primacy of touch over vision, that persons "know, and develop their knowledge as much through their capacity for feeling as by using their senses," that is, "sense depends upon feeling in a way in which feeling does not depend upon sense."[21] The functional difference between feeling and sense, he claims, is that

> sense enables the reaction to anticipate contact, and this is especially true of visual consciousness. By substituting, as stimulus, light reflected from an object for actual contact with the object, it makes possible an anticipatory adaptation on the part of the organism, without any cognition of the object.[22]

That is, through the sense of sight, one "imagines" or anticipates what contact with the Other would be like, but one does not make contact with it in any way ("feel" it as existent). Thus knowledge of this object (may) take on a different character than if we actually come into physical contact with it.

However, if a feeling is strong enough, it generates its own images in accordance with the (past) experiences of the lived body.[23] The growth of a fetus and therefore its movements increase with maturity; therefore, stronger movements may induce stronger images (i.e., of a healthy baby), whereas fluttering, minute movements indicate the mere stirrings of life. Within this process, imagination and emotion come into play in direct response to the feeling that initiates them and then they begin the process of constructing the image—feeling exists *simultaneously* with the construction of the image and is responsible for its emergence. But in contemporary society we no longer wait for these movements or give them the requisite attention. Squier notes that

> the different stages of embryonic/fetal life are increasingly mediated by—and thus constructed by—ultrasound and other fetal visualization technologies. And while this has received less emphasis or analysis, it is also arguable that the increasing gynecological and obstetrical uses of visualization technologies have catalyzed a similar shift in our conception of the Mother.[24]

Squier concludes that visualization technologies have made the pregnancy "more real" and motherhood therefore "more immanent." The image, "seen" at a "distance" from the body, is constructed before the mother has any feeling or resulting emotion regarding that image. There is a gap (however slight) between receiving the "representation" of the fetus via technological means and the attachment of thoughts and emotions to that image. Squier suggests that the cultural imaginary inserts itself into this gap. She argues that the fetus has been given more "concrete social space and more subjectivity" than the gestating woman because attached to the *image* of the fetus (which is projected *at* the mother, not *from* the mother) are the dominant cultural metaphors (see note 13).

Before technological intervention, the woman's feeling of the fetus was primary. It was *her* subjective experience that was paramount and *her* experience that enabled the fetus to have any kind of identity at all. Thus the "unseen" was granted a reality through the communicated experience of the mother, which also may have legitimated the unseen emotions that attended such physical feelings. In addition, the mother's feeling the fetus within her contributed to her awareness of the fetus taking up space in her body—of the fetus and herself residing within one *physical* boundary—an awareness of their relation and its implications for their *individual* developments.

Although physical feelings exist for the technologically focused pregnant woman, they no longer hold any significance for her and do not play a part in her reflection on the experience of pregnancy, other than as an inconvenience. As Squier notes, "we have no customary term that captures the in-between subject that is the gestating woman. There is no quick, specific term for her complex, liminal subject position."[25] Unable to deal with the ambiguity that a pregnant woman's body presents, medical science now posits two individuals—the fetus and the mother—and places them in an antagonistic position, a position that Squier notes has all but erased the mother's subjectivity. This is facilitated by the ability to "see" the fetus and idealize that imperfect visualization into what we perceive to be a *normal*[26] baby, attended by the culturally acceptable (or "normal") emotions. However, if we want to circumvent this antagonistic paradigm, desiring instead to see the mother and fetus as interdependent for their individual fortunes on the existence of each other, we can fall prey to a form of biological determinism. Terminating a pregnancy will remain a concept with which we have to struggle. John Macmurray saw the dilemma that framing the world within these two paradigms— the material (technological) and the organic—would create, and we now turn to his theory of personhood.

The "Form of the Personal"

Within our project, Macmurray's theory of the self assists us in understanding why the feeling body is important, and what relevance it has for addressing ethical issues. Since he conceived of persons as primarily agents who act with intention, his endeavor, in part, was to explore how the subjective aspect of the self fit in and contributed to the actions of persons in the world. Within the field of action, knowledge has its place, as it shapes our *intentions* to act, and thus guides our ensuing actions, but knowledge has many facets. Knowledge is of two kinds, embodied knowledge and theoretical knowledge, but theoretical knowledge is (or should be, so he thought) derived from the actions of concrete, specific bodies in the world.

Macmurray contends that "knowledge . . . in its primary form, is the theoretical determination of the past in action."[27] "New" knowledge is a theorizing of previous experience that can be used in a different context. However, thought must include within itself a "receptivity," or what we call sense perception. This "embodied" knowledge has feeling as its primary sense, as it is physical feeling that gives us a direct awareness of the world—both of ourselves and what is not ourselves. In "feeling," one is *directly* aware of the other and the self "bumping up against each other" within a common space. Therefore knowledge, in its fullness, is an "objective awareness," Macmurray claims, as it is "awareness of the Other and the Self in relation."[28] "Feeling" functions as a selective element, in that "I" feel "You," and such a feeling provokes the awareness that "You and I" have come into contact, and through this contact we have knowledge of the relation we now are part of and cannot escape. As individual selves we can cooperate within the common space of our relation or we can choose to battle for our individual rights, but we *cannot* remain immune to the effects each of our actions produce.[29]

There is another important aspect to the knowledge that we create, one that is often ignored. "Knowing in action is possible only through an active ignoring of most of what is presented, that is to say, by a *selection of attention*. [However] I can only ignore what I am aware of . . . so we say that we are 'unconsciously' aware of a thing when our attention was focused on something else."[30] Macmurray notes that the significant quality of *persons* is that they act with *intention*. Nevertheless, he emphasizes that the negative aspect, or receptive quality, to intention is *attention*. That is, wherever our attention is focused informs the knowledge we accumulate and therefore forms the subsequent intentions for action. However, the focal point on which our attention rests is influenced by many things. First, it is influenced by bodily feeling; if we are in pain, inevitably our thoughts will tend to focus on that pain until we find relief. Second, it is influenced by external sources, such as education and media, that condition us to respond "unconsciously" or automatically to certain stimuli. This response is not a given, however, since it is a habit and is therefore learned (and thus can be unlearned). Nevertheless, unless we make a conscious effort to do otherwise, we will respond habitually to specific ideas or thought patterns within our culture, that is, accepting them somewhat thoughtlessly as "the way things are" when that is not necessarily the case. For instance, in the examples summarized by Davis-Floyd regarding the habits of "attending" of two different groups of women, one group chose to "pay attention to" the dominant discourse of our culture—the technological one. The so-called organic group consciously avoided this discourse and focused on an alternative method of birth giving that required different kinds of knowledges and thus a different focus for their attention.

Shifts of Attention

Michael Lipson and Abigail Lipson have articulated clearly how this shift of focus works in ethical development. They explore the role of *attentional dynamics*—"how our capacity to attend underlies our ethical abilities."[31] In their investigation they do not advocate any particular set of values but endeavor to reveal how "the capacity to attend can be exercised in the service of all the major theories of ethics as they currently exist."[32] Like Macmurray, they advocate an understanding of the "intrapsychic and interpersonal conditions under which persons affect one another's moral development *for the good*."[33] Attention in this context refers to directing one's *awareness* to a specific person or thing. Lipson and Lipson affirm the value of "objective awareness," a term Macmurray also uses. It requires some self-abnegation on our part to shift attention to the Other, they claim, but by eliminating the focus on the self, we have more room to take in information about the Other. Hence our knowledge of the Other is enhanced or increased in proportion to our limiting attention to the self. Therefore, our actions will be more "moral" the more understanding we cultivate, since such understanding shapes our intentions and hence our actions toward the Other. The self-abnegation that Lipson and Lipson are talking about is the choice to limit attention to oneself and focus on the Other.

Macmurray views this process a bit differently. For Macmurray, "objective awareness" constitutes the awareness of the Other and self in relation, which of necessity must also be an awareness of the *difference* between self and Other. Within this awareness we cannot ignore knowledge of our own (general) needs, as we are one term of the relation that "You and I" belong to. Neither can we ignore our knowledge of the "space" we both inhabit. Although Macmurray contends it is right that we focus attention on the Other, he introduces a concept he calls the process of "withdrawal and return," which constitutes the "form of the personal." Moral autonomy emerges from the process of withdrawal and return; in each encounter, we are invited to overcome our self-centered, egoistic motivations and act instead on our understanding of the Other and the self in relation. In the process of withdrawal, we withdraw into (individual) reflection[34] and return to action with the intention to act in terms of what our newly accumulated knowledge of the other informs us that they require. After engagement with the Other, we withdraw again to reflect on our actions to see if the intention that preceded them became manifest in those actions, that is, was our knowledge accurate and did our response suffice?[35] Macmurray makes it explicit that increased self-awareness will contribute to our ability to understand the other. Implicit in this process is that our understanding is always incomplete and is shaped by other sources of knowledge. Thus, in thinking of the Other, we must also keep in mind the other knowledges we have of the world in which this Other and I inhabit. Additionally, through his concept of withdrawal and return, Macmurray also allows for the changeability of the Other, the environment, and the self. Knowledge of the Other or of our shared world is not fixed in any sense—it is always open to revision, which Lipson and Lipson claim is a by-product of reflecting on our attending habits. The focus of our attention is generally influenced by habits, by external occurrences or actions, by new ideas, and by an already existing hegemonic worldview. Our capacity for transforming our ethical understanding lies (at least in part) in our ability to shift attention from the "common" or "habitual" center of focus to an alternative one, a process that has the potential to alter formerly held worldviews. We suggest that shifting our focus away from the ultrasound screen and onto the felt experience of the pregnant body provides an alternative understanding of that body, an understanding that may reframe the experience of pregnancy for Western women.

The "Personal" Body

In this section we return to the research of Davis-Floyd and Squier, keeping Macmurray's theory of personhood in view. As already noted, Squier comments on a disturbing aspect of technological representations of the fetus: they increasingly imply that the fetus and the mother are two separate "selves" that are in conflict. Within this conflict, either the fetus or the mother gains the dominant subjective position, depending on the desired end result. The fetus can be viewed as mere "cells" or the mother can be seen as merely a "container" for the fetus.[36] Davis-Floyd found similar views present within the group of women who embraced the technological paradigm. They saw their blooming bodies as "uncontrollable," their pregnant state introducing complications into their lives that made them uncomfortable, since "the medical interpretation of the best interests of the baby demanded that their own needs and desires be subordinated to the all-important product of this manufacturing process."[37]

However, the women who acted under the holistic paradigm saw the mother and the fetus (or baby to be) "as one integral and indivisible unit until birth." They did not perceive themselves as "passive containers" but felt themselves to be passionately involved in a creative act, comfortable with the notion that they themselves were being simultaneously "created" in the process of giving birth.[38] Alternatively, the women adopting the technological paradigm were unhappy with such "uncontrolled" creation and were unwilling to undergo change if they, themselves, did not initiate and control that change. These two disparate worldviews—the material (or technological) and organic—are important for the remainder of our discussion. We will suggest that both worldviews are insufficient for women's needs. Although we cannot ignore the material and organic aspects of human life, they are nevertheless insufficient in themselves to describe human life and human dilemmas, and particularly the experience of pregnancy as a whole—which includes the possibility of the termination of that pregnancy.

As we already pointed out, women adopting the "technological" worldview in Davis-Floyd's study drew sharp distinctions between "mind" and "body." The body was merely matter that needed to be controlled by an educated and self-disciplined mind. Matter behaves mechanically—its behavior is absolutely uniform, doing the same thing in the same circumstances, and is completely consistent. It is *not* unique and individual in its actions.

On the "organic" view however, mind and body are seen as interconnected and interdependent. The organic body "is conceived as a harmonious balancing of differences, and in its pure form, a tension of opposites; and since the time factor—as growth, development or becoming—is of the essence of life, the full form of the organic is represented as a dynamic equilibrium of functions maintained through a progressive differentiation of elements within the whole."[39] Unlike material bodies, living bodies do not always behave in the same way in the same circumstances. The ideas bound up with our consideration of the nature of living beings are

> the ideas of growth, development and evolution; the idea of adaptation to environment, of fitting in to one's place in a complex organization or community; the ideas of progress and purpose, of the end to which the whole creation moves; the idea of the service of the species and its development. These are all ideas which express the nature of living beings, of plants and animals.[40]

The organic paradigm adopts a teleological view of the world. Each person has a specific function within the whole, fulfills that function to the best of his or her abilities, and the whole moves forward. On this scenario, a pregnant woman fulfils her function by making it possible for the fetus to develop unhindered. In addition, it is understood that it is a woman's duty (to the whole) to be a mother, and if she is unable to bear children, she is "defective" in that function. However, Macmurray denies that persons can be reduced to a function. If only the well-being of the whole is taken into account, the autonomy of the individuals who constitute that whole is sacrificed. What he claims *is* characteristic of human persons is that they "have the capacity to know other things and other people and enjoy them. And when we are completely ourselves we live by that knowledge and appreciation of what is not ourselves, and so in communion with other beings."[41] There are three important points here. First, we have the capacity to gain some understanding or knowledge of a world outside of ourselves—a world of infinite variety that demands heterogeneous methodologies of knowing. Second, we use the knowledge we gain to act in terms of the Other whom we have gained understanding of—whether or not we act to their benefit, our own benefit, or toward a mutual benefit—and we then take responsibility for what we do. Humans can recognize the needs of others, which in turn give us reasons for acting—acting in terms that we judge "right" or "wrong" in accord with our vision of how the world should be. We have the ability to act purposefully according to that vision. Third, we must *be ourselves*, that is, we must claim and cultivate our self-awareness or subjectivity in order to expand our agency. Claiming full subjectivity (i.e., using the knowledge of body *and* mind) would enable us to address the ambiguity and uncertainty that conflicting knowledges may present.

What was most "real" for the women who adopted the technological worldview was the picture on an ultrasound screen, the medical report, and so on. The *thing seen* had a more objective reality than the *person who felt* the thing being seen (even, it seems, when the feeling person was themselves). The women who adopted the organic worldview, however, did not deny any of the knowledges that they were exposed to, either that of their body, that of their midwife or doctor, or that of technology. However, they appeared to trust their body first and foremost as the primary source of knowledge—their body was most "real" to them. We would argue that the women who adopt what Davis-Floyd calls the "organic" worldview actually claimed a "personal" worldview, or a "personal" body. They acknowledged the fetus inside them—they consciously "felt" its movements and its dependence on them—and recognized that the existence of that Other being might well transform their lives. Living with the uncertainty of entwined existences, they appeared to be comfortable within the "liminal" space Squier notes is so characteristic of pregnancy. They *claimed* personhood (in Macmurray's sense) through understanding the "relational" quality of their individual lives. And with *awareness* of self, Other, and the context in which self and Other are located, they intentionally shaped the character of that relation.

But what, we ask, if circumstances were such that one of these women, for whatever reason, decided she should end her pregnancy? How would she come to terms with such a decision, since she sees the life of her fetus and her own life as already mutually influential and connected, *as one*? We think that in the case of abortion, the customs of other cultures can inform our own thinking about this problematic issue, as other cultures have focused on aspects of personhood that North American culture has ignored.[42] In the attempt to achieve a deeper understanding of this particular issue, we will shift our attention to Japan and the ritual of *mizuko kuyo*. Japan is a highly technological society, like North America, but its culture has been heavily influenced by Asian religions such as Confucianism, Shintoism, and Buddhism. None of these religions or worldviews has affirmed the mind/body split that characterizes North American culture.

Terminating a Pregnancy: Abortion in Japan

Bardwell Smith, in his essay "Buddhism and Abortion in Contemporary Japan: Mizuko Kuyo and the Confrontation with Death," addresses the difficulty that moderns experience in dealing with death, particularly "the mother's experiencing of death, whether or not this death has been willed by her."[43] But Smith also considers factors within Japanese society that contribute to the dilemma surrounding abortion specifically. Smith investigates a Japanese Buddhist response to the widespread phenomenon of abortion in modern Japan—a response embodied in a ritual exercise called *mizuko kuyo. Mizuko* means "water child or children, referring normally to an aborted fetus (induced or spontaneous) but also to stillborn infants and those who died soon after birth."[44] The term *kuyo* means to offer and nourish. "In this sense, it is the offering up of prayers for the nourishment of the spirit of the aborted or stillborn child. Also . . . it is intended to console the parents, especially the mother, though not infrequently one finds fathers coming with the mother or even by themselves."[45] The ritual addresses a significant dilemma that Japanese women face. On the one hand, the Japanese place immense weight on the mother-child relationship, in which, Smith claims, the average woman still seeks to find her "deepest identity."[46] Additionally, one of the dominant religions, Buddhism, teaches that life begins at conception.[47] On the other hand, Japanese women have little access to family planning methods or sex education.[48] "The result is naivete, embarrassment, misinformation, and an alarming rate of unwanted pregnancies within marriage and, increasingly in the past ten years, outside of marriage as well."[49] A conservative estimate of abortions in Japan states that there are about 1 million abortions per year, more liberal estimates putting the figure at 1.5 million.[50] Smith notes that women's limited procreative choices contribute to frustration on their part, as well as considerable resentment. How do they cope?

Japanese women have responded to their quandary by participating (often secretly) in the Buddhist ritual of *mizuko kuyo,* which is used to heal the "broken connection" that these women feel when they abort a fetus. Studies that take the life process seriously, as well as the individual's feelings, such as anxiety, guilt, rage, and violence, which often accompany the confrontation with death or any of its equivalents, indicate that images of continuity, or life equivalents such as connection, integrity, and movement, heal the severing of connection that happens in situations such as abortion.[51] However, in order for these images to be successful, there is a need to confront issues within the human community that resist facing death or death equivalents; an *attitude of realism* needs to be adopted. Buddhism, despite teaching that human life begins at conception, is also

the endorsement of a profoundly human experience, namely, that nothing less than a human life is at issue. One question revolves around the symbolic nature of what are called *mizuko*, for in the case of *mizuko* there is obviously a fundamental inversion of the typical and expected sequence in the ancestor-descendant continuity. A child here dies before its parents. This naturally raises religious questions in Buddhism about what happens to the *mizuko*, as well as psychological questions as to how one experiences the loss, how one grieves. Even the prospective experiencing of family bond becomes an avenue for discovering hidden connections in life . . . and a source of deep meaning. If so whenever ambivalence exists in the decision to abort, mourning becomes the acknowledgement that something of consequence has occurred, that one is never quite the same again. It is therefore to acknowledge death, even a death which one has willed. . . . In the words of Magda Denes, "That . . . is the dilemma of abortions."[52]

Although no "recommended form of service" exists, Smith notes that a number of common elements are found among the many rituals of *mizuko kuyo*. These involve invoking the names of one or more forms of the Buddha and various boddhisattvas, chanting parts of sutras, or songs of praise, and offering food, light, flowers, and incense to the Buddha on behalf of the child and as tokens of the larger offering of one's life.[53] In many cases, "some sculpted representation of Jizo[54] or of an infant symbolizing a mizuko is brought by the family and left in a specially designated place within the temple grounds" and often a "posthumous Buddhist name is given the child and this is inscribed on an *ihai* or mortuary tablet, which is left in a special chapel within the temple or taken home and placed in the family . . . Buddhist shrine."[55] It is precisely the point, Smith claims, "to put [the mizuko] into the ancestral lineage."[56] Thus this act is a refusal to deny the fetuses' existence and the connection they share with those who created them. He also claims that this is a *redressive ritual*, a "means of confronting situations of frustration caused by broken connections of one sort or another. . . . In the process, people are assisted to confront threatening situations or broken connections both more deeply and more constructively."[57]

We believe this ritual has significance for our discussion of the "personal" body and personhood because in the process of addressing the act of terminating a pregnancy it acknowledges the physical feelings (and the attendant emotions, etc.) of the mothers and family members affected by that decision, without denying them the choice of terminating the pregnancy. That is, *in this aspect at least*, it recognizes the physical and emotional feelings of the mother as an important part of her subjectivity. By addressing the bodily, emotional, and intellectual needs of the mother, the ritual does not minimize her experience or sentimentalize it. The woman, in her turn, takes responsibility for shaping the character of her relation to the fetus that no longer exists in physical fact but has its place in her memory.[58]

One of Macmurray's consistent themes is that "personhood" is a *relational* concept:

> Human experience is, in principle, shared experience; human life, even in its most individual elements, is a common life; and human behaviour carries always, in its inherent structure, a reference to the personal Other. All this may be summed up by saying that the unit of personal existence is not the individual, but two persons in personal relation; and that we are persons not by individual right, but in virtue of our relation to one another. The personal is constituted by personal relatedness. The unit of the personal is not the "I" but the "You and I."[59]

We are persons in virtue of the social character of our human makeup, but, we would argue, we *claim* personhood when we acknowledge this character, cultivate it, and seek to shape our world accordingly. The technological worldview denies us this opportunity. It affirms a sharp mind/body split, designating some things as "mind" and others as "matter" in order to pursue the ends it desires. The organic model, on the other hand, affirms the interconnectedness of mind and body, and this is its strength, but it denies us the intentionality (and therefore autonomy) of our actions in creating our world, hence limiting our responsibility for that creative act at the same time. Additionally, with its emphasis on the biological, it potentially reduces human persons to their biological function, which women are (rightly) wary of. Claiming personhood maintains the value of organic life, yet one can intentionally seek to develop understanding regarding that life and its interconnected nature and act accordingly. We gain such an understanding in and through the location and perceptions of a specific existent body.

As already noted, whether we form images out of a significant individual (bodily) feeling, or whether the image as presented to us already encompasses cultural concepts, these images shape the paradigm within which we act and think and form the choices we construct for ourselves when making decisions regarding prospective actions. To adopt uncritically images projected at us is to make ourselves even more vulnerable to distortions in thinking. By shifting attention back to the body and its knowledge-providing capacities, we claim some advantage in our efforts to subvert the dominant paradigm (if we so desire). When the "location" and information of the individual body transmits different knowledge than that of the hegemonic view, the interface between these two understandings (the individual and the social) creates room for transformations of knowledge to occur within the dominant paradigm. When we claim a "personal" body, we use our body's knowledge along with the understanding we possess of our specific body's relation with the world, aware that in our actions we play a part in shaping the character of that relation.

Concluding Thoughts

It is highly questionable whether a fetus can be granted the status of a person on these terms. Certainly the fetus is an organism that would be a person if left to develop unhindered. Squier states that one of the fetus's most powerful attributes is its "pure potentiality." "As pure potential, it is powerful precisely because it never comes into being. At birth, it ceases being that fetal subject; it becomes, instead, a baby, with the specific positionalities of class, race, sex, and all so on, that constitute the human individual."[60] However, the mother of the fetus already belongs to a specific race, class, and culture, factors that influence her life and within which she must live and act. Smith's essay indicates that Japanese women who participate in the ritual of *mizuko kuyo* use it to address the frustration of some of those factors (i.e., the lack of birth control, adequate education on sex, religious beliefs, a patriarchal society, etc.)—factors that limit their agency in other ways. In doing so, however, they acknowledge the fetus as one part of a "potential" relationship but, nevertheless, one who has not attained the full subject position of the mother. Japanese women deny neither the reality of the fetus as existent nor their own reality—a reality that makes it impossible (at least through their interpretation of their environment) for them to bring a child into the world at the present time. They do not deny their feelings of anger, sadness, and frustration at the broken connection of a relation but rather acknowledge them. And in doing so, they accept another reality—that in a grossly imperfect world we are constantly compromised in our efforts to do good.

Macmurray notes the paradox of the personal: "The problem that faces us when we seek to do what is right is the impossibility of doing it without some admixture of what is wrong."[61] The process of reframing the dilemma of abortion, though, raises different questions for our consideration. It redirects the question of whether a woman is "right" or "wrong" in seeking to terminate her pregnancy to a consideration of the social fabric in which unwanted pregnancies occur. In so doing, it does not deny anyone's emotions or feelings, nor does it demand specific emotions or feelings—it merely leaves room for such a possibility and allows for women to attend to the ambiguity of emotions that may occur when a pregnancy is terminated. What it does not do is reduce the fetus to "matter" or the mother to a "mind" that cannot recognize the life she has the potential to give, or assign the mother the status of "vessel" for a developing fetus. This is the value of the "form of the personal" that seeks to integrate mind and body into one knowing person. We are reminded that in order to shift our attention to the Other, and thus achieve "objective awareness," we need to be aware of the images that influence our thinking and "order" and "filter" the information we take in from the world. "Objective awareness" demands "subjective awareness."

In this sense, it is thought provoking to construct the pregnant woman's body as a metaphor for the *hope* that infuses Macmurray's "form of the personal." As the woman's body circumscribes a boundary within which she and an other exist, so all of humanity exists within the boundary of the planet we inhabit. As most relationships existing in the world are unequal, so is that between mother and fetus. In addition, as in most relations (defined as such by the fact that they exist within and acknowledge a common environment), a deepening of the relation is achieved only by the *intention* of both persons to do so. Either one can turn away and reject a deepening of the relationship for several reasons, one of which may be that the present environment is not conducive to forming such a relationship at this time. To some extent, all of human life belongs in that "liminal space," which Squier contends is so distinctive of mothering, as we ceaselessly "give birth" to one another (through the shaping of ideas, attitudes, knowledge, etc.) while remaining open to rebirth (through the same process) ourselves. This is the inherent hope that resides within the form of the personal: that we desire to give birth and do not resist being reborn.

If we shift our attention from the ultrasound screen to the "feeling" body of the pregnant mother, another scene unfolds before us that allows us to acknowledge the primacy and full subjectivity of the mother, the potential of the fetus, and the environment within which the relation must survive and flourish. Neither the mother nor the wider society and world can be excluded from the "big picture." Neither is innocent of responsibility for the choices she will make. The human dilemma presents itself when we seek to improve one state of affairs yet find we cannot do so without inflicting damage somewhere else. The response, though, is not to ignore the existence of that damage but to recognize it and seek to heal its wounds in alternative ways. And for women, it sets a dangerous precedent when the *thing seen* is more real than the *person who feels* the thing seen. *Persons* exist within a context that limits their choices. That is the human dilemma, but it is profoundly, in the instance of abortion, a woman's dilemma.

Sandra Harding notes in one of her essays that "new philosophies ask how and what kind of local knowledge 'travels' and—because cultures are tool boxes and prison houses for the growth of knowledge—what is lost and what is gained when it does."[62] Knowledge in the Western world has been constructed on the model of vision and manifests itself through concepts and categories that are often structured in sharp opposition to one another (the "seen" and the "unseen"). In the nondualistic perspective of some Eastern cultures, the moral questions that their knowledge seeks to address reside on a continuum. Although clarity may be sought, it is recognized as an elusive entity. Shifting attention to the lived body avoids harsh judgments and circumvents the cultural imaginary, or at least avoids further entrenching it. To return to the quotation at the beginning of this chapter, Finzi's request for a theory of mothering, we advocate investigating norms regarding what constitutes personhood that are omnipresent in other cultures before constructing that theory. We may find that some knowledge "travels" better than another and that we, as North Americans, also have "knowledge" that can assist women in other cultures to develop other aspects of their subjectivity. It is to our advantage, as women, to continue the pursuit of knowledge that "travels," knowledge that affirms our embodied experience as women.

Notes

1. Silva V. Finzi, "Female Identity Between Sexuality and Motherhood," in Gisela Bock and Susan James, eds., *Beyond Equality and Difference: Citizenship, Feminist Politics, and Female Subjectivity* (London: Routledge, 1992), p. 140.

2. Ibid., p. 141.

3. John Macmurray, *The Self As Agent* (London: Faber & Faber, 1957), p. 104.

4. Buddhism, one of the predominant religions of Japan, as well as Shintoism, its native religion, do not adopt the perspective of mind/body dualism that manifests itself within Christianity, which is the predominant religion in the Western world. For another East Asian view of mind and body, see Shigenori Nagatomo and Gerald Leisman, "An East Asian Perspective of Mind-Body," *Journal of Medicine and Philosophy* 21, no. 4 (1996): 439–466.

5. Macmurray's "form of the personal" incorporates both the technological and the organic worldviews within itself. Thus he does not ignore them or abandon them but claims that they each manifest only one aspect of human life or human experience.

6. In contrast to an "organic" body or a "technological" body.

7. Barbara Duden, *Disembodying Woman: Perspectives on Pregnancy and the Unborn* (Cambridge: Harvard University Press, 1993), p. 79.

8. Ibid., p. 81.

9. For an interesting discussion of "medicalized subjectivity," see K. P. Morgan, "Contested Bodies, Contested Knowledges: Women, Health, and the Politics of Medicalization," in The Feminist Health Care Ethics Research Network, Susan Sherwin, coordinator, *The Politics of Women's Health: Exploring Agency and Autonomy* (Philadelphia: Temple University Press, 1998), pp. 83–121.

10. Macmurray, *Self As Agent*, p. 111.

11. Ibid., p. 108.

12. Ibid., p. 110.

13. The moment or awareness of contact, the "feeling" simultaneously introduces an awareness of the Other, who impinges on us and we on them. This

awareness, according to Macmurray, is the stimulus (or ground) for what we call moral action—or what theorists such as Zygmunt Bauman (*Postmodern Ethics* [Oxford: Oxford University Press, 1993]) have called the "moral impulse."

14. Vangie Bergum, *A Child on Her Mind* (Westport, Conn.: Bergin & Garven, 1997), p. 146.

15. Robbie Davis-Floyd, "The Technocratic Body and the Organic Body: Hegemony and Heresy in Women's Birth Choices," in Carolyn F. Sargent and Caroline B. Brettell, eds., *Gender and Health: An International Perspective* (New Jersey: Prentice-Hall, 1996), p. 123.

16. Ibid., p. 129.

17. Ibid.

18. Ibid., pp. 134–135.

19. Ibid., p. 143.

20. Ibid., p. 144.

21. Macmurray, *Self As Agent*, p. 126.

22. Ibid., p. 125.

23. Macmurray claims that "feeling . . . forms the matrix of consciousness within which presentational consciousness is occasioned. The simplest explanation of this seems to be that a feeling is present which would generate an image if the stimulus were a little stronger; and the character of the feeling, as a result of experience, enables us to anticipate the image, and so functions, in the control of behaviour, as the image would if it were formed" (*Self As Agent*, p. 123).

24. Susan Squier, "Fetal Subjects and Maternal Objects: Reproductive Technology and the New Fetal/Maternal Relation," *Journal of Medicine and Philosophy* 21, no. 5 (1996): 517.

25. Ibid.

26. Squier notes that what is generally considered "normal" is constituted by the cultural imaginary. In Euro-American culture, the imaginary subject is white. Furthermore, the fetal subject is the "impossible subject" because it never comes into being and is therefore powerful because it remains "pure potential." Because the fetus has "neither specificity nor voice" it becomes "a magnet for both advocacy and representation" ("Fetal Subjects and Maternal Objects," pp. 533–534).

27. Macmurray, *Self As Agent*, p. 135.

28. Ibid., p. 129.

29. In summary, Macmurray succinctly states, "*My* freedom depends on how *you* behave" (and vice versa). This has strong implications for action. "What limits the freedom of agents is the presence of other agents in the same field of action. However in determining a future one determines an environment which itself provides a limitation to further action. This is the principle of the irreversibility of action" (Macmurray, *Self As Agent*, p. 135). Our actions shape a world, and within that world take on meanings, meanings which then play their part in constructing our (new) worldview (through their integration with other, already present thoughts or beliefs) and hence influence future actions (our own and others'). Thus our identity is in a continual process of renewal—however slight and insignificant.

30. Macmurray, *Self As Agent*, p. 130. In their recently published book, *Philosophy in the Flesh* (New York: Basic, 1999), p. 18, George Lakoff and Mark Johnson

elaborate on this idea. They claim it is an inevitable result of how humans "categorize" information. They state that "a small percentage of our categories have been formed by conscious acts of categorization, but most are formed automatically and unconsciously as a result of functioning in the world."

31. Michael Lipson and Abigail Lipson, "Psychotherapy and the Ethics of Attention," *Hastings Center Report* 26, no. 1 (1996): 17.

32. Ibid.

33. Ibid.

34. Although reflection is noted here as "individual," such reflection does not exclude dialogue with others. Such dialogue, however, is viewed as an "action" that would take place in a social environment and would then contribute to one's private reflections.

35. We use the terms "knowledge" and "understanding" interchangeably. Although we acknowledge that there are slight differences in their meanings, we contend that "understanding" a thing *is* knowledge, and that knowledge leads to a fuller understanding—therefore we believe that to conflate the two terms is not problematic.

36. In her chapter, "The Power of 'Positive' Diagnoses: Medical and Maternal Discourses on Amniocentesis," in K. L. Michaelson, ed., *Childbirth in America: Anthropological Perspectives* (South Hadley, Mass.: Bergin & Varvey, 1998), p. 103, Rayna Rapp cites a woman she interviewed: "When we walked into the doctor's office, both my husband and I were crying. He looked up and said, 'What's wrong? Why are you both in tears?' 'It's our baby, our baby is going to die,' I said. 'That isn't your baby,' he said firmly, 'it's a collection of cells that made a mistake.'" On the other end of the spectrum, Hilde Nelson in her article "The Architect and the Bee: Some Reflections on Postmortem Pregnancy," *Bioethics* 8, no. 3 (1994): 247, argues against sustaining the pregnancy of women who die during the first or second trimester of pregnancy, as postmortem pregnancy "is a destructive icon that undercuts women's agency." In the first case, the fetus is reduced to mere matter, in the second case it is the mother who is reduced to matter.

37. Davis-Floyd, "Technocratic Body," p. 147.

38. Ibid.

39. Macmurray, *Self As Agent*, p. 33.

40. John Macmurray, *Freedom in the Modern World* (1968; reprint, New Jersey: Humanities, 1992), p. 123.

41. Ibid.

42. W. De Craemer, in his essay "A Cross-Cultural Perspective on Personhood," *Milbank Memorial Fund Quarterly/Health and Society* 61, no. 1 (1983): 19–34, makes it clear that the Western vision of the person is a minority viewpoint in the world. The majority viewpoint manifest in most other societies, both technologically developing and technologically developed (e.g., Japan), does not reflect the North American perspective of radical individualism or adopt logical-rational dichotomies (e.g., opposing body and mind, thought and feeling, the conscious and the unconscious, etc.). In contrast, the Japanese vision of the person is quite different. In the Japanese context, it is not emotion but rather cold, rational calculation that distances one from empathic identification with others (which is regarded as indicative of inner pollution).

43. Bardnell Smith, "Buddhism and Abortion in Contemporary Japan: *Mizuko Kuyo* and the Confrontation with Death," in Jose Ignacio Cabezon, ed., *Buddhism, Sexuality, and Gender* (Albany: State University of New York, 1992), p. 65.

44. Ibid.

45. Ibid., p. 73.

46. Ibid., p. 82.

47. Ibid., p.˙72.

48. Samuel Coleman's essay "Family Planning in Japanese Society" uses primarily Japanese sources along with his own research conducted over a twenty-eight-month period in Tokyo. His analysis articulates the lack of adequate family planning methods and sex education in Japan, the consequences of which appear in the general unavailability of modern contraceptive methods, but also the lack of reliable information provided to men and women about birth control and sex. The topic of sexual relations is still a taboo subject for discussion in most schools and in family circles (quoted in Smith, "Buddhism and Abortion in Contemporary Japan," pp. 70–71). Recently the Toronto *Globe and Mail* reported that after nine years of deliberation, the Japanese government has finally approved the use of the birth-control pill (*Globe and Mail*, June 3, 1999). Thus Japanese women's agency has been hindered in ways that are different from the limitations that North American women contend with. This chapter is intended to increase awareness of the limitations placed on women in both cultures, and what we can learn from one another in regard to addressing those limitations. Factors that affect how Japanese women use ultrasound technology are no doubt diverse, yet their manner of acknowledging the emotional component of a pregnancy speaks to their ability to refrain from falling into a pattern of either ignoring the existence of the pregnancy or oversentimentalizing it.

49. Smith, "Buddhism and Abortion," p. 71.

50. Smith states that the figure of 1 million abortions per year is twice the officially reported number. He also notes that obstetrician-gynecologists have an enormous economic stake in abortions, as they derive a large share of their income from the practice (Smith, "Buddhism and Abortion," p. 70).

51. Smith, "Buddhism and Abortion," p. 67.

52. Ibid., pp. 72–73.

53. Ibid., p. 74.

54. *Jizo* is a boddhisattva in Japanese Buddhist cosmology. He is considered the foremost protector of children, particularly those who die early. Thus he is intimately identified with those who have been aborted, who never came into this realm of existence. Smith notes that Jizo identifies with those who are suffering and hence is an apt paradigm for worlds in which strife, discouragement, and passion reign. "In such a world he represents the possibility of hope; he is the epitome of compassion in a realm where this is rare" (Smith, "Buddhism and Abortion," pp. 80–81).

55. Smith, "Buddhism and Abortion," p. 74.

56. Ibid., p. 82.

57. Ibid., p. 77.

58. Even when there are no cultural rituals that assist women to cope with circumstances of broken connections, such as may be experienced in the termina-

tion of a pregnancy, researchers found that Canadian women create their own rituals to validate the loss of the potential child (P. Marck, "Unexpected Pregnancy: The Uncharted Land of Women's Experience," in Peggy Anne Field and Patricia Beryl Marck, eds., *Uncertain Motherhood: Negotiating the Risks of the Childbearing Years* (Thousand Islands, Calif.: Sage), pp. 82–138; J. Straszynska, "Tending the Garden: Restoring Wholeness: Coping with the Abortion Experience" (master's thesis, University of Alberta, 1999).

This suggests that there is a stronger connection between the physical and the emotional (or mental) aspects of human experience than medical science would like to admit. Viewing the fetus as "matter" appears to be difficult for women. In addition, viewing themselves as "one" with the fetus would tend to preclude terminating a pregnancy. There appears to be a need to deal with the emotional "hangover" that terminating a pregnancy may leave a woman with.

59. John Macmurray, *Persons in Relation* (London: Faber & Faber, 1961), p. 61.

60. Squier, "Fetal Subjects and Maternal Objects," pp. 533–534.

61. Macmurray, *Self As Agent*, p. 100.

62. Sandra Harding, "Gender Development and Post-Enlightenment Philosophies of Science," *Hypatia* 13, no. 3 (1998): 160.

7

Normalizing Reproductive Technologies and the Implications for Autonomy

Few nations are immune to the lure of reproductive technologies. Although there are national differences in the particular types of technologies that become commonplace, and significant differences in the role of national governments in promoting or restricting each sort, most societies support development and use of at least some forms of reproductive technologies. For example, most governments have specific population targets in mind, and they encourage use of the reproductive technology that facilitates those goals. Most governments also seek to ensure a "healthier" population and value technologies that can support that goal as they understand it. Even where local cultures are inclined to be suspicious of technology generally as representative of a new form of Western imperialism, we can still generally find encouragement of some types of interventions in reproductive processes. As various reproductive technologies take root in particular societies, they alter the reproductive experiences, opportunities, and duties of women. In this chapter I consider how the routine use of various forms of reproductive technology may affect women's autonomy.

I take the term "reproductive technology" to refer to any technological intervention in the social and biological processes of human procreation. As such, it covers such diverse activities as those associated with the prevention and interruption of pregnancy (contraception and abortion) as well as the facilitation of pregnancy through assisted conception (in vitro fertilization and its variations, artificial insemination, embryo transplants, cloning). It also includes the many activities that constitute medical surveillance and management of pregnancy and childbirth (including prenatal monitoring and diagnosis, fetal surgery and transfusions, use of electronic fetal monitors, surgical delivery) and the technology-assisted support of endangered newborns (via incubators, neonatal intensive care units, neonatal surgery). In addition, since human reproduction includes not only biological procreation but also the socialization and education of the young, reproductive activity extends throughout the period of childhood, providing many more opportunities for medical and other scientific experts to monitor and intervene in parenting practices through technological and other means. For the purposes of this chapter, I shall follow the usual convention and restrict my discussion of reproduction to the social and biological activities associated with producing babies (or preventing their birth).

Both the avoidance and the pursuit of pregnancy are now commonly construed as medical events, and, because medicine is heavily oriented toward the use of technology, they have become sites for extensive technological involvement. Indeed, throughout the industrialized world (and in many other parts of the globe), nearly all stages of pregnancy and childbirth are now inextricably bound up with technological monitoring and intervention. Significantly, there is widespread social agreement that technology is a desirable resource for the pursuit of procreative goals. Although some cultures resist the attractions of reproductive technology, most have come to accept the value of at least some types of reproductive technologies; even societies that strongly distrust the impact of Western technology on traditional cultural values and practices frequently manage to accommodate certain forms of reproductive technology.[1]

In this chapter I wish to pursue the sorts of pressures that cause cultures to think that technology is inevitable. I am concerned with puzzles about the role of personal autonomy in determining appropriate medical and technological care surrounding reproductive decisionmaking within particular cultural understandings of reproduction. To understand the range of autonomy issues involved, I shall explore a variety of activities related to reproductive decisionmaking: some examples are drawn from areas where personal autonomy is clearly and explicitly restricted and others from areas where personal choice is apparently respected, although participation in the practice may seem required.

Technologies to Prevent Births

To understand how the most familiar notion of patient autonomy functions in debates about reproductive practices, I first turn to some that are highly contested in many societies. Most prominent among the reproductive technologies now subject to heated public debate in Canada and the United States are those designed to allow women the means to avoid bearing children. Abortion and, in some circles, contraception are the focus of intense political campaigns to restrict their accessibility. Anti-abortion campaigners try to defend the lives of fetuses by demanding restrictive abortion policies while pro-choice activists commonly appeal to the autonomy ideal, demanding unlimited access to abortion services by stressing women's right to choose whether or not to bear children. Most of the technology involved in preventing and terminating unwanted pregnancies is relatively commonplace and straightforward; it is legal and political policies, not technological restrictions, that often keep them out of the hands of women who might choose them. But, since abortion is classified as a medical procedure, and the most effective forms of contraception (though this may change in the United States) (the Pill, IUDs, and sterilization) still require medical action or supervision, the necessary technology is available only by action of licensed physicians; hence, women are dependent on the technical intervention—and, therefore, the sympathetic cooperation—of medical practitioners. Activists on both sides of the abortion debate understand that social and political campaigns that dissuade physicians from providing this service will interfere with women's autonomy to fully control their procreative lives.

In North America, many of those who oppose abortion also object to the use of "artificial" contraception and seek to limit its availability as well, though objection to contraception is much less common. Those who oppose contraception generally cite religious and cultural reasons to restrict personal access to any technology that separates sexual from reproductive activity. In other societies (e.g., Japan) contraception is considered more objectionable and is less accessible than abortion.[2] Although proponents of choice on abortion can be expected to support voluntary contraceptive use, many observe that contraceptive use is frequently coerced. For example, some government-sponsored population-control policies are aimed at compelling members of certain disadvantaged groups to accept permanent or long-term forms of contraception. In the United States, for instance, Latina women in New York have a rate of sterilization that is seven times higher than that of women of European descent, and there is reason to doubt that all sterilized women provided fully informed consent to the procedure.[3] In contraception, as in abortion, policies can be either coercive or permissive; that is, they can restrict women's autonomy or promote it in very explicit ways.

Although abortion and contraception are especially visible sites of political struggle, they are certainly not unique in this regard. Other very clear political battles are being waged over the uses of other sorts of technologies, such as the looming possibility of cloning human beings and contractual pregnancies. More subtle power struggles are associated with changing norms and expectations of family size, composition, and genetic links. Because the political, social, and economic significance of reproduction extend well beyond their effects on the immediate family, the impact of reproductive technologies may be felt not only by those directly involved in their use but by many others as well. As a result, many forms of reproductive technologies raise important questions of freedom and control. All are potentially subject to challenge and social conflict.

Accepted Technologies

In the West, most public attention in regard to reproductive technologies is directed toward technologies identified as "new," namely, those concerned with assisting conception and with genetic screening and manipulation. But before exploring these headline-grabbing technologies, I want to situate them more fully in their social context—a world in which procreation is already heavily medicalized and subject to pervasive technological intervention. It is much easier to appreciate the ways in which the "new" reproductive technologies have been accepted in our society and to understand the fears many people have about their growing use if we recognize that the new reproductive technologies are not an entirely new phenomenon; rather, they represent additional steps along an already well-established continuum. The prevailing social acceptance of existing technological intervention in so many aspects of reproduction makes the treatment of infertility and the prevention of genetic defects seem familiar and appropriate. Reproduction has been widely accepted as an event requiring extensive medical involvement, so it seems "natural" to look for medical solutions to any problems that arise in this sphere.

The defining events of procreation are pregnancy and childbirth. In the developed world (and increasingly in many parts of the developing world) both events are subject to ongoing medical surveillance and control. From the initial perception of possible pregnancy, women are expected to present themselves to medical experts for certification of their pregnant state and a schedule of regular prenatal observation and advice. Physicians use technology to date the time of conception (rather than rely on a woman's estimate), monitor fetal development, evaluate routine blood tests, and perform ultrasounds ("baby's first pictures"); where deemed appropriate, they conduct various genetic tests through amniocentesis or chorionic villus sampling. During this period, medical authorities advise prospective parents on the value of genetic screening, instruct them on the changes that should be made in the woman's diet, lifestyle, sexual activity, work schedules, and so on, and direct them to prenatal classes to help train them in the techniques of "natural" childbirth. Doctors interpret, evaluate, and set the standards of normalcy for the various changes associated with the different stages of pregnancy.

It is worth noting that this sort of intense surveillance is not limited to the distinctive values of North American life. In Japan, ultrasounds are "given routinely three or four times during each pregnancy and up to seven or eight times at certain institutions."[4] In China, where concern is to ensure both a lower birth rate and a "high quality" of offspring, many married women are subjected to semiannual gynecological exams and "even before marriage, some women are required to undergo examination to detect any visible structural problems with their reproductive organs and/or family history of genetic abnormalities which might lead to the birth of disabled children."[5] Medical surveillance of pregnant women and fetuses has become accepted practice throughout most of the world.

The effect of granting medical experts authority to manage pregnancies is significant. As Barbara Katz Rothman documents, such surveillance trains women to distance themselves from their pregnancies and to rely on medical interpretations of their experiences. The widely accepted emphasis on medicine's power to avert potential disaster ironically contributes to women's heightened sense of anxiety throughout their pregnancy and makes them increasingly dependent on physician reassurance. Rather than trust their own sense of well-being and excitement, most defer to medical authorities and await expert assurance of healthy outcomes before celebrating a pregnancy or allowing themselves to begin significant emotional bonding with their fetuses. In such a climate, women are well conditioned to comply with medical advice and direction about prenatal care and their own behavior.[6]

The basis of such deference is questionable, however. Although pregnancy and childbirth have become far safer events for women who are subject to technology-based prenatal care, medical monitoring and intervention are not the only factors to be credited with these improved statistics. Nontechnological measures, such as improved nutrition, fewer (and better spaced) pregnancies, more hygienic conditions, better education, and mature mothers (i.e., those past adolescence) also have helped reduce the incidence of maternal and childhood mortality and morbidity. Moreover, dependence on technology to improve maternal and fetal health may actually be quite dangerous in the developing world, if efforts are primarily geared to importing Western technological expertise and equipment instead of improving the social conditions of women.[7] Everywhere, the emphasis on technological surveillance tends to distract from the significance of social and economic conditions for the outcomes of pregnancies. In a political climate in which the basic necessities of healthy living are severely threatened for large segments of the population, concentration on the benefits of technology supports neglect of other factors, with potentially devastating consequences.

Despite the well-documented and uncontested importance of social and economic conditions for healthy pregnancies, many countries, both rich and poor, make technology the major focus of medical attention. There are several reasons for this. First, technology is profitable for those who produce it and those who deploy it; particular technologies are often aggressively marketed by companies very skilled at creating demands for their products. In addition, physicians are well trained in the use of technology, whereas most have little formal training in the relation between social conditions and health. And even if they do recognize the value of social changes, as individuals they lack the power to make such changes. Moreover, by deploying sophisticated technological instruments that provide them with data that are otherwise unavailable to women, physicians are able to establish expertise that is considered superior to a woman's intimate and unquantifiable feelings of pregnancy. Although much of the needed information can be obtained by the use of traditional technology such as stethoscopes, ultrasounds and electronic fetal monitors have vastly expanded the scope of medically mediated knowledge about the fetus in a form that fits neatly within current cultural habits of learning.

Example 1: Ultrasound

Let us look more closely, then, at these two commonplace technologies. Ultrasonography was introduced into obstetrical care in the 1960s. The technology of ultrasounds, like much of the technology used in medicine, was originally developed for military uses, in this case, the detection of submarines. When it was discovered that this visioning technique could also be used on soft tissues in the human body, medicine quickly began to explore biological uses. Once medical researchers established that ultrasounds could give them visual information about fetuses, they sought reasons to employ it; they have settled on its usefulness for dating fetal age, assessing fetal functioning, and detecting anatomical anomalies. Ultrasound is a powerfully attractive technology in a modernist culture that values visual information above all other kinds. By allowing trained personnel to gain visual access to a fetus, to record its movement and anatomical shape, ultrasounds provide medical practitioners with a highly prized "window on the womb." This visual knowledge can then be offered to the prospective parents, who are happy to have access to this new way of "getting to know" their fetus (once interpreters help them to make sense of the fuzzy images).

As Rosalind Petchesky observes, this technology serves a political purpose as well as a medical one. It "disrupt[s] the very definition, as traditionally understood, of 'inside' and 'outside' a woman's body, of pregnancy as an 'interior' experience" and "allows the fetus to be viewed and *treated* as if it were outside a woman's body."[8] Visualization helps make the existence and status of fetuses far more real to physicians and the public than anything a pregnant woman may report. When fetuses can be viewed as separate beings, they can be treated as such and pregnant women can be reduced to "uterine containers" or "fetal environments." Visual imaging allows obstetricians to treat fetuses as patients and it thereby helps to support cultural images of fetuses as independent beings, existing in isolation, rather than as entities intimately connected to the women whose bodies nurture them. Or, as Rothman succinctly puts it, "The technology that makes the baby/fetus more 'visible' renders the woman invisible."[9]

Hence, even though this technology has been well received by both patients and practitioners, and despite the fact that it sometimes plays an important role in identifying and potentially correcting certain sorts of problems in pregnancies, its effects are not all positive. As it is presently understood and used, ultrasound technology contributes to further entrenching medical control over pregnancy by increasing women's sense of dependency on scientific experts. By making frequent observation and evaluation of fetuses possible, it also makes this activity desirable, for it is now the norm in industrialized countries for pregnant women to have and to share visual images of their fetuses, along with reports of the demonstrated "healthy status" of the developing embryo. By now a routine part of pregnancy, the use of ultrasound has created a new set of expectations about the experience and customs of being pregnant.

It is worth reflecting on the history of this now commonplace use of a form of reproductive technology. Of particular concern is the fact that use of this technology became routine in the medical management of pregnancies despite the fact that its long-term safety for mothers and fetuses had not been established.[10] In this it follows a pattern common to many other medical interventions in pregnancy, a pattern that has sometimes led to dire results. Two notorious examples of medical treatments widely prescribed to pregnant women prior to exhaustive testing and evaluation are thalidomide and DES. In the case of thalidomide, the damaging results were almost immediately apparent: in about 15 percent of cases, women who took the drug during the first trimester gave birth to children born with limbs missing. The damage of DES use was slower to become evident, showing up only some twenty years later in the form of unusual genital cancers in some of the children whose mothers took DES during pregnancy. The tragedy of DES use is especially poignant because the drug did not even achieve the goal it was prescribed for, namely, reducing the rate of miscarriage; significantly, while it was thought to have this effect, it was widely prescribed even to women at no particular risk of miscarriage.

I do not want to be alarmist about this. Ultrasounds have been in use for decades and they do seem to be far safer than thalidomide and DES; they are certainly safer than the fetal X rays that they replace. Nonetheless, it is still too early to be certain that they involve no long-term risk. Moreover, studies by the major American regulators in the early 1980s showed "no improvement in pregnancy outcome" from routine use; in fact, the FDA specifically recommended against routine use of ultrasounds. And yet, despite unanswered questions about long-term effects and the fact that there is no clear clinical benefit, they have become a routine part of prenatal care. In fact, many centers prescribe multiple ultrasounds throughout the course of a single pregnancy. The apparent overuse of this technology has become so significant a problem that both the Canadian and American Societies for Obstetrics and Gynecology issued practice guidelines in the early 1990s, recommending ultrasounds only at eighteen to twenty weeks gestation in the hope of reducing the use of this technology at other stages of pregnancy. Still, many patients and their physicians seek more frequent "looks" and find these limits hard to accept. Nor is the popularity of multiple tests confined to the West; as already noted, multiple ultrasounds are also the norm in Japan and represent the ideal in China.

Even though there is no statistical benefit in pregnancy outcomes associated with the performance of frequent ultrasounds, most women understand that their use in any particular pregnancy can still be valuable to them as individuals. Modern societies seem inevitably to constitute ablist cultures; as such, they urge women to have only "healthy" babies and they hold women accountable and responsible for the care of any child who is less than "perfect." Aware of these responsibilities, most women seek this easily available confirmation of the health of their fetuses. Prenatal surveillance provides them with both a means of improving "quality control" and, in most cases, the opportunity to obtain reassurance that all is normal. Obstetricians, for their part, fear expensive malpractice suits if they fail to detect fetal anomalies and so they are strongly motivated to recommend use of ultrasound testing. Moreover, in a modernist culture that highly prizes visual knowledge, women understandably welcome access to the visual images this technology provides; it helps them feel more intimately connected to a fetus they can "see" as well as feel. It also allows them share with their partners, as well as with family and friends, this culturally expected way of getting to "know" their fetus, thereby increasing everyone's sense of anticipation about the coming birth.

In the ordinary sense of autonomy, the use of ultrasound would have to be said to be a matter of autonomous choice. In most nations, no laws forbid or mandate ultrasound for pregnant women. No woman is explicitly coerced by her physician or anyone else into accepting ultrasound; rather, most pregnant women are eager for the opportunity to have such exams. Still, there are questions to be asked about the degree of autonomy available to a woman regarding use of this technology. It is so commonly used and so generally valued that it is difficult for anyone to resist its use without being judged irrational and irresponsible. Now that ultrasound has become established as the normal standard of obstetrical care—despite unresolved questions about its efficacy and safety—most who are asked to decide upon its use in a particular case do not feel truly free to decline. In health matters, and especially in the realm of reproduction, in which the interests of future persons are thought to be at stake, normalization of technology places an enormous burden of proof on those who would refuse it. Hence, with each use, it becomes ever more established as part of routine prenatal care and thus helps consolidate the significant power and control that attaches to those who provide services deemed essential elements of good prenatal care, whether or not they want such power.

Example 2: Fetal Monitors

A similar story exists in the development and deployment of electronic fetal monitors. Also drawing on sonograph technology, this equipment allows medical personnel to monitor the heartbeat of a fetus throughout labor, providing a warning if fetal stress reaches dangerous levels. The technology was developed in the 1960s to provide information to assist in the management of high-risk labors (roughly 10–15 percent of cases). After an aggressive marketing campaign by the manufacturer, it was quickly taken up for use in all hospital deliveries. Fetal monitors are attractive to hospitals, for they provide more complete scientific data than earlier methods. They also reduce hospital costs, since they allow fewer staff to keep track of more patients.

Although the information they provide can be very valuable in quickly identifying problems in certain sorts of high-risk deliveries, these benefits come at a price. For one thing, this technology requires a birthing mother to remain prone and strapped to the machine, which increases her stress and discomfort. Further, the monitors distract attention away from the actual woman in labor and redirect it to machine readouts. Moreover, they support a crisis atmosphere in childbirth, which has the effect of further increasing physician control and reducing a woman's sense of her own right to control events.[11] Also, the data provided can be easily misinterpreted, appearing to signal fetal distress where none exists and unnecessarily triggering medical recommendations (sometimes demands) for surgical intervention by way of cesarean delivery, a risky procedure for both women and fetuses. In fact, once hospitals adopted these monitors for routine use, cesarean delivery rates increased by up to 50 percent.[12] Nonetheless, like ultrasounds, fetal monitors became the standard of obstetrical practice in North America long before they were subjected to controlled clinical trials to establish their efficacy and safety. When appropriate studies were finally done, some fifteen years after the introduction of this technology, no benefit could be found for their routine use. Indeed, careful clinical review suggests that better care can be achieved through alternative practices that involve a dedicated midwife attendant at each birth.[13]

The pattern represented here is common to many forms of reproductive technology: a technology that is produced to assist in a limited number of special cases becomes the standard of practice for all cases. Once available, such technology becomes subject to an overwhelming sense of technological imperative: birthing women and obstetricians face the burden of refusing (instead of requesting) their use, not feeling sufficiently confident to refuse its use in any particular case. Moreover, the environment in which this technology is employed is designed to encourage its use: in North America at least, maternity hospitals are set up to deal with deliveries that pose serious risks of complications, although this category of birth is a minority of cases seen. Procedures are followed that treat all deliveries as potentially high risk.

Under the best of conditions, childbirth is an emotionally charged event; when it is conducted within a system poised for crisis, dangerous outcomes loom large and opportunities for informed personal choice are of little use to individual patients. Only careful statistical study and general practice guidelines can assist consumers and physicians in making decisions about whether or not to partake of any particular technology in such a climate. Individual patients are asked to give their informed consent to the use of technology, but since few are in a position to truly weigh relevant risks and benefits, most are not really well situated to execute autonomous choice.

Such conundrums might tempt us to romanticize the freedom of women in less industrialized nations, where use of ultrasound and fetal monitoring machinery is much less common. In general, sophisticated biomedical equipment is much less accessible in nations with low health care budgets, which is not to say that childbirth there is free of technological imperatives. As Maria De Koninck documents, international efforts to reduce maternal and infant mortality rates in very poor countries often amount to efforts to transfer the biomedical expertise and orientation developed in the West to local experts who are trained to intervene at the moment of delivery if childbirth has been designated as complicated or high risk. Although such interventions surely save some lives, they do so by focusing on problems in isolation of their causes. For example, cesarean sections are a means of saving the lives of young women who become pregnant before their pelvises have fully matured, although efforts to change social custom to postpone pregnancy until the end of adolescence would save the lives of even more women.[14] Yet in many poor countries economic pressures are forcing the age of marriage even further downward. Even in nations like the Sudan, where high-tech machinery is virtually unavailable, Western experts have transformed local birth customs and practices and introduced the values of privileging visual knowledge and favoring the comfort of medically trained birth attendants over that of the birthing women.[15] Women in many non-Western countries lack education, social status, economic independence, and recognized authority over their own lives, which means that most have very little power to influence decisions about the role of biomedicine and technology in their pregnancies and childbirth experiences. In such a climate, even the appearance of autonomy may be lacking as women struggle to situate themselves in belief and value systems that do not place much value on individual choice (especially on the part of women).

Assisted Conception

I have reviewed these various examples of the extent of current technology use and biomedical values in reproductive activities to clarify the context into which the so-called new reproductive technologies are being introduced. I am, finally, ready to turn to high-profile reproductive technologies, namely, efforts to assist couples experiencing infertility to procreate. Although the media tends to approach these technologies as if they are entirely distinct from current practices, I have tried to make clear that they are being developed and introduced in a cultural milieu where many other aspects of reproduction are already subject to extensive, and virtually inescapable, technological monitoring and intervention. As a consequence, the medical community and the public are well conditioned to expect further expansion of the range of reproductive technology into new areas: it would seem very odd indeed if medical researchers were to fail to seek technological innovations to address unwanted barriers to conception.

At the same time, appreciation of the history of some existing reproductive technologies provides a basis for understanding why many feminists seem so suspicious about the possible future deployment of many of the new reproductive technologies. Even though at the moment, most new reproductive technologies are being used to treat only a minority of cases considered "high risk" or "problematic," they could become the norm for all pregnancies in the future. If that were to happen, we would again have to contend with serious questions about the degree of choice and control available to prospective parents. In reproduction, as in other areas of life, technology created to meet special needs tends to slide quickly into becoming normalized and routine for all possible cases, leaving little room for the person most directly affected to weigh its appropriateness and, perhaps, to refuse participation. Hence we must evaluate each technology for its potential impact on not only the currently targeted group of patients but all patients in the future.

Consider the technologies designed to address infertility. The most prominent of these technologies is in vitro fertilization (IVF) and its many variations. Like most reproductive technologies, new and old, IVF involves intervention in women's bodies even when the source of the problem (in this case, infertility) is associated with the male partner. In order to conduct IVF, physicians need access to gametes from both a man and a woman. It is usually a simple (technology-free) matter to collect sperm from men through masturbation. Egg collection is a much more invasive procedure, requiring careful timing (and hence frequent monitoring by ultrasound) and surgical access to the ovaries; this involves potential risks of infection, bleeding, and damage to other organs. In fact, egg collection is such an invasive and risky procedure that the specialists involved prefer to collect several ova at once. In order to facilitate this, they begin by inducing superovulation in the woman through injection of powerful hormones (which likely increase risk of future ovarian and breast cancers). If physicians do manage to collect some viable eggs (the process often fails at this stage), the next step is to introduce those eggs to the collected sperm (in vitro) and see whether or not fertilization occurs. Physicians monitor the course of the fertilized eggs for a day or two, sometimes taking the opportunity to remove a cell from each to test for genetic anomalies. Then they either freeze or transfer the eggs that appear to be developing normally. At this point, the hope is that one transferred egg will implant in the woman's uterus and develop into a (healthy) fetus. Since approximately 80 percent of IVF attempts fail to produce a live baby at the end, physicians usually transfer a few fertilized eggs at once to increase the chances that one will continue to develop. (Three is the current norm in Canadian clinics, but it is not uncommon for clinics around the world to transfer several fertilized eggs at once in an effort to boost their pregnancy rates.) Not infrequently, these procedures result in multiple births, putting added strain on the health of both mother and fetuses.

Even though IVF technology is expensive, dangerous, disruptive, emotionally demanding, and usually unsuccessful, there is a long waiting list of anxious couples hoping to gain access to it as the preferred means of responding to infertility. Originally designed for woman with blocked fallopian tubes, it is now used for other kinds of infertility, including low sperm count in male partners.

Again, this is not a technology reserved only for rich countries. In many societies, the social pressure to reproduce is intense. Even in nations that face problems of excessive birth rates, there is significant demand for treatment of infertility. Although the plight of the infertile may easily be overlooked in countries struggling to reduce population density, there is evidence that childlessness is treated as a suspicious anomaly rather than a valued social contribution. The very practice of concentrating efforts on reducing birth rates helps to emphasize the normalcy of multiple pregnancies and renders "unnatural" the state of being childless. Hence, while China struggles to restrict all couples to a single child, those with no children face discrimination on every front; not surprisingly, many demand access to reproductive technologies.[16] And in Pemba, Tanzania, where the fertility rate is among the highest in the world and standards of living are low, there is a strong demand for technologies that can help infertile couples produce children.[17] In many less developed countries, where IVF is beyond the financial means of most, interest in reproductive assistance is probably even greater than it is in the more affluent West. In countries that focus on limiting population growth, there is a particularly strong sense that having children represents "the norm" for women, whose worth is likely to be measured in terms of their reproductive achievements.

Given the expense and risks associated with IVF, it seems unlikely that it will replace "natural" or sexual fertilization as the normal way of conceiving a child, but some practitioners have mused about a future when this will indeed become the norm for all who can afford it. They base this prediction on the fact that IVF provides the opportunity to detect genetic anomalies at the earliest possible stage of embryo development, thereby reducing the emotional and physical costs associated with the late-term abortions that are required by alternative methods of genetic screening.

I do not really expect that IVF will end up becoming the preferred method of conceiving a child for couples who have nontechnological alternatives—after all, it is expensive, invasive, and risky, and there are undeniable pleasures associated with the more established, nontechnological methods. Nonetheless, in the industrialized world, IVF has already become established as a routine treatment for those who experience unwanted infertility, a sizable group now composing roughly 10 percent of the population interested in procreating. Moreover, the technology has been widely publicized with approving media coverage of "miracle" babies and happy parents, and this has contributed to a climate in which the widespread use of IVF makes most infertile couples feel a need to "try" it in their ongoing pursuit of producing a biologically related child. North American society is highly pronatalist (even if it seems rather uninterested in and even hostile to actual children). Having children is the norm for adults, and childbearing is romanticized and promoted in a multitude of ways, both explicitly and indirectly.

A few decades ago, infertility was likely to be viewed as a sad fact of life for certain couples. But the existence of IVF and numerous other fertility-enhancing technologies has made acceptance of infertility seem unnecessary and correspondingly more difficult; people are told that no one needs to accept a diagnosis of infertility as final. When success stories are reported, other couples can see the rewards of trying all available measures in the face of involuntary childlessness. Ever since this technology was first successfully used on humans, significant medical and social resources have been directed at circumventing infertility (IVF does not "cure" the condition), and these investments provide further evidence of the high level of social importance assigned to the pursuit of biological reproduction. Hence those who are involuntarily childless experience increased pressure to conform to such clearly important social expectations and do what is necessary to reproduce.

The growing use of such technologies has already become "normal" for (relatively affluent) couples experiencing infertility. The burden of proof in decisionmaking about participating in such technologies often rests with those who contemplate declining them rather than with those who seek access. Rejecting technological options tends to be especially complicated for women, since women's worth is largely defined in terms of their role as mothers. In such an environment, it is difficult for anyone to truly weigh the risks and costs of such highly prized assistance.

I do not doubt that women who pursue IVF deeply want to bear children; my worry is about a culture that demands and so readily accepts such sacrifices of its women. Moreover, when so many resources are invested in meeting the seemingly inexhaustible demand for IVF, other sorts of available responses to infertility become eclipsed. New reproductive technologies, like many of their predecessors, tend to absorb medical attention and detract from exploration of other sorts of resolutions to problems identified. Now that involuntary childlessness has been socially constructed as a medical problem, attention is shifted away from nonmedical alternatives such as acceptance of childlessness, adoption, foster parenting, change of partner, alternative family structures, and changes in lifestyle; these sorts of accommodations seem to pale in comparison to the socially privileged status of technological solutions. The priority given to technological solutions to infertility becomes even more problematic when we consider that many dollars are spent to help relatively affluent couples produce genetically related children while millions of other children are left to suffer malnutrition, abuse, and neglect. Moreover, comparably little effort is directed at the prevention of infertility (e.g., by preventing the spread of sexually transmitted diseases and becoming more proficient at diagnosing them and treating them when they occur). As in so many other areas of medicine, when technological solutions are offered, prevention seems a far less urgent priority.

Conclusion

What seems called for is a new interpretation of the ideal of autonomy. I suggest that we turn to a concept of relational autonomy that is intended to supplant the prevailing individualistic conception of autonomy and address some of the puzzles we have identified. Where the traditional conception envisions the individual as existing separate from and independent of society, a relational ideal recognizes the essential complexity of the relation between persons and their culture. It is rooted in a relational concept of the self which recognizes that selves are social beings significantly shaped within a web of interconnected social and political relationships. In relational theory, individuals are understood to engage in the events constitutive of identity and autonomy (e.g., defining, questioning, revising, and pursuing projects) within a configuration of relationships, both interpersonal and political. Thus autonomy is recognized as a capacity that can be enhanced (or repressed) by one's social position (e.g., the degree of internalized oppression one experiences).[18]

A conception of relational autonomy helps explain why the expression of an informed preference is not an adequate measure of autonomous choice, for it makes visible the ways in which social norms often condition preferences and also make alternative choices inconceivable. It helps us see the political dimensions of circumstances where decisions may at first appear to be primarily matters of personal choice. In so doing, this concept helps explain why personal preference is not an adequate measure of autonomy. Within the context of reproductive technologies, an ideal of relational autonomy reveals the importance of evaluating the political climate in which reproductive choices are made before determining whether or not some reproductive decision is autonomous.

For many of the forms of reproductive technology reviewed in this chapter, important social programs have been developed and promoted in the West as if they were merely opportunities for the exercise of individual choice. Use of patient autonomy language and the implementation of informed consent procedures foster the sense that we are simply dealing with private decisionmaking. As a society, however, we are currently engaged in a process of transforming reproductive activities and setting new norms of reproductive behavior that individuals may soon be in no position to resist. In a context of medicalized procreation, the appearance of personal choice may well become more illusionary than real.

In nations that are less committed to the value of individual freedom and autonomy than Canada or the United States, practices aimed at controlling the "quality" of offspring may be so forcefully imposed that even the illusion of private choice is absent. Women are always caught within social forces that constitute public policy about the ways in which their reproductive functions are best pursued. Although there is often apparent space for them to make some choices within those structures (such as whether to seek assistance from biomedical or traditional caregivers), their choices are inevitably structured by the prevailing value system and the rewards and punishments it provides for the results of their reproductive practices. Typically, women everywhere make pragmatic choices within the governing frameworks that adapt (rather than docilely obey) dominant values and expectations. Whereas they may negotiate some space for alternative values and exercise agency in the ways in which they interpret the dominant values, their choices generally reflect and often support the existing power structures.[19]

Therefore, simply observing that women choose to use a technology is not a sufficient test to determine that they are exercising autonomy in a given aspect of reproductive practice sphere. Moreover, once a technology becomes routine, its very familiarity can undermine a woman's realistic chance of refusing its use. Hence, we must be very careful to evaluate each technology that is introduced and not consider the issue settled by data on how frequently women use that form of technology. Only by questioning and examining the goals and achievements of each particular technology will we be able to tell if it is something that should become routine in the reproductive lives of women. To date, that step has largely been missing in the implementation of many reproductive technologies. We cannot afford to omit this level of discussion in the future because the emerging new technologies promise to have an even greater impact on the shape of every society than have those in the past. Nor can we afford to let ourselves be so absorbed by the glitter and promise of technology as to forget that nontechnological programs will always be essential elements of healthy reproductive practices. Adopting a nuanced, contextualized, politicized understanding of autonomy as relational can help guide these necessary, but difficult, discussions.

Notes

Earlier versions of this essay were read at the University of Manitoba and the University of King's College. I am grateful for the thoughtful comments received on both occasions. Barbara Parish was particularly helpful in responding to the earliest drafts. The final draft was prepared at the Bellagio International Study and Conference Center.

1. Margaret Lock and Patricia A. Kaufert, eds., *Pragmatic Women and Body Politics* (Cambridge: Cambridge University Press, 1998).

2. In Japan, for example, the Pill did not become legally available until 1999. Apparently there is concern about the health risks of artificial hormones and social worries that a truly reliable contraceptive would encourage promiscuity among both men and women. (Margaret Lock, "Perfecting Society: Reproductive Technologies, Genetic Testing, and the Planned Family in Japan," in *Pragmatic Women*, pp. 206–239.) More cynical commentators ascribe the long resistance to the power of a large gynecological lobby dependent on the fees they receive for performing abortions.

3. Iris Lopez, "An Ethnography of the Medicalization of Puerto Rican Women's Reproduction," in *Pragmatic Women*, pp. 240–259.

4. Margaret Lock, "Perfecting Society," in *Pragmatic Women*, p. 228.

5. Lisa Handwerker, "The Consequences of Modernity for Childless Women in China: Medicalization and Resistance," in *Pragmatic Women*, pp. 178–205.

6. Barbara Katz Rothman, *The Tentative Pregnancy: Prenatal Diagnosis and the Future of Motherhood* (New York: Viking, 1986), p. 86.

7. Maria De Koninck, "Reflections on the Transfer of 'Progress': The Case of Reproduction," in The Feminist Health Care Ethics Research Network, *The Politics of Women's Health: Exploring Agency and Autonomy* (Philadelphia: Temple University Press, 1998), pp. 150–177.

8. Rosalind Pollack Petchesky, "Foetal Images: The Power of Visual Culture in the Politics of Reproduction," in Michelle Stanworth, ed., *Reproductive Technologies: Gender, Motherhood, and Medicine* (Minneapolis: University of Minnesota Press, 1987), p. 65.

9. Rothman, *Tentative Pregnancy*, p. 113.

10. Murray Enkin, Mark J. N. C. Keirse, and Iain Chalmers, *A Guide to Effective Care in Pregnancy and Childbirth* (Oxford: Oxford University Press, 1989).

11. As Enkin, Keirse, and Chalmers observe, "Use of continuous electronic monitoring changes the delivery room into an intensive care unit. . . . The presence of a monitor may also change the relationships between the woman and her partner on the one hand, and the woman, midwife, and doctor on the other" (*Guide to Effective Care*, p. 198).

12. Judith Kunisch, "Electronic Fetal Monitors: Marketing Forces and the Resulting Controversy," in Kathryn Strother Ratcliff, ed., *Healing Technology: Feminist Perspectives* (Ann Arbor: University of Michigan Press, 1989), p. 54.

13. Enkin, Keirse, and Chalmers, *Guide to Effective Care.*

14. De Koninck, "Reflections," pp. 150–177.

15. Janice Boddy, "Remembering Amal: On Birth and the British in Northern Sudan," in *Pragmatic Women*, pp. 28–59.

16. Handwerker, "Consequences of Modernity," pp. 178–205.

17. Karina Kielmann, "Barren Ground: Contesting Identities of Barren Women in Pemba, Tanzania," in *Pragmatic Women*, pp. 127–163.

18. Susan Sherwin, "A Relational Approach to Autonomy in Health Care," in *Politics of Women's Health*, pp. 19–47.

19. Lock and Kaufert, *Pragmatic Women*.

8

Autonomy and Procreation: Brazilian Feminist Analyses

JUREMA WERNECK
FERNANDA CARNEIRO
ALEJANDRA ANA ROTANIA
WITH
HELEN BEQUAERT HOLMES
MARY R. RORTY

As citizens of Brazil, a country that does not offer conditions for making full use of our citizenship, we are active witnesses of the perverse effects of population control policies on women's physical and mental health. Sudden changes occur in our cultural values, which are caused not only by the thoughtless acceptance of new contraceptive methods but also by new technologies in "assisted reproduction" offered to address the stress of infertility among women who desire motherhood. In our view, both bioethics and the Western women's movement have failed to help us avoid the brunt of these policies and may even have exacerbated their effects.

Our theoretical studies and ethical questions arising from contacts with feminists from the Northern Hemisphere have resulted in fruitful critiques. Thanks to this interchange we became aware of a remarkable ethical challenge, a challenge with no prior experience: the possibility of techno-scientific extracorporal procreation affecting men and women in the Brazilian North and South. Further, unequal socioeconomic contexts do not separate us from the ethical questions common to us: what moral values should guide our conduct when we exercise the power of procreation and create the subjective experience of maternity? What common cultural values can we resort to in the existential choice between adoption and assisted reproduction?

First we analyze ethical and social issues raised by population policies that have promoted the surgical sterilization of women in Brazil. Then we present a narration about a possible way for a woman to intensively deal with and decide about the dilemmas created by access to reproductive technology. Finally, we frame an examination of adoption through a meditation about the Yerma tragedy. We hope that these specific descriptions can stimulate bioethics and global feminism to envision ways to ameliorate our distress.

Surgical Sterilization of Women: A Challenge for Feminist Bioethics

My voice (J.W.) is the voice of a woman from the Brazilian black women's movement, the voice of a woman who has reflected on racism, sexism, health, fertility, body cycles, and birth control policies for some time. My voice is the voice of a black woman from a country both capitalist and peripheral. Among all women there is great diversity of race, language, history and traditions, culture, ideas, and so on—diversity that creates tension. Any woman's specific kind of diversity could be considered an example of a handicap by someone somewhere. Despite this, I hope we can dialogue.

Principles in Bioethics

Autonomy, beneficence, and justice are highlighted as important principles in bioethics. To make some choices in health, environment, procreation, and human rights we must consider them. But in some ways these principles are too complex to use in understanding and defining the limits of human actions.

For example, what are the limits to individual and collective autonomy? How do social and political factors influence the extension of autonomy to individuals and to communities? What is the precise meaning of the very important word "autonomy" to us as human beings and as black women?

To talk about autonomy is to try to describe our desire, rational or not, to live without domination and tyranny. It is to express our desire to negotiate with the "other" even as we express our need for self-determination and liberty. Yet this subject incites many hot debates. Are we ready to make a primary ethical agreement and simultaneously consider self-determination, individual rights, rights of the other, and the future of hu-

manity? Many of these questions also apply to the concepts of beneficence and justice.

Surgical Sterilization of Women in Brazil

In Brazil, tubal ligation, severing the fallopian tubes, is now the primary
method of contraception available to and used by women between the
ages of fifteen and forty-nine. It is important to note that there is no Brazilian governmental policy or program to explain this phenomenon. In our
country, surgical sterilization is illegal and can be done only for medical
reasons, for instance, when a woman's life is in danger. In 1986 a feminist
researcher said that at that time the population of reproductive-age sterilized women in Brazil was as large as the entire population of Belgium.[1] To
repeat, millions of nonwhite sterilized women from one country in the
South equal to the total white population of one country in the North. This
was 1986. Fourteen years later, I can guarantee, based on the daily experiences of many people, mainly women, that those figures have increased.

Brazil is a huge country in South America with a huge population, and
its fertility rates are higher than the fertility rates of people in the North.
Let us imagine the worries and fears of some politicians and scientists in
agencies, offices, and parliaments in the North. Let us also imagine the
political and economic interests behind their eyes when they think about
this so-called population bomb. I do not think that female sterility is disturbing their sleep.

Since the 1970s the population of Brazil has been considered a major
foe of population balance on earth. Some Malthusian bureaucrats have
considered us potential hungry mouths, guerrillas, and destroyers of biodiversity. We are barbarian people who must be controlled. And they
have done it. We now stand first in numbers of sterilized women. We
now have a negative fertility rate. What has happened to us?

Feminism and Sterilization

Feminism brought to us, women of the Western countries, a new kind of
relationship between ourselves and our bodies. It also brought the idea of
self-determination. The body, an important part of ourselves, has itself
special meanings and rights. Our recent history and our slogans show
that. For a woman to control her own body cycles, as an expression of nature inside us, is a demand, a struggle, and a victory. Our fertility, our
pregnancies, and our abortions are facets of our own right to choose and
of our power to do so. Many women have welcomed surgical sterilization as a method of contraception. Democracy has been interpreted as the
right to choose our own mutilation.

There has been much debate on why a woman would choose surgical sterilization. For many, this is a pure expression of a woman's power: a woman can choose this procedure if it seems good for her. It is like a trip to a contraceptive supermarket that offers many products of many different flavors and colors and prices. This is the right one to choose. To question this scenario is to question the basis of a liberal feminism spread around the Western world. Who could do this? Who would dare?

But for many black women this situation has different meanings. In our part of the world contraceptive choices are subject to different interests from different actors. First are the transnational corporate interests to sell this and not that contraceptive method. Second are foreign governments' interests to promote birth control among dangerous populations of blacks, indigenous, poor, and all the outsiders on earth. And finally are the needs of modern societies which, like medieval Europe, do not welcome children.

In countries like Brazil, delivering a baby is not an easy process: we do not have the means to guarantee the security and peace we need for giving birth. On the contrary, we face neglect, disrespect, and danger, with high rates of maternal mortality. Coloring this scenario are hunger, poverty, and epidemic diseases, as the heritage of the welfare capitalist states in the North.

Women's suffering in giving birth is only senseless if we do not desire pregnancies. If we do not want children, our right to choose is useful if we select the choices under the birth control policy. I call this situation black women's reality.[2] The consequence is millions of sterilized women, black women, for whom there is no concern after that about their health, their psychological state, or their happiness and life. The important thing is that fertility rates should decrease.

In Brazil the majority of women who want to avoid pregnancy have themselves sterilized or use contraceptive pills without medical prescriptions. Under these circumstances, can this be considered a choice? When this involves mainly black women from the very poor areas of the whole country and from the cities—slum-dwellers, unemployed or abandoned women—what can we call this? With millions of sterilized women, what can we say about their health, their experiences with side effects, their suffering from an irresponsible, externally imposed program. Is it possible to speak of beneficence?

What good springs from surgical sterilization? And for whom? I claim that sterilization is a "choice" for those without choices, an expression of despair for those who do not want or cannot find a solution for sexuality without liberty or for an unhappy life with economic and emotional problems. For these reasons can a surgical end to fertility be considered a good? And just because there is a strange coincidence between some women's choices and some racial, social, and gender-based characteristics, what is the right motivation for these choices? Can a birth control policy based on the surgical sterilization of black and indigenous women be considered ethically acceptable?

Racism and sexism still operate in both northern and southern societies and influence many scientific and political programs and policies at national and international levels. In a world where women's choices are overridden by the drive for modernity, how can we justify using female sterilization as a contraceptive method? Is this how justice is extended to us?

Ethics and Sterilization

What should be the consequences of every human's choices? What is the extent of human responsibility? What is the fallout from the contraceptive choices of some bureaucrats and scientists in some agencies, offices, and parliaments? Let me point out that they are the same choices made by some liberal feminists from the North and the South in the name of self-determination and the right to choose. Feminist discourse is very important because it can not only influence but also legitimate actions from eugenics policies. This happens in Brazil and maybe everywhere.

What conclusions can we draw? The questions posed above raise serious concerns and confirm the need to discuss and understand the limits of all human actions. Tubal ligation demonstrates that social and political inequalities are still alive in democratic and capitalist countries. When women's bodies, their cycles and functions, can be considered something to throw away in the name of liberty or self-determination, we can claim that feminist demands are still unfulfilled.

It is urgent for every woman, for every human being, to consider the political and social consequences of all our daily decisions and actions, to hold them up to ethical judgment. All feminists must question our own victories and our so-called liberty, and not just when we are talking about contraceptive choices. For a global discourse we must understand that our choices are choices for the future and that our responsibility extends from ourselves and our neighbors alive today to those in the future whom we shall never see. As an example, let us look at the following narrative about Aline, an infertile woman, as she considers the consequences of her decisions.

Aline's Decision: Free and Informed Consent

Aline was young. Her sensuality was inherited from the 1970s winds of freedom. She lived the lightness of her youth and the "weight and the resistance of being." She lived in "a room of one's own."[3]

She worked and knew the public world. She lived the challenges of a body exposed to the sweet happiness linking transgressions, desires, fears, and intense pleasures.[4] Catholic morality was not a burden for her in the least. Sex was happiness. She felt no guilt.

She learned how to avoid pregnancy: Science offered pills and surgical sterilization. Aline took pills but, fortunately, she learned that she could also use the diaphragm or make a seductive demand for using a condom, or could even combine the famous "rhythm" method with the mucus perception method. As for eroticism, "my body belongs to me" was her favorite motto.

One day she met André. She felt all possible passions and the humanizing sensation of reciprocity.[5] Though she came from a generation eager to be free, to enjoy, and to be sovereign in the erotic living of daily life, she felt an imperative to marry and to procreate. But time passed and she did not get pregnant.

It is as if she had come "to a castle wall where freedom, fun, and sovereignty end, and then was stuck with a mighty no: a denying or a subtraction as if it had come from somebody else's wish or from some evil genius."[6]

Alarmingly, she believed she saw less love in her partner's eyes. She felt inadequate, dissatisfied, and excessively lonely. No descendant was announcing itself as the future and a real alterity. She needed help. "Going to the other" was a necessity.[7] She needed ways and means, but which ones? Now she felt the threat of getting lost in this new situation in which fundamental elements were no longer taken for granted. She perceived her own vulnerability.

After six months of tests and consultations, her doctor recommended that she try in vitro fertilization. The idea of an assisted reproduction took Aline by surprise. She heard whispered promises. She no longer owned her body. To most women it is essential to feel themselves fertile. But that is not the promise she heard. Technology promised to supplant the entire reproductive process. She knew it was an experiment guided by scientific methods with the best intentions. The techno-scientific power created an ethos in which instruments were emancipated from natural limits and inherent kindness. Science would impose moral criteria and behavior.[8] She only needed to agree. A big dose of confidence was essential: Aline wrestled with this difficulty.

How can her acts of procreation be free acts, that is, affirm her rights? How can Aline become autonomous in this tragic encounter between the feminist ethos[9] and a techno-scientific process that is autonomous itself?

How could she feel herself reaffirming the principle of "free and informed consent" from the Nuremberg Code of 1947, a guarantee of autonomy to anyone subject to a specific experiment?

She lived with the ambiguities of identification and alienation. Where was her power to decide? Will she be "misunderstood, ill-treated, bent and reduced to impotence and to slavery?"[10]

Autonomy and the Difficulty of Being

The concept of autonomy, as conceived by feminist groups concerned with health and reproductive rights, can humanize women when they assume an ethical attitude in their erotic, sexual, and reproductive lives through reflection on the experience of becoming a person.[11] If this process happens inside institutional medical practice, it is much more complex. When individuals (men and women, clients and professionals), are mediated by high technology, they are divorced from conditions that could make them autonomous, that is, conditions in which they are inseparable from humanity and at the same time are holding one singular person in an I-Thou relationship.[12] Humans cease to exist when they are mediated by an impersonal apparatus in an institutional world. Relationships between subject and doctor/researcher are swallowed by this institutional anonymity, without a trace of the special relationship in which the other is presence, limit, and opportunity, that is, alterity. Also without a trace is any perception of the future as an alterity. Reproductive autonomy is confined to the "choice among technologic market options" and thus discarded. The split between ethics and rights is complete, and the difficulty of being is totally and fundamentally lived.

Difficulty of being is an existential human condition; for Lévinas it happens in a corporal way. The body is an ideal to conquer.[13] This corporal conquest does not let the self fly magically as in a fairy tale. Lévinas teaches that in aiming to overcome this difficulty, we may find new sources of alienation and new inadequacies. Meeting with the other becomes impossible, which brings on loneliness.

When a woman who wants to get pregnant faces techno-scientific power, her autonomy may turn into antinomy—a blind alley, extreme loneliness, or slavery to the heteronomy of the chains of laboratories, institutions, and political alliances that make decisions about research projects. Women's rights in these settings are certainly questionable.[14]

The gravity of the orientation of these processes is still not clear to Brazilian women's organizations concerned with health and human rights. Who is responsible for reproductive decisions? Not women and men and their sovereign, sensual, anguished, and willing bodies and their ethical capacity from authentic I-Thou relationships. In the new engineering of baby production, the actors are doctors, laboratory workers, ethics committees, semen owners, donors, semen banks and "stored" embryos, specialized clinics, lawyers, contracts, and judges. Not only infertile but also sterilized women are a potential market. Women serve as source material. Eroticism, the meeting of bodies, woman and man, is dispensed with. Is the laboratory-processed creature a human being or an artifact?

Is there a consistent ethics in each moral agent in this chain of techno-scientific practices? Is it possible to build up an empirical consensus about these proceedings? The emerging biotechnology industry extends fertility control policies to "biopolitics in their scope of application and also micropolitics . . . in the molecularization of reproductive control."[15] "A woman's right to choose [so dear to feminism] has lost much of its authority."[16] The familiar world of procreation has expanded and become a property of big business. The rights of other generations are also challenged.

The Decision

Aline lived the dialectics of an ethical and political being. But in her education she had learned the value of questioning deeply the reasons for living. She noticed that the right to information, so familiar a requirement for us, cannot be simply access to techno-scientific knowledge but must include the capacity to comprehend what is happening, as well as the capacity to judge events and actors in their alliances and singularity.[17] She realized that access to services or to information is not the same as acquisition of "well-being."

Aline's discernment and moral conscience did not come from reading codified research protocols or from listening to technical explanations. She reflected deeply over her wishes and motivation for motherhood, with the support of women's self-help groups. Objectives of experimental trials are not always "meritorious enough." Individual rights would be, in these situations, problematic. Pain and risks of participation in an experiment as a "source of ovum capture" or a host uterus, for example, can be denied, minimized, or seen as something "natural" and unavoidable, that is, not as resulting from an ethically questionable cultural construction of motherhood/fatherhood. Aline saw herself in a modern biotechnology adventure—an emerging process that would deeply disturb future generations. Who has the right to decide for them?

Aline had time, room, and somebody to shelter her and listen to her. She lived in an I-Thou relationship. She could listen to herself and could perceive the other in full integrity, recovering her ethical competence. She became free and autonomous, deciding the best for herself in her relationship with the world. Responsibility, thought Aline, comes before freedom and is not grounded in technology but in virtue. Freedom is not an arbitrary choice of objects, proceedings, and apparatus dragged in to support one's desire.[18] She began to visit the nursery of the hospital without knowing why.

One day an assistant called her to see a newborn baby whose mother, a teenager, had just died.[19] Aline's reasoning expressed itself through a cuddling gesture. She took the baby in her arms and said, "You are my beloved Thou."

She felt the internal subjectivity of becoming a mother—she named her baby Esperança![20] She was happy. She was born again, took hold of herself, and lived her ethical autonomy. She called André, "I am taking our baby home," and she heard, "Come! I am here waiting for you." Then they started living the sweet and tender experience of becoming mother and father. Justice was complete.

It is said that Aline got pregnant and had two other children. But life could have taken other turns and nevertheless she would continue to be ever conscious in making ethical and inspiriting decisions.

Between the Blood and the Act

John: Why don't you bring in your brother's son to take care of? I'm not against it.

Yerma: I don't want to take care of anybody else's son. I feel that my arms would freeze from holding him.[21]

Yerma, a tragic poem in three acts written by Federico Garcia Lorca in 1934, is about a woman who desires a child but cannot bear one. The reason for her inability is not made clear. We do not know if she is infertile or if he is sterile. Typically, however, it is implicit throughout the text that she is the one to assume the disability. Her self-image is that of an arid desert "surrounded by a natural world where everything seems to be in its place and life pulses in rhythm, showing the harmony between heaven and earth."[22]

Why the act? Why blood? An act is a gesture, a movement of the body expressing something beyond the physical. It may be an expression of an idea, of feelings; it is an image of the unspoken, the symbol, the culture. Blood is a vital component of the material world. It is nature, biological life. It is between the blood and the act, the material and physical and its cultural meaning, that Yerma's tragedy unfolds. It is a human tragedy, the obstinacy of the species.

In claiming "I don't want to take care of anyone else's son," Yerma rejects the possibility of being a nonbiological mother by refusing to adopt a child. Suggesting that her arms would freeze if she were to embrace her brother's son, she sees her vitality paralyzed within a "natural world where everything seems to be in its place." Thus she reveres matter, despite the way the material world is thwarting her desire to conceive. In fact, she reinforces her limits, enacting through her gesture both nature and culture. She becomes immobile exactly where humanity and all the Yermas at the beginning of the new millennium are facing a crossroad: the scientific and technological developments of contemporary biology.

New Reproductive Technologies

It was thought that this dominion (over nature) was to be used for the sake of human life, to promote abundance . . . but instead, progress may become a curse.[23]

Extremely complex ethical problems are developing in the wake of conception by the new reproductive technologies (NRTs) and human genetic research. These new technologies challenge guidelines for human action. The familiar contrast between nature and culture has been shattered, and new ethical principles are urgently needed to help us confront the dazzling scientific "progress" that faces us.

A woman's desire for a biological child can be met in many ways, and the NRTs increase the options.[24] Not only the possibility of a child but even some characteristics of that child can be controlled. In today's scientized and technologized world, cryogenic preservation of embryos and expanded diagnostic capacities allow artificial reproduction to be associated with "quality" standards for embryos. The new technologies promote a spiral of manipulation in search of biological "perfection." According to Bernardo Beiguelman[25] we are emerging from an industrial era into a biotechnological one, in which we apply to living beings methods developed in industry for inert materials. Just as in engineering, we have projects, product planning, and quality control.

NRTs and genetic research support the revalorization of the ideal of a human norm and an ideological/scientific manipulation of biological material to attain that ideal, a path termed neonaturalism or genetic essentialism. The medical practice of instituting IVF treatments for either male or female sterility only confirms this tendency.[26] All the scientific advances that NRTs represent take place in women's bodies. Natural biological procreation was a basic component of the oppression of women manifested in patriarchal theoretical works and philosophy, and that situation does not alter with the new technologies. In IVF services, women are subjected to aggressive hormone treatments and a variety of tests, controls, and procedures—all for a treatment that according to international estimates has only a 10 percent chance of success.

Never before has the desire to exercise knowledge and the power it can bring produced so many unprecedented situations. The natural is no longer valued in its own right, but only insofar as it can be a means to power. We are challenged to create a new ethic to guide humanity's present and future actions in relation to all living beings, and to humans in particular, taking into account the question of gender. It is more important than ever that women redefine what it is to be human, taking into consideration what we are and what we want to be. We can only know what must be done when we are clear about who we are.

Adoption: Cultural Reflections

On the top of the neighboring mountain, the Alipinagle village was sadly impoverished. The next generation would not be sufficient to populate the land. The Alitoa people sighed, saying "Oh! Poor Alipinagle! After these people have gone, who will take care of the land, who will stay under the trees? We should give them some children to adopt, so that the land and the trees will have someone after we are gone."[27]

Adoption is an ancient custom that is practiced in different cultures and in diverse ways. In the neonaturalistic context of contemporary biological science and technology, this custom produces inevitable opposition. According to Margaret Mead, adoption was common among the Arapesh and Mundugumor of New Guinea, but the context was different. In the preceding quotation it is clear that adoption is part of a worldview in which "the people belong to the land, not the land to the people." A story is told of a priest who asked an Iroquois why he was willing to adopt a child of uncertain paternity. The Indian answered disdainfully, "You Frenchmen love only your own children. We love all the children of the tribe."[28]

In our culture adoption seems to be an alternative for sterile couples, for single women, and as an alternative to abortion or to NRT. But it is also a vehicle for exploitation, where the commercialization of children can be seen as a solution to poverty. Solidarity and cooperative values no longer predominate; we have moved far from the values of the Arapesh or even the ill-tempered Mundugumor described by Mead. In the contemporary attitude of neonaturalism or techno-scientific manipulation, there is no particular value accorded to adoption for social, rather than individual, purposes. According to Malin Bode, in 1987 in the then German Democratic Republic, 8,000 adoptions took place. Half (4,000) were incognito adoptions, the adopted child having no family relationship to the adopting family. Of those, 1,000 came from Third World countries.[29]

The other 3,000 were born in the GDR, 80 percent of them illegitimate—born to low-income mothers, prostitutes, prisoners, or mothers dependent on social welfare. Ninety percent of the adopting parents required a child less than a year old, and 20 percent specified a child free of any serious health problems. Anonymity for both the birth mothers and the recipient parents is guaranteed by law.[30] Analyzing these statistics, Bode concludes, "The starting point for adoption or for NRT is a deep desire for children, which ends up becoming a demand for child-merchandise. This demand can be met by technological medicine or by market forces—both are different modalities of the same policy."[31] Adoption as a personal and an ethico-political alternative to the use of NRTs cannot be analyzed by taking into account only the aspects that Bode mentions. It is necessary to incorporate new dimensions in our reflections.

What Is It To Be Human?

According to Hans Jonas, we know a lot more about what we don't want to know about than we know about what we want to know. Thus philosophy should first consult our fears, and only then our desires. A social critical perspective alerts us to the fact that "to face the crucial dilemma of contemporary scientific-technological power, we must avoid manichean reductionism, [or] any fragile consolation for laziness and cowardice."[32] An ethical route to facing these challenges must specify what is "natural." We must establish what we understand about ourselves and what we want to be, reexamine human nature, before decreeing what we ought to do.

Different conceptions of the nature of woman determine different options for reproduction, whether through NRT or adoption, and also determine different ethical attitudes toward those options. The following responses of women asked about NRT illustrate this point.[33]

I think it will be marvelous when we are able to produce children in a glass womb. A woman will be able to order a child. She will have options. If she wishes the pregnancy to take place within her body, she will be able to do that. If she wishes, she can use other technologies.[34]

Is it possible that we are . . . purely cultural? . . . Are we completely social beings? . . . Is the fact that a desire exists sufficient to justify its becoming a reality? Is the realization of any desire unquestioned? . . . I think about the need to resacralize life. It is not important whether it is God or not. We need to find something, at some point in our existence, which is considered untouchable, sacred.[35]

The first quote reveals a vision of nature as subject to domination and control and presumes a degree of knowledge and possible range of action that can transform the species itself into an object of engineering. It assumes infallibility of knowledge and expresses an attitude of enchantment by technology, through which our autonomy is mediated. In this perspective, human control over human nature itself, as well as over other living beings, is restricted only by the limits of science and technology. The phrase "glass womb" encapsulates the separation of the body's functions from its material and its reduction to mere tool. Such radical technological transformation, still only possible in science fiction, points to the modification of our species into something else, changing as it does not only reproduction but the social and historical identity of the species, its own self-understanding. The human subject in this vision constitutes itself exclusively as rational and dominating, observing and manipulating nature so as to control it. This perspective imbues the ideology (and practice) of the majority of scientists and specialists in human reproduction.[36] Such action for the sake of control lies at the root of the "ethic of the possible," technology at the service of desire, the normalization, a posteriori, of the utilitarian-instrumental character of scientific discovery, and a radical disjunction between culture and nature.

The second quote speaks of doubt, expresses fear, and points to limits. It is an effort to establish a reflective distance between the subject and the perspective of objectification. It expresses a need to rethink what we are, to rethink the idea of nature and of the human, a recurring and fundamental theme in all ethical discussion. Perhaps we have forgotten the knowledge of Being in its fullness. Treating the body as a machine and assembling machines with our body, we extrapolate from it the human capacity of making. Making and power are not questioned but are linked to the desire for knowledge. The quote opens this linkage to doubt and fear, and urges the elaboration of an ethic of limits, solidarity, and responsibility. Hans Jonas proposes that "now the duty of the human being is to include responsibility [toward] nature as a condition of his own survival and as an element of his own existential integrity. The communion of human destiny and of nature, rediscovered in danger, leads us to also rediscover our own dignity and [demands] attention transcending the utilitarian perspective."[37]

The desire for something sacred in our existence in the second quote can be understood as the recognition of a limit on action set by respect, a feeling born from the conviction that "to risk what is mine also means to put at risk something which belongs to others [be it the integrity of the species, future generations, or human identity] over which I have no right."[38] Women are understandably reluctant to invoke the sacred, in light of the oppressions and injustices historically invoked in its name. However, the philosophical sentiment behind Jonas's proposal does not necessarily spring from belief in a transcendent authority, and he opens the possibility of rethinking the grounds of human limits. It may be necessary to recontextualize the image of nature and humanity. Bartholo suggests, "The modern human adventure of desacralization of the cosmos disconnects human action from its traditional coordinates, opening the possibility of a 'purely' human freedom. With the dissolution of the sacred, lessening the fear of divine punishment, the human condition becomes the only useful foundation for the construction of ethical imperatives of a new type."[39]

Bioethics: Frontier or Everyday?

Scientific and technological developments that enable ever more sophisticated manipulation of living beings for assisted reproduction, recombining DNA, hybridization between species, and the improvement and modification of genetic patrimony raise ethical questions which, according to Berlinguer,[40] are characteristically "frontier cases," extreme situations that occupy the majority of ethical discussions in First World countries. The impact of the latest techno-scientific advances, their implementation and their implications for the future, provoke an upsurging of moral impulse and intense scientific, legal, and philosophical reflection, constituting what he terms "frontier bioethics." But he notes that little work is being done, either in research or in practical applications, on the most common sources of sterility, for example, either in determining its causes, which are mainly psychological, affective, and social, or in broadening the search for alternative therapies. For Berlinguer, politics, the scientific and commercial relations between industrialized and underdeveloped countries, justice, and the impact of cultural habits and behaviors need to be included in the scope of bioethical debate, opening the space for an "everyday bioethics."[41] Such a broadened bioethics would address more adequately the reality of poorer countries and might actually contribute to the issues that they face.

Examples of the situations that need to be included in bioethics debates about social and political options are not hard to find: the abandonment of thousands of Latin American and South American children; the lack of governmental and social support for the children as well as their mothers; indifference to single mothers, low-income adolescent pregnancy and maternal mortality rates; and the misery, hunger, and burdens of poor rural and urban women. Garrafa points out that "all situations of social exclusion are directly related to the ethics of solidarity, which must become one of the pillars of everyday bioethics."[42]

To speak of an "ethics of limits, solidarity and responsibility," of an "everyday bioethics," is to propose categories of analysis and approaches that allow a greater clarity and range of applicability in our deliberations. But it is important to realize, as Bode suggests, that the NRT and genetic manipulation and the invisibility of the plight of women and abandoned children of which we have spoken are interlinked, are but two sides of the same contemporary problematic, the model of a civilization in crisis, interlinked aspects of the same economic, political, and cultural problematic. Perhaps Bode's claims can become the starting point for a more courageous reflection between northern and southern feminists. It is impossible to reconceptualize thought and action without also addressing the understanding of human nature and the material world in light of the contributions of those historically excluded.[43]

Adoption or Assisted Conception?

Is the suffering caused by sterility sufficient justification for the use of NRT? Is the adoption of an abandoned child a more ethically acceptable answer than the invocation of technologies that promise to meet the need for motherhood? How would we begin to answer such a question?[44]

Abandoned children are already in the world, and the reasons why they were not cared for are varied and complex. Their very abandonment constitutes a reason for adoption; and such children are in need of, and can respond to, gestures that encourage them to value their lives. Approaching adoption, we must penetrate at least two different realities: she who has a child and gives it away and she who does not have a child and receives one. I (A.R.) do not wish to ignore the multiplicity of causes that provoke the abandonment that makes a child available for adoption at a given cultural moment. But here I wish to dwell on the reality of the recipient: her longing for a child and her options to gratify it through reproductive technologies or through adoption.

It requires courage to reflect on the ethical implications of two such weighty options, but some of the considerations surfacing in recent bioethics debates help me in my reflections. Hans Jonas suggests that nature might be thought of as a good in itself. What is, has a right to be; nature merits respect. Applying these considerations to the choice in question suggests that the use of biotechnology in human reproduction could be seen as a threat to the material integrity of the species, as an intervention in the environment, as a threat to human identity for the sake of power. This broader perspective must be taken into consideration in determining the good to be obtained through any particular action. To search for a child born by others, a life already existing but not accepted, furthers several desirable ends: protection, solidarity, and affection for another, but also a restraint on someone's power to dominate nature, an exercise of responsibility toward what is fundamental to one's being and that of others. Tubert claims that from a psychoanalytic point of view "to adopt a child requires the recognition of castration," that is, the acceptance of an incapacity with respect to one kind of need.[45] In our terms, what is needed is the recognition of nature, and the reformulation of our desires within the framework of self-knowledge and relationship with the Other.

To suggest that accepting a natural limit in the specific case of sterility is ethically acceptable for women might seem contradictory. After all, women have only recently emerged from a historical and cultural order where we were considered socially and morally inferior, where we could not exercise responsibility as subjects, where we were forbidden, on the basis of a respect for the natural order, to avoid or interrupt pregnancy. The exercise of human capacity has long challenged the chance of nature; that is what makes us human. Carniero points out that women do not remain subjugated by the natural order.[46] Because they are human, women can intervene in that order and modify it through knowledge and action. The possibility we have of either accepting or transgressing the natural order is a source of autonomy and self-determination for women as responsible subjects, and it must be accommodated to contemporary alternatives. The recognition of these new dilemmas, of limits and lacks and the new forms that desire takes, can help locate us as responsible subjects in respect to power and the desire for omnipotence, compulsion, covert oppression, and the transgressions of others.

It is common to justify the current limitless and inexorable commitment to scientific and technological progress by assuming a continuity with our human past, and thus to elide the difference between a manipulation of nature and an alteration of it. Traffic accidents don't stop the use of automobiles. We clone babies just as we make bridges: because we can, as one more extension of our capacity to make. The extension of this capacity effectively happens at the expense of the forgetfulness of Being. Because we don't recognize this difference, we risk that which makes us unique as a species—our exercise of responsibility. And it is this risk that makes technologies of conception ethically unacceptable. It is in self-limitation that we find the source of women's autonomy, in the deconstruction and reconstruction of the meaning of our actions, in nature's own affirmation.

Adoption can be seen as a starting point for the deconstruction and reconstruction of gestures, of human action. To adopt is not to presuppose unlimited power, to exercise omnipotence, but rather to be conscious of the intrinsically dangerous nature of unlimited power and to recognize another who is not the product of my dehumanization. This requires that there be no self-deception. To take care of other people's children is not the same as biological motherhood, and the quest for freedom need not lead to pretense or denial. The blood, the material substratum, is not frozen in sterility—it is simply absent. But all children, biological or non-biological, need to be "adopted," accepted into the symbolic context of a family, of history and culture, accorded the status of an object of human responsibility. This is as true for adopting as for procreating. The infertile woman's acknowledgment of this material incapacity, this lack, creates the space within which she can exercise her agency, can originate a gesture that will lead to a reencounter with her own subjectivity, and to an encounter with the Other. This encounter will not be the result of a technological objectivization of the human, through which the very identity of the human and the future of human life is placed at risk. Rather, it will simply be the human reaching out to the human in one more act of the drama of fulfilling human needs. It is her reformulation of her desire through the concrete exercise of responsible autonomy, which becomes ethically acceptable when she shows respect to the being of which she is a part.

Conclusion

We have shown how the bioethics principle of autonomy and the feminist "right to choose" cannot be appropriately applied to certain issues in reproduction that concern Brazilian feminists. First we examined conditions under which women in Brazil "choose" surgical sterilization. After noting that this method is pushed by northern commercial interests and not by the Brazilian government, we pointed out the remarkable coincidence that those making this "choice" are mostly black, indigenous, or poor. Furthermore, concern for these women's subsequent psychological and emotional health is nonexistent.

Next we examined infertile women's "choice" of adoption or NRTs. In Third World countries NRTs are readily available to high-income women, an example of global overmedicalization, technologicalization, and commodification of life. Human fertilization is not a simple biochemical process that can be controlled by science. The body is a vulnerable knower of feelings and passions. The "neonaturalism" of the scientific worldview has corrupted not only natural reproduction but also adoption; for the sake of the future of humanity and to atone for the complicity of northern and southern feminists in this corruption, we need to affirm our humanity and the humanity of abandoned children by incorporating them into a social world rather than threaten the future of the species by NRTs.

To become a mother is not enough; it is necessary to be responsible, to have human integrity. Bioethics, as a social movement and as a field of knowledge production, should valorize the symbolic universe and women's and men's concrete cultural lives in order to find common cultural values. Feminists need to consider "the right to choose" in its global ramifications, for we must transform bioethics in a direction very different from that taken by northern developed countries.

Notes

Jurema Werneck is the author of the "Surgical Sterilization" section; Fernanda Carneiro, of "Aline's Decision." Earlier versions of these sections were presented in San Francisco in November 1996 at the first conference of the International Network on Feminist Approaches to Bioethics. Alejandra Ana Rotania is the author of "Between the Blood and the Act," which she presented at the Latin American and Caribbean Bioethics Congress in Sao Paulo in October 1995. Paulo Macedo and Ana Regina Reis translated "Aline's Decision" from Portuguese into English; Dayse Abrantes and Peter Howard Wertheim translated "Between the Blood and the Act" from Portuguese into English. Helen Bequaert Holmes edited the first two sections and Mary Rorty, the final one. We thank Francis Holmes for secretarial assistance.

1. Elza Berquó, "A esterilização feminina do Brasil hoje," in *Quando a paciente é mulher—relatório do encontro nacional saúde da mulher: Um direito a ser conquistado* (Brasília: 1989), p. 79.

2. In *Black Feminist Thought* (New York: Routledge, 1991), Patricia Hill Collins discusses autonomy in a world that black women do not recognize as theirs, since, being occupied and colonized by racist power, they cannot own their bodies. She also emphasizes "the power of self-definition" (pp. 34, 91–94) for black women's survival as a group and for their resistance to efforts to control their reproduction and sexuality (pp. 50–51). She argues that black women have forged a sense of self and bodily integrity that is rooted in strong dyadic relationships with their children. Motherhood becomes here a source of self-determination that is integrative, extended, and communal. "We are together, my child and I." Alice Walker, "One Child of One's Own: A Meaningful Digression Within the Work(s)," *Ms* 8, no. 2 (1979): 75.

3. Luis Carlos Susin, *O homen messiânico: Uma introdução ao pensamento de Emmanuel Lévinas* [The messianic man: An introduction to the thought of Emmanuel Lévinas] (Petrópolis: Vozes, 1984), p. 113.

4. George Bataille (*O erotismo* [Porto Alegre: L & PM, 1987]) says that life is an erotic game between transgressions and interdictions, and eroticism is a sensitiveness linking desire, fears, anguishes, and intense pleasure.

5. Martin Buber, *I and Thou*, trans. Ronald Gregor Smith (Edinburgh: T. & T. Clark, 1937); *Eu e tu* (São Paulo: Editora Moraes, 1974) teaches that the sensation of reciprocity is a reinvigorating factor of humanization.

6. Susin, *O homen messiânico*, pp. 111–112.

7. A concept of Lévinas meaning the necessary process of going to the other and excessiveness of the "self" as a threat to it. Susin, *O homen messiânico*.

8. Henrique C. de Lima Vaz, *Escritos de filosofia*, vol. 2, *Ética e cultura* (São Paulo: Edições Loyola, 1993), pp. 62–65.

9. To de Lima Vaz (ibid., pp. 13–15) the *ethos* has a home place, a safe shelter, a space from which the world becomes livable for humans through their uses and habit, and a second place for the realization of goodness and the development of praxis. In the praxis developed in the contemporary women's movement are peculiarities that will translate into particular ways in the *ethos*. Here I (F.C.) consider that an individual woman is socialized in a particular ethos in habits and sexuality. Nowadays she is also socialized in the sphere of culture that introduces other values, uses, and habits, thus leading to ethical conflicts.

10. Susin, *O homen messiânico*, p. 113.

11. This concept is inspired by the Brazilian philosopher Marilena Chaui, *Cultura e democracia: O discurso competente e outras falas* (São Paulo: Cortez Editors, 1985).

12. According to Martin Buber, "Through the *Thou* a man becomes *I*. That which confronts him comes and disappears, relational events condense, then are scattered, and in the change consciousness of the unchanging partner, of the *I*, grows clear, and each time stronger." Buber, *I and Thou*, p. 28, and *Eu e tu*, p. 32.

13. Susin, *O homen messiânico*, p. 172.

14. Simone Novaes and Tania Salem, "Recontextualizando o embrião," *Revista de estudos feministas* IFCS/UFRJ-PPCIS/VERJ 3, no. 1 (1993).

15. Sarah Franklin, "Postmodern Procreation: A Cultural Account of Assisted Reproduction," in Faye Ginsburg and Rayna Rapp, eds., *Conceiving the New World Order* (Berkeley: University of California Press, 1995), pp. 326–327.

16. Ibid., p. 325.

17. Hannah Arendt, *A condição humana* (Rio de Janeiro: Relume Dumará, 1993), p. 123.

18. Susin, *O homen messiânico*.

19. Certainly due to a lack of attentive medical care during pregnancy and delivery.

20. Esperança is the Portuguese word for "hope," a common woman's name in Brazil.

21. Federico Garcia Lorca, *Yerma*, trans. Cecília Meirelles (Rio de Janeiro: Livraria Agir Editora Coleção Teatro Moderno, 1963), p. 10. English translation by Dayse Abrantes and Peter Howard Wertheim.

22. Ibid.

23. Hans Jonas, "Dalla filosofia alla scienzia," *Lettera internazionali (Roma)* 30 (1991): 66.

24. NRT technical procedures include hormonal induction for oocyte capture, artificial insemination-husband, donor insemination, in vitro fertilization (IVF), other methods for uniting gametes, and cryopreservation of sperm and embryos. Jacque Testart, *L'oeuf transparent* (Paris: Flammarion, 1986), is concerned about "perversion" in the use of these, that is, leading to egg fusion, female parthenogenesis, tissue banking, male pregnancy, and artificial wombs. See also Silvia Tubert, *Mujeres sin sombra: Maternidad y tecnologia* (Madrid: Siglo XXI, 1991); Tom Wilkie, *O projecto genomo humano: Um conhecimento perigoso* (Rio de Janeiro: Jorge Zahar, 1994); Cynthia de Wit and Ann Pappert, "Current Developments and Is-

sues: A Summary," *Issues in Reproductive and Genetic Engineering: Journal of International Feminist Analysis* 4, no. 1 (1991): 53–72.

25. Bernardo Beiguelman, "Genética e ética," *Ciência e cultura* (Revista da Sociedade Brasileira para o Progresso da Ciência) 42, no. 1 (1990): 61–69.

26. Consider, for instance, some of the treatments being developed for male sterility. If the sperm count is low, a sperm can be directly injected into an ovum by micromanipulation, a technique known as intracytoplasmic sperm injection (ICSI). This technique has now been used for injecting not only a sperm but also its precursor, the immature spermatid without a flagellum. ICSI is used in France and Brazil in cases of male sterility. It is worth nothing that it is the woman with no physiological obstacles to procreation who undergoes the process of superovulation, ovum harvest, IVF, and embryo transfer.

27. Margaret Mead, *Sex and Temperament in Three Primitive Societies*, 3d ed. (New York: Morrow, 1963), p. 43.

28. Tubert, *Mujeres sin sombra*, p. 50.

29. Asia and Latin America were the primary sources, not only Brazil but also Guatemala, Honduras, and Paraguay. Approximately 14,000 children from Korea were "sold" annually in the United States and Europe, until a change in governmental regulations curtailed those adoptions. Malin Bode, "Adopción: La alternativa a la tecnologia reproductiva?" in Paula Bradish, Eva Feyerabend, and Uta Winkler, eds., *Mujeres contra las tecnologias reproductivas y ingeniería genética* (Frankfort: Ponencias del II Congreso de Feministas, 1988).

30. Bode, "Adopción."

31. Ibid., p. 38.

32. Roberto dos Santos Bartholo Jr., *A dor de fausto* (Rio de Janeiro: Revan, 1992), p. 99.

33. The following quotes come from a debate about new reproductive technologies that took place in São Paulo in 1991. The testimonies illustrate ways of thinking, including some conceptions of nature and what it means to be human, which have been culturally introduced (translated by Dayse Abrantes and Peter Howard Wertheim). ECOS, "New Reproductive Technologies," in *New Reproductive Technologies: The Conception of New Dilemmas* (São Paulo: ECOS, 1991), p. 18.

34. Ibid.

35. Ibid., p. 22.

36. Roger Abdelmassih, "Tudo por um bebe" [Anything for a baby], *ICAPS Bulletin* (Informativo do Instituto Camiliano de Pastoral da Saúde e Bioética) 13, no. 123 (1995): 4–5; Alejandra Rotania, "O projecto genoma humano: Desafios éticos da biologia moderna" [The human genome project: Ethical challenges of modern biology], *Revista da sociedade Brasileira de historia da ciência* 9 (1993): 3–16.

37. Hans Jonas, *Ética, medicine e Teeniz* (Lisboa: Vega, 1994), p. 176.

38. Ibid., p. 44. Examples within the brackets are mine (A.R.).

39. Bartholo, *A dor de fausto*, p. 75.

40. Giovanni Berlinguer, "Bioetica quotidiana e bioetica de frontiera," in A. DiMeo and C. Mancina, eds., *Bioetica* (Roma: Editori Laterza, 1989).

41. Note Virginia Warren's similar concern, in which she contrasts "crisis" and "housekeeping" issues. Virgina L. Warren, "Feminist Directions in Medical Ethics," *Hypatia* 4, no. 2 (1989): 73–87.

42. Volnei Garrafa, "Bioethics, Responsibilities, and Solidarity," *ICAPS Bulletin* (Informativo do Instituto Camiliano de Pastoral da Saúde e Bioética, São Paulo) 13, no. 123 (1995): 12.

43. Leo Pessini appropriately focused on the greatest challenge in Latin American bioethics as mediating between exaggerated opposing perspectives in order to redeem what is unique and singular in Latin culture, thus developing a truly alternative perspective that would enrich the multicultural dialogue. In Latin America, he pointed out, bioethics has adopted a partisan alliance with poverty and exclusion; the presence of women is still minimal. Bioethics needs to contribute to the fight against the oppression of gender, and it needs the participation of people acting more directly against racism. Leo Pessini and Cristhian Barchifontaine, "O desenvolvimento da bioética na América Latina: Algumas considerações," in *Fundamentos da bioética* (São Paulo: Paulus, 1996). See also Fátima Oliveira, *Genetic Engineering: The Seventh Day of Creation* (São Paulo: Moderna, 1995).

44. This question is not, as might initially appear, distant from and distorting of the reality of Third World countries. Reproductive technologies are readily available to high-income women and couples. Further, their availability is symbolic of a questionable overmedicalization that affects the whole population. It is related to the growing technicalization and commodification of life and incorporates the democratic assumption that any and all technological commodities should be available to all social classes, suggesting that fertility treatments, for instance, should be offered in public health services.

45. Tubert, *Mujeres sin sombra*, p. 182.

46. Fernanda Carneiro, "Aborto: Da solidão ao diálogo," in Haidi Jarschel, Mara Regina Vidal, Nancy Cardoso Pereira, eds., *Mandrágora: Direitos reprodutivos e aborto* (São Paulo: NETMAL, 1993), p. 66.

9

Friendly Persuasion? Legislative Enforcement of Male Responsibility for Contraception

NAOKO T. MIYAJI

Men play a key role in bringing about gender equality since, in most societies, men exercise preponderant power in nearly every sphere of life, ranging from personal decisions regarding the size of families to the policy and programme decisions taken at all levels of Government. It is essential to improve communication between men and women on issues of sexuality and reproductive health, and the understanding of their joint responsibilities, so that men and women are equal partners in public and private life.[1]

The concept of reproductive health and its attendant rights is increasingly recognized internationally. Article 7.2 of the Programme of Action of the International Conference on Population and Development (ICPD), as well as Article 96 of the Beijing Declaration and Platform for Action (BDPA), declare that "reproductive health ... implies that people are able to have a satisfying and safe sex life and that they have the capability to reproduce and the freedom to decide if, when and how often to do so."[2]

Nonetheless, women globally are gravely impacted by unwanted pregnancy and its consequences. Every year 50 million abortions are carried out, some 20 million of them under unsafe conditions. Between 70,000 and 80,000 women die from unsafe abortions every year.[3] Major international documents quite reasonably emphasize the importance of education, access to information, and adequate health care to improve this situation, but until such measures produce changes, many women will continue to suffer.

135

In this chapter, I discuss the possibility of imposing a legal duty on men to practice both safe and contraceptive sex. Such a measure would serve to deter men from violating women's sexual and reproductive rights. Specifically, it would have a significant and quick impact on reducing the number of unwanted pregnancies, abortions, and deaths from them. Thus I view legal sanctions against men not as an end but as a means to change social norms and men's behavior with respect to sexual and reproductive issues. In a narrow sense, the end is simply responsible behavior by men regarding safe and contraceptive sex. In a wider sense, however, it is nothing less than a gender equal society that supports such responsibility.

Unwanted pregnancy is caused by and results from the unequal power relationship between women and men. Fear of both the imagined and the actual consequences of an unwanted pregnancy oppressively burdens women by restricting women's behavior and reminding women that many men lack respect for women's concerns.[4] Women's self-awareness and empowerment are important and necessary but not sufficient to eliminate unwanted pregnancy or to achieve gender equality. It is the man's involvement that causes pregnancy. As the introductory quote states, men play a key role in bringing about gender equality, since they have more power. It is thus important to shift our attention from women to men in order to raise men's consciousness on sexual and reproductive issues, and cause men to think more seriously about these matters.

To achieve this end, I propose two possible legal formulations for imposing a legal duty on men to practice both safe and contraceptive sex; one is a "women's assertion" model, the other a "men's protection" model. Although I favor the second model in principle, in practice, I suggest using both models, employing one or the other depending on a woman's actual vulnerability at the social and individual level.

I expect criticism of legal enforcement as the best or most useful means to change men's behavior toward women, since I realize the kind of law I envision will not become a reality anywhere in the world without major changes in societal attitudes. Thus I view my proposal as a provocation, an opportunity for men and women everywhere to reflect on the patriarchal nature of current social arrangements, the use of male-female biological differences to control women, and the employment of social prejudices to bolster misconceptions about men's and women's supposed "nature." As I see it, exploring the possibility of making it men's rather than women's legal duty to practice both safe and contraceptive sex makes men's instead of women's behavior the object of social scrutiny, destabilizes current unexamined premises about reproductive issues, and promises a new way to achieve equality between women and men, thereby eradicating the suffering of women.

Although my argument is based on the situation in Japan and to some extent in the United States, I try to keep my perspective global. After all, women suffer from unwanted pregnancies throughout the world, with especially grave consequences in developing countries. Since I am well aware of how cultural complexity and variety shape sexual and reproductive issues differently in different areas of the world,[5] I realize some of my specific arguments on sexual norms and legal arrangements might be peculiar to Japan. Nevertheless, I believe the basic mechanisms producing unwanted pregnancy are quite universal, and that a global consensus, as expressed in international documents, exists on the path toward gender equality. Much of the experience of women that I have found described in ethnographies of both developing and developed countries[6] is quite similar to that of Japanese women. Therefore, strategies to change the situation of women in Japan should be of some use to women in other parts of the world eager to develop their own strategies to improve their status.

Legal Formulations

Women's Assertion Model

In this model, if a woman has not taken contraceptive measures, does not want to get pregnant, and clearly requests her male partner to use contraceptive measures, then her male partner should face legal sanctions for causing a "forced pregnancy" if he fails to comply with her request, engages in noncontraceptive sex, and impregnates her. The term "forced pregnancy" has been applied to a rape, the intentional aim of which is to impregnate a woman so that the child she carries will be ethnically mixed.[7] In other words, the purpose of such a rape is for one nation to "ethnically cleanse" another nation. However, even in intimate, supposedly consensual sex, a pregnancy resulting from a male's practice of noncontraceptive sex in spite of his partner's request can be considered forced. In fact, the sex here is not truly consensual but is analogous to rape. Only sex that includes agreement as to the type of sex, the desirability or undesirability of pregnancy, and the use or nonuse of a specific method(s) of contraception is fully consensual in my estimation.[8]

I call this legal formulation a "women's assertion" model because it is based on the idea that, under ordinary circumstances, women can and should be able to protect themselves against an unwanted pregnancy, either by employing contraception themselves or by asserting their preferences for contraceptive sex to their male partners and refusing to have sex with them if such preferences are not respected. As in a traditional rape case, a woman in an unwanted pregnancy case would have to prove that she did not consent to noncontraceptive sex. In Japan, evidence concerning the degree to which the female partner resisted an act of noncontraceptive sex would probably be required. (Article 176 of the Japanese penal code defines rape as intercourse forced by a man on a woman by either physical violence or the threat of it.) Among other defenses, it could be argued that the woman could have protected herself with contraceptives if she had really wanted to avoid pregnancy rather than take the riskier course of asking the man to take contraceptive measures. It is a weakness of this model that I return to in my discussion of liberal legal individualism.

Men's Protection Model

Many questions arise from the "women's assertion" model, since not all women have access to safe and affordable contraceptives or have the power to say no to men pressing for noncontraceptive sex. Why should *women* have to use contraceptives that may be unsafe, ineffective, and expensive? Why should *women* have to explain the danger of pregnancy and ask men to take precautions against pregnancy? And why should *women* bear the burden of proving their resistance against noncontraceptive sex in order to pursue a legal remedy in case of pregnancy? Men should know that women are usually fertile and that intercourse without contraception very often results in pregnancy.

Because of these questions, I propose a second formulation, a "men's protection" model. Under this model, unless a woman expresses explicitly her desire for a reproductive outcome, in the event of impregnation her sex partner would face legal sanctions for his practice of noncontraceptive sex. A man must thus protect not only his partner from unwanted pregnancy but also himself from the aftermath of noncontraceptive sex.

There are at least two justifications for such a measure. The first one is a shared responsibility argument. Major international documents emphasize that men and women should share responsibility equally in sexual and reproductive matters.[9] Among other things, men and women should share the burdens of an unwanted pregnancy equally. These include the burden of avoiding it (i.e., contraception) and the burden resulting from the failure to use contraception (i.e., pregnancy and its consequences). Since women are disproportionately burdened when a pregnancy occurs, it would seem only fair that men assume the burden of contraception. Without this kind of rebalancing of the "natural" burdens of reproduction, responsible action by men is unlikely, and women and men won't achieve equality. Consider how burdensome the impact of noncontraceptive sex is to women: the fear of getting pregnant; the physical and psychological consequences of pregnancy, including the visible signs of pregnancy, the resultant social stigma, and the loss of educational and career development opportunities; the physical and psychological consequences of abortion, including not only the actual complications of abortion but also fears about such possible complications as infertility and even death; and the physical and psychological consequences of unwanted delivery and unwanted motherhood.[10] Because men do not have to bear any comparable burdens, most men are largely indifferent to these problems. Only by requiring men to take full responsibility for contraception is there any possibility of coming even close to equalizing men's and women's sexual and reproductive responsibilities.

The second justification for a "men's protection" model is a harm-to-others argument. If men practice noncontraceptive sex, it can cause serious harm to women, but the converse is not true so long as men are not criminally sanctioned or civilly liable for the harm of an unwanted pregnancy. Men may negotiate with women about contraceptive measures, but they should have no right to expect or require that women protect themselves from unwanted pregnancy. Of course, women may use their own contraceptive methods, but they would be under no legal obligation to do so since, unlike the case with men, noncontraceptive sex may cause harm to women but, as it stands, not to men. Similar and more detailed discussions of these justifications are found in Numazaki,[11] who argues that intravaginal ejaculation constitutes sexual violence against women.[12]

The basic rule of such a statute would be that, in order to avoid complete liability for a pregnancy and the resulting legal sanctions, a man must take contraceptive measures or obtain explicit consent from his partner for noncontraceptive sex. Consent may be given when she wants to become pregnant, prefers to use her own contraceptive measures, or chooses to take a risk. Even in these situations, if a man has no intention of becoming a father, is unsure of the safety and reliability of his partner's contraceptive measures, or does not wish to cause another a risk of harm, he has the right to use contraception. Explicit consent might take a written form if either partner anticipates trouble with the other in the future.

Compensation for Forced Pregnancy

If the concept of forced pregnancy is accepted under either the "women's assertion" or "men's protection" model, pregnancy resulting from a man's engaging in noncontraceptive sex without the partner's consent could be subject to either criminal or civil penalties, or both, providing tort remedies for negligent and/or intentional violations of the law, and/or criminal penalties to punish commission of a sexual assault–type offense. A woman who suffered an unwanted pregnancy would be able to claim compensatory and perhaps punitive damages from the man who failed to employ contraception. Such damages would compensate the woman for all of the injuries—including psychological, social, and economical harm—suffered from the forced pregnancy and birth or, should she choose, the abortion.

In any given case of unwanted pregnancy, the woman should be completely free to choose abortion or birth. If a woman decides not to abort the fetus, her decision should not entail any obligation on her part to raise the child. If she wishes, she may play the role of a surrogate mother, with responsibility for raising the child borne by the man causing the unwanted pregnancy. If the woman instead chooses to bear and raise the child, she would be entitled to receive compensation for child-rearing expenses from the genetic father. As I discuss more fully below, the welfare of the child should be considered an issue separate and distinct from that of who is responsible for raising the child.

The Two Legal Formulations
and Women's Vulnerability

In my view, the shared responsibility and harm-to-others arguments would justify using the second legal formulation based on the men's protection model, but in order to avoid contributing to the view of women as powerless and dependent on men this model might reinforce, I would propose using one or the other formulation depending on the degree of vulnerability of women at the social as well as individual level.[13]

The proposed two legal formulations are both based on the idea that a man should pay a price for impregnating a woman by noncontraceptive sex when the woman has not consented to such sex.[14] The difference between the two is the assumption of consent. The women's assertion model presumes that a woman has consented to noncontraceptive sex unless she makes it known that she does not want it. This model might work well enough in societies where (1) sufficiently safe and reliable contraceptive measures are easily accessible to women, (2) women's status is reasonably equal to men's, (3) women's assertiveness is viewed positively, (4) women's desire for sex is openly acknowledged and women can initiate sexual relationships (i.e., a free sex ideology is strong and a double standard for men and women does not exist), (5) safe abortion is available, and (6) men's responsibilities for child rearing as fathers are well recognized.

In contrast to the women's assertion model, the men's protection model, which presumes the woman's lack of consent to noncontraceptive sex and requires the man to prove that the woman consented, seems more appropriate in societies where (1) women do not have adequate information about and/or access to safe and reliable contraceptive mea-sures,[15] (2) differences between men and women are significant both on the educational and economic level, (3) women are encouraged to be obe-dient to men, (4) men are supposed to take the initiative in sexual rela-tionships, (5) abortion is either prohibited by law or dangerous, and (6) pressure on women to assume a traditional maternal role is strong. On an individual level, the men's protection model would, no doubt, serve so-cially vulnerable women,[16] such as adolescent girls and young women (the exact age might differ slightly depending on the nation or commu-nity), and women who are poor or with limited education, especially when their male partner is an adult,[17] is richer, and is more educated.

Although the men's protection model is the more difficult one for cur-rent societies to accept, paradoxically, I think a male sexual and repro-ductive responsibility argument has a better chance of being heard and being accepted in a strongly patriarchal society than in a society that is more gender egalitarian. In a society where men's authority is largely un-contested, a "male responsibility" argument can be phrased in terms such as "if men are wiser than women, then men should take more re-sponsibility for sex than women"; "if abortion is a sin, then the men who cause unwanted pregnancy and compel women to end pregnancy are the sinful ones"; "if sex should be only for procreation and contraception is against God's will, then men should control their sexual behavior"; and "if fathers have rights to their children, then they also have responsibili-ties for all their children, including those who are the products of an un-wanted pregnancy." Without close knowledge of a given culture, these examples remain speculative and could be counterproductive if they re-inforced paternalistic attitudes. But, at least in the short term, a male re-sponsibility argument may afford to women their best chance to reduce unwanted pregnancies in precisely those strongly patriarchal societies where the notion of women's control over their own bodies is weak.[18]

Prevention of STDs, Including HIV/AIDS

In a society (or relationship) in which the possibility of contracting sexu-ally transmitted diseases (STDs), especially HIV/AIDS, exists, the second approach, which imposes a heavier responsibility on men, is more logical from a public health standpoint. Since a condom is the only effective tool to prevent the infection, and since it is virtually impossible for a woman to force a man to wear a condom, it is men who must take the responsi-bility to protect women and/or themselves from STDs, especially HIV/AIDS. Men should have the duty to wear condoms, particularly if they choose to have sex with sex workers whose risk of contracting STDs, especially HIV/AIDS, is high and with respect to whom there is a presumption of no reproductive intent. Although sex workers can use their own contraceptives to protect themselves from an unwanted pregnancy, there is no widely accessible female contraceptive that they can use to protect themselves from an STD or HIV/AIDS. For this reason, it is clear that condom use by men is literally vital for sex workers. Sex workers, either male or female, should have a right to safe and contraceptive sex that is not waivable through the use of money.

Concerns About the Two Models

The kinds of laws I am proposing are, of course, subject to major concerns about their implementation, including (1) proof of paternity, (2) dependence on biotechnology, (3) emphasis on biological connection, (4) emotional resistance to obtaining explicit consent in an intimate relationship, (5) individualistic liberal legal thinking, and (6) child welfare. Analysis of these problems will illuminate current social arrangements and conceptions that have contributed to the perpetuation of gender inequality, as well as the implications my proposed laws have for feminist strategy.

Proof of Paternity

The primary technical difficulty under such legislation would be proving that a particular man engaged in unlawful, noncontraceptive sex and that he is the father of the fetus (or child). This difficulty, however, has been substantially reduced by advances in the technology of genetic analysis. In the near future, a woman will be able to have fetal DNA analyzed through her own blood. If a woman suspects that the man with whom she has had sex will refuse to cooperate and provide a blood sample, she can preserve his semen after noncontraceptive sex. In the event of pregnancy, she can request genetic analysis of the semen sample and have it matched against that of the fetus. In possession of such powerful evidence, legal authorities will find it easier to obtain the man's cooperation in subsequent fact-gathering and legal proceedings.

Dependence on Biotechnology

As is apparent from the preceding discussion, the proposed legal scheme requires heavy dependence on biotechnology. Feminists and others have long cautioned against being controlled by biotechnology, especially in matters of reproduction. Since the advance of biotechnology is unlikely to stop, however, those who have concerns about its being used in ways that harm women should work to regulate it so that it is used to benefit women. Moreover, they should encourage the development of biotechnologies that positively benefit women.[19] The legal framework proposed here might have the consequence of directing biotechnology toward the goal of gender equality by stimulating the development of many good male contraceptives. Current research and development of contraceptives is confined mainly to those that affect the functioning of the female body. The gaze of medicine and science has focused on people who are easily— in a social, not a biological sense—controllable.[20] The important issue may not be the advance of biotechnology itself, but rather who controls its direction. However, severe limits still exist; in countries where such advanced techniques are not available or for individuals who cannot afford their cost, the proposed statutory scheme has little or no real use. In some countries, assuring the availability of affordable condoms to everyone might be the first difficult step in the direction of such a scheme.

Emphasis on Biological Connection

When the biological father can be identified scientifically, many issues arise as well. First, despite the imposition of legal liability based on the father's act of noncontraceptive sex, and not on his biological link to the fetus as such, such liability may contribute to perpetuating the importance given to the biological link between parent and child.

Second, the fact that the biological father can be identified may in itself be a great incentive for men to employ contraceptive measures. No longer will men have the option of evading responsibility for an unwanted pregnancy by denying having had sex with the woman or by asserting that some other man is the biological father. Biological fathers will have to assume responsibility for their biological fetuses and children. However, the same technology that can identify the biological father may make it difficult for women to exert power based on their more obvious biological link and/or to secretly choose a social father regardless of his biological link to the child or fetus.

Third, patriarchal systems and the surveillance of women's sexual behavior are said to exist in part to safeguard the biological link of father and child. The use of biotechnology may help free women from such sexual surveillance, but this might be too optimistic. Patriarchal systems have also tried to evade the biological link of father and child in some contexts. By categorizing women as Madonna or whore, wife or prostitute, and by forcing some women into monogamy and assuming others to be promiscuous, men have controlled the evidence and claims of the biological link made by women.

Depending on the rules governing who may initiate an analysis of the biological link, with whose cooperation, and who may have access to the results, greater or lesser surveillance of women's sexual behavior will be the outcome. How such rules would affect patriarchal systems needs further analysis, and legislative provisions regulating these matters must be drafted with great care.

Emotional Resistance to Obtaining
Explicit Consent to Noncontraceptive Sex

Some would feel awkward requesting explicit, especially written, consent for noncontraceptive sex in order to be free from the risk of legal sanction. Sexual conduct is usually considered an act of passion, desire, and biological urge rather than a rational and calculated action. It is also considered intimate, informal, and implicit rather than formal and contractual. This is the case even where the idea of family planning is widespread. Thus emotional resistance to explicit consent may be hard to overcome.[21]

Some may argue that explicit consent should be necessary in the case of contraceptive sex because it requires extra effort over "natural" sex, which is noncontraceptive. In practice, however, it makes more sense to require that such consent be required for noncontraceptive sex. After all, in most societies the vast majority of sexual encounters are those in which pregnancy *is not* desired. Moreover, encounters in which pregnancy *is* desired are more likely to take place in the context of a firmer, probably more rational relationship between the partners. In such circumstances, meaningful consent can be established through ongoing communication and thus is less of an issue.

Marriage has historically been considered a contract, implying mutual consent to sex and procreation. However, marriage quite often exists in the context of unequal power relationships. As a result of this awareness, the concept of marital rape has acquired greater legal recognition in some countries, mandating that the marriage contract does not entail the obligation to comply with the partner's sexual wishes all the time. And, of course, sex in marriage (except in some religious traditions) is not always for procreation. Thus obsolete notions of the marriage contract should not be used as a substitute for explicit consent to noncontraceptive sex in couples.

Liberal Legal Individualism

For a feminism espousing liberal legal individualism, what has been at stake is the woman's right to her own body, as well as autonomy. Since an unwanted pregnancy can be avoided without the man's cooperation, and since many women do not trust men to take their contraceptive duties seriously, a self-protection strategy seems the easiest and most reliable course of action for a prudent woman. Since such a strategy meshes well with an ethic of individual autonomy, which includes the idea of preventing the state from interfering with women's (and men's) privacy, it is not surprising that feminists (especially in the United States) have favored it and put a high priority on ensuring their right to contraception and safe abortion.[22] On the surface, this self-protection strategy seems to maximize women's autonomy. The woman can, if she wants, choose to protect herself from or end an unwanted pregnancy without letting anyone, including her partner, know that she has made this choice.

However, for all its apparent advantages, there are severe limits to the self-protection approach. Sexual and reproductive issues are deeply relational: intercourse and pregnancy arise in the context of a relationship between a man and a woman. Furthermore, they contain the possibility of creating a relationship not only between a woman and a fetus but also between a man and a fetus. In downplaying the relational aspects of intercourse and pregnancy, certain liberal feminists have bolstered women's autonomy but have weakened men's sense of relational responsibilities in regard to their female partner and their fetus. If feminists want to achieve relational equality between men and women, they cannot do so simply by emphasizing pregnancy as under women's control; they must also stress men's responsibilities. Demanding that men be more responsible in "private" relations does not negate women's autonomy or weaken women's power of self-protection. The autonomy of women can be truly realized only when it is conceptualized in terms of their relationships, and only when the men to whom they are related value women's autonomy as much as men's autonomy. The possibility of communicative and trusting relationships between women and men should be more envisioned and promoted.

As for state interference with individual freedom, all law contains this danger, to which we must be alert.[23] But as cases of domestic violence and child abuse show, appropriate social and legal intervention plays an essential role in preventing abuse in private relationships inappropriately protected by a "sanctity of the family" concept.[24]

Child Welfare

The major concern about the legal remedy proposed here has to do with the consequence of pregnancy: the child. What will happen to the child if it is given to a biological father who did not voluntarily choose to become a father? To be sure, some children might suffer from being given to men who did not want to be fathers. But such children might not fare any better in the custody of women who did not want to be mothers. Just because women in most countries might be, on the average, better and more responsible caregivers than men does not mean that all women are better carers than men. Nor does it mean that women are by nature better carers than men. Cultural ideology and social pressure are probably the main reason why women rather than men are children's primary caregivers.[25] Because this is so, if human beings wished, they could transform cultural ideology and social pressure, directing men rather than women to be children's primary caregivers. Men's ability to love and care for children may be vastly underestimated; these abilities should be promoted.[26]

Burdened with an unwanted pregnancy, a woman who does not want her life changed coercively but detests sacrificing the fetus's life should have the choice of passing the child to the father, whose responsibility would be to provide good care for it. Blame and social disapproval should be directed at the man who fails to practice contraceptive sex and refuses to take responsibility for the care of the child, not at the woman if she chooses abortion. If women, including sex workers, start leaving babies with the babies' fathers, men may finally realize the serious effect of noncontraceptive sex and begin to shoulder their sexual and reproductive responsibilities.

I expect this argument to be criticized on the basis of cruelty and irresponsibility to a child in terms of using a child as a mere means in a power game between women and men. In response, I would say that I am quite optimistic that most men will act responsibly once they are forced into the situation of taking care of the child, although I am pessimistic about men's behavioral change in matters of contraception and child care without any compulsory measures. First of all, taking care of a child is not a "punishment" but can be a great fulfillment, as many women have been enjoying up until now. To be sure, there will be some men—hopefully very few—who will be unable or unwilling to take responsibility for the consequences of their actions. In such cases, some societal measures other than relying on the mother's care will need to be taken, as has been done for the support of single mothers in various countries. No woman should be forced to rear a child that a man forced her to have by his failure to use contraceptives. The child is the man's and society's "problem," not the woman's.

Conclusion

Although the difficulties and concerns linked to enforcing legal responsibility for men's contraception are numerous and serious, I hope the analysis here provides a clearer and more precise vision of the abstract moral claim of "shared responsibility of men and women in sexual and

reproductive issues" and a more specific agenda for changing men's behavior and social attitudes.
   Even if legal enforcement is not achieved, once the concept of male responsibility for contraception is understood and accepted, many things
will change. Male contraceptives will be more aggressively developed.
Research in population control, AIDS prevention, and child health will
focus more on men's sexual behavior and paternity bonding than on
women's reproductive behavior. Sex education projects will target boys
rather than girls, male clients rather than female sex workers, husbands
rather than wives. If a state is aggressively working on population control, men's abstinence, contraception, or voluntary sterilization will be
more seriously considered as an alternative to women's forced sterilization or forced abortion. Statistics on male contraceptive practice will become an important part of indicators of gender equality. (They might be
even better and more sensitive indicators than the Gender-Related Development Index [GDI] or the Gender Empowerment Measure [GEM],
indexes the U.N. Development Program offers for each country's status
of gender equality.)[27]
   Not only the political but also the medical and the scientific gaze has
been fixed on women. Those who have more power, and thus are able to
resist becoming the target of education and training for behavioral
change, were often left alone, even though changing their behavior
would have been very effective in the long-term prevention of unwanted
pregnancies and the spread of STDs such as HIV/AIDS. In addition to
the traditional moral view that reproductive issues are *women's* issues,
this supposedly scientific gaze needs to be changed in the interests of attaining true equality between women and men.

Notes

This paper is a revised version of my arguments published in Japanese. Naoko T.
Miyaji, "Haramaseru sei to haramu sei: Hinin sekinin no jittaika no kanousei o
saguru" [Impregnating sex and pregnant sex], *Gendai Bunmeigaku Kenkyu* 1 (1998):
19–29; and Miyaji, "Haramaseru sei no jikosekinin wa dou jittaika shiuruka" [How
can responsibility of impregnating sex be substantiated?], *Impaction* 108 (1998):
144–151. They were written as a critique of Ichiro Numazaki's paper, "Haramaseru
sei no jiko sekinin" [The self-responsibility of the "impregnating sex"], *Impaction*
105 (1997): 86–96. A draft of this paper was presented at the Second Conference of
the International Association of Feminist Approaches to Bioethics (FAB2) in 1998. I
thank participants of FAB2 for their valuable comments. I also thank Jack Tobin for
his insightful comments and linguistic as well as legal advice.

   1. *Programme of Action of the International Conference on Population and Development* (ICPD), Art. 4.24 (Cairo: September 1994).

2. *Beijing Declaration and Platform for Action* (BDPA), Fourth World Conference on Women, September 15, 1995, United Nations; and *Programme of Action of the International Conference on Population and Development*.

3. World Health Organization, *Life in the 21st Century: The World Health Report, 1998. Report of the International Forum for the Operational Review and Appraisal of the Implementation of the Programme of Action of ICPD*, Netherlands Conference Centre, The Hague, Netherlands, February 8–12, 1999.

4. BDPA, Art. 94, states that "the limited power many women have over their sexual and reproductive lives and lack of influence in decision-making are social realities which have an adverse impact on their health." Art. 95 notes that "young men are often not educated to respect women's self-determination and to share responsibility with women in matters of sexuality and reproduction."

5. Malcolm Potts, Peter Diggory, and John Peel, *Abortion* (Cambridge: Cambridge University Press, 1977).

6. For example, see Faye D. Ginsburg and Rayna Rapp, eds., *Conceiving the New World Order: The Global Politics of Reproduction* (Berkeley: University of California Press, 1995); and Emily Martin, *The Woman in the Body: A Cultural Analysis of Reproduction* (Boston: Beacon, 1987).

7. BDPA, Arts. 13, 115.

8. The meaning of consent in unequal power relationships is developed from my research on informed consent and truth telling in medicine. Naoko T. Miyaji, "The Power of Compassion: Truth Telling Among American Doctors in the Care of Dying Patients," *Social Science and Medicine* 36, no. 3 (1993): 249–264.

9. *Programme of Action of ICPD*, Arts. 4.27, 7.8, 7.14(e), 7.34, 7.41, 8.27. For example, Art. 4.27 reads, "Special efforts should be made to emphasize men's shared responsibility and promote their active involvement in responsible parenthood, sexual and reproductive behaviour, including family planning; prenatal, maternal and child health; prevention of sexually transmitted diseases, including HIV; prevention of unwanted and high-risk pregnancies . . ."

10. See M. Koblinsky, J. Timyan, and J. Gay, eds., *The Health of Women* (Boulder: Westview, 1993); and Robert Desjarlais et al., *World Mental Health* (New York: Oxford University Press, 1995), pp. 179–206.

11. Numazaki, "Haramaseru sei" [The self-responsibility of the impregnating sex].

12. I use the term "noncontraceptive sex" instead of "intravaginal ejaculation" because extravaginal ejaculation is not necessarily contraceptive.

13. Numazaki invokes a "vulnerability thesis" in support of the men's protection model. See Ichiro Numazaki, "The Moral Responsibility of the Impregnating Sex: An Autocritique of the Sexual and Reproductive Ethics of Men" (paper presented at the second international Feminist Approaches to Bioethics Conference, Japan, 1998).

14. Here I discuss only instances in which pregnancy has occurred because of the greater evidentiary difficulties where noncontraceptive sex has not resulted in pregnancy, although strictly speaking, forced noncontraceptive sex itself needs to be outlawed because it causes fear of pregnancy by women even if it does not actually result in pregnancy.

15. Where both men and women lack access to accurate knowledge on sexual and reproductive issues, dissemination of information would be necessary before the law is brought into force.

16. BDPA, Art. 99, states, "They (adolescent girls and young women) often do not have the power to insist on safe and responsible sex practices and have little access to information and services for prevention and treatment. Women, who represent half of all adults newly infected with HIV/AIDS and other sexually transmitted diseases, have emphasized that social vulnerability and the unequal power relationships between women and men are obstacles to safe sex, in their efforts to control the spread of sexually transmitted diseases."

17. Boys and young men need to be educated at an early age about the possibility of their harming women by noncontraceptive sex, so that they would not face legal sanction unknowingly.

18. Here I am considering how the social situation can be changed in Japan. Using the above mentioned vulnerability criterion, Japan should choose the first formulation based on (5) and the second stricter formulation based on (1) and (6) (transitional state on [2], [3], [4]). In Japan, abortion is still a criminal act but is allowed under a broad interpretation of "physical or economic reasons." See the Penal Code, Arts. 212–216 and the Maternal Protection Law (former Eugenic Protection Law), Art. 14.1. The spouse's consent is required for abortion, (Maternal Protection Law, Art. 14) although in practice no inquiry is made as to who signed the consent as a spouse. The rate of contraception use is reported as 60–70 percent, with the most common contraceptive being male condoms (70–80 percent). See Teruko Inoue and Yumiko Ehara, eds., *Women's Data Book* (Tokyo: Yuhikaku, 1995), p. 69. Low-dose contraceptive pills were not available for women with the official reason that releasing of the pill might increase the prevalence of HIV/AIDS. The pill was finally approved for use in late 1999 after criticism of the differential and quick approval of Viagra. According to the official record, the number of abortions is gradually decreasing, but still about 340,000 abortions are carried out a year (338,867 in 1996). For the overview of maternal and child health in Japan, see Naoko T. Miyaji and Margaret Lock, "Monitoring Motherhood: Sociocultural and Historical Aspects of Maternal and Child Health in Japan," *Daedalus* 123, no. 4 (1994): 87–112.

19. Genetic diagnosis of the fetus is now much debated, and methods of determining the father-child biological link are already commercially available in many developed countries. Careful monitoring and regulation of such commercial activity may be necessary with respect to access to the information analyzed.

20. Development of antisperm vaccination as a contraceptive is a good example of this bias, since it is safer and simpler to kill sperm than to create a vaccination against it.

21. This also applies to rape. Most of the time, couples understand each other's consent through interpretation of nonverbal communication. The problem arises when the gap between the two partners' interpretations is large.

22. Anita L. Allen, "Privacy in Health Care," in Warren T. Reich, ed., *Encyclopedia of Bioethics* (New York: Simon & Schuster/Macmillan, 1995).

23. One of the possible forms of the state's abuse of the law envisioned here would be disallowing some types of men, I would call them "vulnerable men," to become fathers based on their socioeconomic and educational level.

24. Frances E. Olsen, "The Myth of State Intervention in the Family," *University of Michigan Journal of Law Reform* 18, no. 4 (1985): 835–864.

25. See Elisabeth Badinter, *L'Amour en plus* (Flammarion: 1980); Donna Bassin, Margaret Honey, and Meryle Mahrer Kaplan, eds., *Representation of Motherhood* (New Haven: Yale University Press, 1994); and Jane Swigart, *Myth of the Bad Mother: The Emotional Realities of Mothering* (New York: Doubleday, 1991).

26. The recent Czech film *Kolya* is intriguing in this sense. A middle-aged man who has enjoyed being single and never thought of raising children is left with a stranger's child. His sudden new circumstance leads to communication and an emotional bond with the child, and he ends up discovering that his responsibilities are meaningful, even joyful.

27. U.N. Development Program, *Gender and Development: The Human Development Report* (Oxford: Oxford University Press, 1995). The WHO Regional Office for the Western Pacific (WPRO) proposes to "gender disaggregate all data collected and collated by WPRO and develop gender sensitive and gender specific indicators of health." See WPRO, *Women in Development: A Position Paper* (Manila, 1997), p. 27.

10

"So Bitter That No Words Can Describe It": Mainland Chinese Women's Moral Experiences and Narratives of Abortion

As I see it, ethical inquiries that fail to address the various and rich moral experiences of individuals are meaningless. If feminist bioethicists want to do significant work, they must be attentive to the diverse moral experiences of women in different cultures, classes, and social statuses; and they must listen carefully to individuals' life stories and narratives. In this chapter, I report the results of my efforts to be an attentive feminist listener. As part of a larger study on attitudes about abortion in contemporary mainland China, I conducted semistructured interviews with thirty mainland Chinese women who had had abortions. What follows is a detailed summary of five of these interviews, some general points about all thirty of them, and the results of several surveys I conducted on abortion while I was in mainland China. Since my approach is humanistic rather than scientific, interpretive rather than analytic, descriptive rather than prescriptive, sympathetic rather than judgmental, phenomenological rather than positivistic, what follows is not an "objective" report but the "subjective" account of one witness—me—to the moral world of abortion in China.[1]

Five Women's Personal Accounts

Qianqian's Story

One of my friends and her colleague, Zichuan (Purple Cuckoo), ushered Qianqian (Beautiful One)[2] into a medical school office for her in-

terview with me. She was about twenty-five years old. Her height was
in the upper-middle range and her figure was definitely more slender
than the average. Her voice was pleasing to the ear and had a soothing
effect. After listening to her talk for a few minutes, I could tell that she,
like many other Chinese women, had a talent for oral narration. As
soon as my friend's colleague introduced Qianqian to me, she and my
friend signaled that they were about to leave the office. But Qianqian
stopped them and said, "It would be no problem at all for me if you
want to stay. Actually, I welcome listeners." So they stayed, and their
encouraging comments and light jokes helped to transform what could
have been a painful interview into a chat among three or four old
friends.

Qianqian began her story:

> It was early April. I was just married. We used the safe period and condom
> for contraception. I was very healthy before. But that month I felt a bit un-
> well all the time. Therefore, I took various kinds of medicine. Soon, I real-
> ized that I was pregnant. From magazines and books, I realized that some
> of the medicines I had taken should not be used during pregnancy. I went
> to the hospital to consult with a doctor at the OB/GYN Department. If the
> doctor had said, "no problem," we would have had the child. But he said
> there *might* be a problem; and so because the population policy allows
> only one child per couple, we had to think about *yousheng* (good birth or
> eugenics).

With thoughts of *yousheng* in her head, Qianqian started to fear giving
birth to an unhealthy child, pondering how sad it would be if her only
child was unhealthy. But she could not decide by herself whether to have
an abortion. She discussed the issue many times with her husband and
her parents-in-law. She consulted not only doctors but also some friends
and colleagues. Finally, she and her family reached a decision to terminate the pregnancy.

For Qianqian, like almost every other Chinese woman who has had an
abortion, the experience can be characterized by the Chinese phrase *kegu
mingxin* (having been engraved on one's bones and heart). Qianqian referred to the aborted fetus as *wode erzhi* (my son), noting that she often
thought about the fetus (him) after the abortion.

> When the abortion was nearly done, it was so painful that I was almost in
> shock. The doctor let me see the bloody tissue. I watched the aborted fetus.
> It looked like a roll of fine air. I sighed, "Oh, my poor son. How miserable
> you are!" I described what I saw to my husband several times. When our
> mood was not too bad, we cracked a joke or made some dismissive remark

about the whole event. But I still think about my son's fate. For all I know he would have been very smart—perhaps the smartest child I could ever bear. But he is gone.

Asked why she used the term "my son" and not "my daughter," she replied that "son" was just a general word for the fetus: "I do not regard men as superior to women. Personally, I would prefer to have a girl." But then she acknowledged that despite her own preference, she had actually wanted to have a boy for the sake of her parents-in-law and her husband. Although Qianqian grieved and mourned her aborted fetus as though she had lost someone extremely special and precious, she said that she would probably feel much worse had she lost a child.

Qianqian's abortion constituted a turning point in her life. After the abortion, she felt her girlhood was gone—that she was now a woman. In many ways she regretted the sudden imposition of "womanhood" upon her, with all its heavy responsibilities:

When I was a girl, I was a naive fool. I had no anxieties and no worries. I wore all kinds of beautiful dresses. There were always boys after me. They gave me a lot of attention. When I got married, I was even happier than before. My husband, who is eight years older than I am, took care of every aspect of my life. Every day was full of sunlight. But the abortion made me lose a lot of my joy and happiness.

For Qianqian, the most significant source of her new worries and anxieties is her fear that she will be unable to bear a healthy child—the number one duty for a woman in Chinese society. Facing increased pressure for a healthy child from her husband and her parents-in-law, Qianqian said she was worried about meeting the expectations of society as well as pleasing her loved ones: she expressed concern that unless she got pregnant soon people in general would say that she was a failure as a woman, that is, a woman unable "to bear a healthy child." As a result, Qianqian felt that she needed to attend to her own health, which had never been very good but became much worse after the abortion. She felt she had to get physically and psychologically stronger in order to produce a healthy child and had to avoid future abortions if at all possible. In her own words, "Abortion is not like going through a cold. In the future, I will be very, very careful about contraception. You really cannot be too careful about this." Stressing how fortunate and grateful she was for the care and love her husband had given her during the abortion process, Qianqian nonetheless made it clear that, if she could help it, she would never have an abortion again: "The love of my husband was indispensable. He was so caring for me that he even washed my underwear after I had the abortion. Without his love, I might not have been able to bear it. However," she added, "no matter how much your husband and family members love you, no one can experience the pain *for* you. I must suffer it by myself."

Yingying's Story

Because mainland Chinese women do not use makeup except for some special occasions, such as parties or wedding ceremonies, the fact that Yingying (Oriole) had some light makeup on her face signaled to me that she was an exceptionally fashionable young woman. I interviewed Yingying while she waited for an IUD insertion—the most common method of contraception for married women in China. Although she and her boyfriend had obtained a marriage license, they had not had an official wedding ceremony yet. Nevertheless, Yingying addressed her boyfriend as *laogong* (the old man)—a term that wives in the North commonly use to refer to their husbands, especially in public. Previously, her *laogong* had asked her to have an IUD inserted, but she had not listened. Subsequently she got pregnant and had to have an abortion. The experience motivated Yingying not to make the same mistake twice and to protect herself from future unwanted pregnancies.

Yingying had an abortion because she and her boyfriend believed they were not ready for a child. She said that among her many college classmates no one had yet had a child. She compared having a child to "being fastened on a rope." For her and her boyfriend, a child would require all their attention and full responsibility. But it never occurred to them to remain childless to escape these burdens. Indeed, Yingying commented that "every family must have a child. Otherwise, life would be too boring." Moreover, she considered it better for the child to have a brother or sister. "Ideally speaking, one boy and one girl is the best. I cannot imagine how boring my parents' life would be now if they did not have any sisters or brothers."

When I asked her how she felt after her abortion, Yingying replied, "I felt *neijiu* (guilty conscience or compunction)." And when I further asked, "To whom?" she replied without thinking, "To the aborted child, of course." She continued: "It was really too cruel. He or she should have been able to be born but was destroyed by her or his own parents." Sometimes, but not very often, she said she thought of the aborted fetus. She occasionally made jokes—sad humor—with her boyfriend that, when they had a child in the future, she would tell that child that he or she would never have been born if she had not had the earlier abortion. "How absurd life is!" Yingying sighed heavily.

Jinglian's Story

Jinglian (the Golden Lotus) had two abortions because she already had one child—the only child she wanted. She explained that if she had two children, she would have to "split her heart into two parts," a state of affairs she could not abide. Particularly sensitive to pain in a society in which women generally report having a hard time bearing even small discomforts, Jinglian described her two abortions as exceptionally painful. In addition, she described these abortions as extraordinarily emotional experiences because she found it difficult to part with her aborted fetuses *(heng kexi)*, viewing them as *maomao*—one of the Chinese phrases commonly used to refer to infants and very young children.

Because Jinglian had a different doctor for each of her two abortions, she was well aware of how much difference it makes for a woman to have an empathetic doctor instead of a unkind, even cruel doctor:

> Some doctors are good; some are very bad. I had my first abortion at the People's Hospital in this city. Because the machine had some problems, the doctors got angry at me. When they performed the abortion, they said some very bad words about me, such as my getting pregnant due to *bu zhenjing* (an affair or extramarital sex, literally this phrase means "not being right" or "not being normal"). They implied that I deserved all the pain. The second time, I had the abortion at a much smaller clinic. The doctors' manners were very good. Before, during, and after performing the abortion, they asked many questions with deep concern and sincere care. I felt much less pain.

In addition, expressing considerable unhappiness with her husband, Jinglian commented that if a husband does not stand by his wife when she really needs his support, "the couple's emotional relationship will be harmed and become unharmonious." Women, implied Jinglian, should not tolerate such neglect from men.

Cuihua's Story

Cuihua (Jade Flower), the mother of one female child, was a biomedical research technician at a medical school. I conducted my interview with her at her place of employment, a biochemistry lab. She had had two abortions—the first due to an abnormality in the fetus and the second, to China's "one-child" population policy. The first time she went to the hospital with her husband; the second time with her mother. She described her first abortion, which had been a surgical one, as painful and bitter. She tried a chemical abortion the second time in hope of avoiding the pain of a surgical abortion. However, the drug was not effective and, once again, she had to submit to a surgical abortion.

Cuihua's two abortions led her to reflect on the fate of being a woman in China. She said her experiences had made her recognize more clearly that "to be a woman is really miserable." Cuihua also expressed sadness that her daughter would have to share her sorry lot in life, claiming that when she had given birth to her daughter she had felt "really sad and terrible" because her daughter would "have to suffer the various pains and bitternesses I do."

Cuihua claimed her abortions had actually damaged her health. "After the abortions, my health was not as good as before. My constitution became weak and fragile. I now catch colds often. Whenever my daughter has a cold, I have one too. I coughed an entire summer in the year following the second abortion." One can only speculate whether her physical health problems directly resulted from her abortions or whether they were somatized symptoms originating from her own experience of suffering as a woman, or both.

On being asked about her feeling toward the aborted fetuses, Cuihua gave a negative answer. "I have no particular feeling. Anyhow, I was not able to have these children. I never think of the aborted fetuses." She seemed to realize that she differed from most other women and thus added, "A colleague of mine aborted a son and cried in great grief. But I was fine [with the aborted fetus]."

Xiaoyan's Story

Xiaoyan (the Little Colorful) was in her forties and had had three abortions after giving birth to a girl. All the medical costs were reimbursed in her *danwei* (the work unit). She explained the three abortions as follows: the first time, no birth permit; the second and third times, contraceptive failure. But having no birth permit was the real reason for all three abortions. Although she and her husband desired to have at least one more child, and although they toyed with the idea of violating state policy, they always came to the conclusion that defying the state policy was not worth the negative consequences of doing so.

All three of Xiaoyan's abortions were performed when the fetus was about fifty days old. Xiaoyan said that she had had four children—her living daughter and her three aborted fetuses. She called her aborted fetuses *xiao wawa* (the little children), observing that she often thought about "how old they would now be if they had been born."

Xiaoyan was satisfied with the medical service she received. She stressed that unlike the typical Chinese woman, she had felt no pain at all during her abortions, partly as a result of her doctors' kind manners.

> Since the doctors were my friends or acquaintances, they were very caring to me. They talked with me about various light topics. Their manners were very good and amiable. Affable manners can help a woman get through the abortion procedure. It is horrible when the doctors' manners are bad. Doctors should be especially caring and amiable if the woman has an abortion not because she wants to, but because of the "one-child" policy.

Women's Reasons for Having an Abortion

The twenty-seven mainland Chinese women whom I interviewed had many reasons for their abortion decisions. Listed in order of decreasing frequency, their reasons included the following:

1. The population policy did not allow the pregnancy to continue (13)
   - interval was not long enough (five years after first child) (3)
   - had not reached the required age (23.5 years) (2)
   - had no birth permit because of having had one or two children (2)
   - was not married (1)
2. My living conditions did not allow for a child (8)
   - family economy was not stable or not good enough (4)
   - family condition was not good (2)
   - no decent living place (2)
3. Did not want the child (8)
4. Failed contraception (6)
5. Still young and wanted to *wan* (enjoy, play) for more years (3)
6. Problems with the fetus (3)
7. Some medicine taken during early pregnancy might cause fetal defects (3)
8. Current work too demanding (3)
9. Wanted to bear a child later (2)
   - at age twenty-six or twenty-seven (2)
   - at nearly thirty years of age (1)
10. Meet the call of the country (government) (2)
11. Not married yet (2)
12. Feeling that a child would be a burden (1)

In general, the women I interviewed offered several reasons for their decision to have an abortion. For example, one university graduate student gave at least three reasons for her abortion. She explained:

> I do not want to have a child too early. I would prefer to have my first child when I am twenty-six or twenty-seven years old. I want to *qin-shong* (relax) for several more years. Moreover, I took many medicines before I knew I was pregnant; I even received an infusion. Those medicines may have had a bad impact on fetal development.

A second university graduate student said she became pregnant because her methods of contraception—the rhythm method and the condom—failed. For her, abortion was the elimination of a child neither she nor her husband wanted to have.

> We have been married for less than one year. We could have gotten a birth permit, but we really do not want to have a child right away. We are too young. Moreover, our living and economic conditions are not good enough. We want to be child free for several more years. I would prefer to have my first child when I am near thirty years old. Although my husband wanted this child, and although he was concerned that the abortion procedure might damage my health, I persuaded him that abortion was in our best interests.

The more I talked to women like the ones above, the more I realized that Chinese women mean very different things when they say that they had an abortion because the state population policy would not permit them to have a child. Some women mean that they would have carried the pregnancy to term had it not been for the state policy. Others mean that they agree with the state policy and that they had not really meant to get pregnant. Many of these women attribute their pregnancies to failed contraceptive methods. Yet others use the state policy as an excuse to hide—particularly from husbands, boyfriends, parents, and in-laws—the fact that they themselves don't want a child or, less frequently, the fact that the fetus is a result of illegitimate sex.

Contrary to common Western perceptions, my survey indicated that most Chinese women support the government's population policy. What is more, and also contrary to common Western perceptions, most of the women I interviewed did not want large families. If Chinese women object to any feature of the policy, it is that it does not permit every woman, rural or urban, to decide whether *one* or *two* children is best for her family. Unable to obtain a birth permit for a second child, one woman said this about her abortion:

If I had been able to get a birth permit, I would not have aborted the child. I like the idea that every family should have two children. In that way, each of them has a companion. They can help each other. If we, the parents, need their help, they can discuss with each other how to resolve our problems. Although three or four children in each family are too many, I do not think that two children per family are too many.

Although this woman and most of the women I interviewed expressed a preference for two children rather than one child, it seems that more and more people, even in the countryside, want only one child. A village woman in her middle twenties said she would prefer to have one child only so that she could provide the child with the best education available. Of course, whether this young woman will actually have only one child is not a foregone conclusion. She may face great pressure from her husband, her parents, her in-laws, and her peers to have two children.

A village woman in her late forties had four abortions in the late 1970s, two after having the first child and two after having the second one. According to her, the state population policy was quite permissive at that time. She claimed that it would have been no problem for her to have four or five children if she had wanted to do so. But she and her husband found that two children were sufficient for them. She remarked, "Why do people want so many children? The other people in my village needed *shixiang gongzhou* (ideological work or policy education or persuasion) [to convince them to follow the policy]. But I never needed that at all." Her tone and gesture indicated feelings of pride that she, unlike her fellow villages, was an enlightened woman who could recognize that it is in people's best interests to have small rather than large families.

Finally, and also contrary to common Western perceptions, no woman whom I interviewed said that sex preference, especially preference for a boy, was her reason for having an abortion. What's more, 86 percent of the people I surveyed said that a woman should not have an abortion if the couple "knows that the fetus is male, but they want to have a girl." And 88 percent said that a woman should not have an abortion if the couple "knows that the fetus is female, but they want to have a boy." Although my survey is a limited one, it does suggest that a remarkable percentage of literate Chinese persons agree with the official prohibition on using abortion for sex selection. Only between 12 and 14 percent of the persons I surveyed would want to abort a fetus that was the "wrong sex."

Women's Major Concerns About Abortion

The abortion experience is a memorable event for most Chinese women, but for varying reasons. For some women the worst part of the abortion experience is the procedure itself. This is evident in the remarks of a very shy thirty-year-old woman whom I interviewed at her doctor's office. At the beginning of the interview, she was reluctant to speak. She said that she had nothing to say. But after her doctor encouraged her to try to answer my questions, she agreed to voice her feelings. She said that after having a son, she had had two abortions. Because she did not want a large family to support and educate, she went to the clinic willingly for an abortion each time she knew she was pregnant. For her the worst part of both abortions, particularly the second one, was the physical pain. She described how she felt during her second abortion in a particularly intense way: "My heart sunk. My *qi* (energy) would not come up."

A very successful and fashionable businesswoman in her late twenties or early thirties echoed the feelings of the shy woman. She used three phrases to describe her abortion experience: *tongbu yusheng* (so painful that she did not want to live), *kubu kangyang* (so bitter that no words can describe it), and *ciqing cijing, jiyi youxin* (that scene and that sight will always remain fresh in my memory).

Since early-stage induced abortion is usually practiced without anesthesia, many Chinese women suffer enormous physical pain, as is evident in several of the previous stories. A university graduate in her early twenties vividly described the pain that accompanies an abortion, and how desperately she needed the presence of her husband or any family member during the process. She strongly opposed the hospital policy that does not permit support people in the operating room, insisting that women need as many comforting touches and words as possible during the abortion procedure.

Over and beyond fear of pain, one of the major concerns of Chinese women is that the abortion procedure will damage their reproductive health and/or general health (fertility). A woman who was waiting for an abortion commented to me:

> I am most concerned about the safety of the abortion operation. I chose to come to this big hospital just due to considerations of safety. I hope there will be not be an incomplete abortion *(buwanchuan liuchan)*. I really worry whether the abortion will be very painful, and whether it will affect my ability to have a child in the future, and whether it will worsen my health. After the abortion, I hope the physician will guide me and tell me how to take care of myself. For example, I want to know what diet to follow in order to regain my strength.

Another woman described her feelings about abortion in these words:

I am somewhat scared. I am afraid of the pain, but I am especially afraid that the abortion will damage my future reproductive capacity. It is said that abortion makes many women barren. In the school at which I teach, one woman became sterile because of abortion.

Few women initially mentioned their feelings about the aborted fetus. Among the nineteen women who responded to being asked whether they thought of the aborted fetus after abortion, fourteen (74 percent) said that they never thought about the aborted fetus. One woman asked me, "Why should I think about it [the fetus]?" She noted that she did not feel anything when she parted with the aborted fetus because "there was no use feeling badly about something that couldn't be otherwise." Another woman, who had had an abortion very early in the first trimester, said she rarely thought of the aborted fetus, since "it was not formed yet [like a human being]. If I had to experience induced birth [the late abortion], my feelings might have been very different."

However, some women did think of the aborted fetus after their abortions, as indicated in several of the stories presented above. In fact, 26 percent of the women I interviewed said they had thought about the aborted fetus. One woman and her husband found it particularly difficult to make the decision to terminate the pregnancy. Although the wife viewed the fetus as "a growing life" in her, she felt that she had to abort it because she took a lot of medicine before realizing it could harm the fetus. She noted, however, that she would have continued the pregnancy if the population policy had permitted them to have two children. To have an *unhealthy* child as one's *only* child would be very difficult—indeed a tragedy.

Personal Reflections

Clearly, Chinese women's experiences of abortion are so rich, complex, and different from one another that any single, overarching generalization about these experiences will unavoidably distort their individual uniqueness. The narratives and stories of the women who have experienced abortions should speak for themselves. Nevertheless, hearers of these narratives and stories will, understandably, seek to interpret them. My fear is that my interpretations of these stories and narratives will fail to capture their cultural complexity and their profound humanity.

Nevertheless, I would like to make a general comment regarding Chinese women's moral experience of abortion. Although women's moral experiences of abortion share some transcultural similarities, important cultural differences remain. A rough comparison of American women's and Chinese women's abortion experiences illustrate how similarly and how differently women experience abortion from one culture to another. A century and a half ago, Henry C. Wright wrote a book entitled *The Un-welcome Child: Or, the Crime of an Undesigned and Undesired Maternity*, in which he published letters from women recounting their abortions. Most of the women who wrote these letters said that they "hated"[3] having to abort their fetuses. Some condemned themselves for having no other choice than to "murder" their fetus:

> I consulted a woman, a friend in whom I trusted. I found that she had per-petrated that outrage on herself and on others. She told me it was not mur-der to kill a child any time before its birth. Of this she labored to convince me, and called in the aid of her "family physician," to give force to her argu-ments. He argued that it was right and just for wives thus to protect them-selves against the results of their husband's sensualism,—told me that God and human laws would approve of killing children before they were born, rather than curse them with an undesired existence. My only trouble was, with God's view of the case, I could not get rid of the feeling that it was an outrage on my body and soul, and on my unconscious babe. He argued that my child, at five month (which was the time), had no life, and where there was no life, no life could be taken. Though I determined to do the deed, or get the "family physician" to do it, my womanly instincts, my reason, my conscience, my self-respect, my entire nature, revolted against my decision. My Womanhood rose up in withering condemnation.[4]

Contemporary American women who have abortions are as conflicted about abortion as their nineteenth-century contemporaries. In Carol Gilligan's study of women going through abortion, Sandra, a twenty-nine-year-old Catholic nurse, reports that she had always thought of abortion, as well as euthanasia, as a "fancy" word for murder. The sec-ond time she became pregnant, she found that "keeping the child for lots and lots of reasons was just sort of impractical and out." She had only two options: terminating the pregnancy or giving up the child for adop-tion. She had previously given up a child for adoption and found that "there was no way that I could hack another adoption. There was just no way I was going through it again." Yet continuing the pregnancy would hurt her parents as well as damage herself. Sandra explained why she de-cided to have an abortion in these words: "I am doing it because I have to do it. I am not doing it the least bit because I want to." For her, "abortion is morally wrong, but the situation is right." So she had an abortion.[5]

For most Chinese women who have had abortions, however, abortion is a bitter experience not so much because they feel they are committing murder (though, as we saw, many Chinese women regret destroying an entity they view as a child that might have been) but because they fear they might be jeopardizing their reproductive health and, therefore, their ability to fulfill what they view as their essential womanly duties. Indeed,

> Chinese women's abortion experiences cannot be properly understood and interpreted without addressing the mainstream Chinese definition of womanhood. If the individual has not usually been highly valued in Chinese society and culture, the woman in China has been especially devalued. The character of "*fu*" (woman) in the traditional way of writing, which has been used for at least more than two thousand years, consists of two parts: "*nu*" (female) on the left and "*zhou*" (broom) on the right. It thus means that the woman's place is domestic and that her social role is to submit to and serve men. The traditional term for a woman to address herself to the other is "*lu*" (slave). Until the early part of this century, Chinese women had not only been spiritually and morally fettered by the Confucian definition of womanhood—i.e., the "three obediences" (to father before marriage, to husband after marriage, to son after the death of husband), and the "four virtues" (woman's morality, proper speech, modest manner and diligent work), they had also been physically bound through practices such as foot-binding.[6]

In this century, especially since the establishment of the People's Republic in 1949, the social role and economic position of Chinese women have undergone many dramatic and positive changes. Chinese women's feet have been liberated, and the Confucian ideology of the "three obediences and four virtues" has been seriously criticized. Yet Chinese girls and women continue to experience gender inequality and discrimination.[7] The dominant understanding of womanhood in contemporary China is not much different from the dominant understanding of womanhood in traditional China. First, the individual woman, like the individual man, must subordinate herself to state, society, country, and collective. Second, the ideal woman should be a *xianqi liangmu* (virtuous wife and good mother). The characters of being a good woman include being considerate, kind, good-tempered, physically beautiful, and so on. But the most important requirement for a woman is still to bear and raise two healthy children (in the countryside) or one healthy child (in the city). Consequently, Chinese women who do not have the requisite number of healthy children view abortion as a risk factor—something that might damage their status as women as well as their reproductive capacity.

Notes

1. Jing-Bao Nie, "Voices Behind the Silence: Chinese Moral Views and Experiences of Abortion," (Ph.D. diss., University of Texas Medical Branch at Galveston,

1999). This is the first in-depth academic effort in any language, including Chinese, that explores contemporary mainland Chinese people's moral understanding of induced abortion. It is built on a pilot study that includes the following subjects: thirty Chinese students and scholars currently living in the United States; a survey with 601 subjects and twelve samples conducted in mainland China; intensive interviews with thirty doctors who routinely perform abortions and thirty women who had abortions; some fragmented personal experiences I had while living in China; and a brief historical review of traditional Chinese perspectives on abortion and policy change in the People's Republic of China. I am developing this thesis into a book.

2. In order to protect privacy and for the sake of confidentiality, the names of all the subjects mentioned in this chapter have been changed. All identifying individual and geographic information has been omitted.

3. Quoted in James C. Mohr, *Abortion in America: The Origins and Evolution of National Policy, 1800–1900* (Oxford: Oxford University Press, 1978), p. 110.

4. Mohr, *Abortion in America*, p. 111.

5. Carol Gilligan, *In a Different Voice: Psychological Theory and Women's Development* (Cambridge: Harvard University Press, 1993), pp. 85–86.

6. For contemporary historical studies on women in premodern China, see, for example, Francesca Bray, *Technology and Gender: Fabrics of Power in Late Imperial China* (Berkeley: University of California Press, 1997); Richard Cuisso and Stanley Johnnesen, eds., *Women in China: Current Directions in Historical Scholarship* (New York: Philo, 1981); and T'ung-tsu Ch'u, *Law and Society in Traditional China* (Paris: Mounton, 1961).

7. On the conditions of women in contemporary China in the English language, see, for example, Christina K. Gilmartin et al., eds., *Engendering China: Women, Culture, and the State* (Cambridge: Harvard University Press, 1994); Emily Honig and Gail Hershatter, *Personal Voices: Chinese Women in the 1980s* (Stanford: Stanford University Press, 1988); Margery Wolf, *Revolution Postponed: Women in Contemporary China* (Stanford: Stanford University Press, 1985); and Margery Wolf and Roxane Witke, eds., *Women in Chinese Society* (Stanford: Stanford University Press, 1975).

11

Cultural Differences
and Sex Selection

MARY MAHOWALD

Health care decisions are often affected by the values and disvalues of the different ethnic groups or cultural milieux in which individuals find themselves. Although men as well as women experience these influences, the gender roles imputed to them are usually both different and unequal. Most cultures assume and reinforce a dominant role for men and a nondominant role for women. A key question thus arises for clinicians who wish to respect the autonomy of women: whether decisions that reflect the same priorities as their culture or ethnic group are truly autonomous. As practiced throughout the world, sex selection raises this question also for feminists who wish to promote gender justice while respecting cultural differences. Different versions of feminism support different responses to the question.

Although feminists concur in opposing gender injustice, our standpoints differ according to the version of feminism to which each of us subscribes. The standpoint from which I develop this chapter is an egalitarian version of feminism—one that gives priority to equality as a social ideal. The ideal, I believe, can be best approximated by respecting differences in gender, race, ability, class, sexuality, culture, and ethnicity while insisting that the individuals who embody these differences are equal to one another. To the extent that differences are associated with gender injustice, an egalitarian version of feminism demands efforts to reduce inequality between women and men.

In this chapter, then, I address the dilemma of respect for autonomy versus respect for cultural values from the perspective of egalitarian feminism. While acknowledging the moral relevance of both principles, I argue against an absolute stance with regard to either. Respect for autonomy and respect for cultural differences may be and ought to be simultaneously affirmed to the extent that they are compatible with justice. The practice of sex selection, I maintain, is morally defensible so long as neither its intent nor its impact entails gender inequality or sexism. If either its intent or its impact is sexist, the practice is morally objectionable to anyone who supports an egalitarian theory of justice.

Respect for Autonomy Versus
Respect for Cultural Differences

Respect for autonomy is a cardinal principle of contemporary medical ethics. It is usually linked with the principles of beneficence, nonmaleficence, and justice as basic to ethical decisionmaking in the clinical setting.[1] However, while it is generally assumed that people are or can be autonomous, just what autonomy means, and whether people really are autonomous, are matters of controversy. In health care, it is often assumed as well that the obligation to respect autonomy is equivalent to the obligation to obtain informed consent from patients for testing or treatment. The latter assumption seems to ignore the fact that health care decisions involve others besides patients. In the health care setting, decisions also involve health care givers and family members and may involve patients who are not autonomous. If respect for autonomy is a moral principle, it requires respect for the autonomy of all individuals; additional principles are applicable to nonautonomous individuals.

The notion of *respect* is also subject to different interpretations.[2] To some it simply means "paying attention to" or "taking account of." To others, respect means something more demanding, such as "giving priority to" or "acting in accordance with." The latter meaning would make respect for autonomy not only a cardinal principle but the supreme principle of bioethics. A less demanding interpretation allows that respect for autonomy is one among other principles of bioethics, all of which represent prima facie rather than supreme or absolute obligations. When respect for cultural differences is considered, the same interpretations of the term are applicable. If respect is to be tendered to both autonomy and cultural differences, however, only the less demanding interpretation is possible. If the more demanding interpretation is operable, respect for cultural differences is incompatible with respect for individual autonomy.

Although the foregoing discussion has assumed that respect for autonomy and respect for cultural differences are distinct expressions of respect, it is possible to view the two as identical. Respect for autonomy is equivalent to, or overlaps with, respect for cultural differences for individuals who autonomously conform to the value systems that their cultures embody. Unless we subscribe to cultural determinism, however, we need to confront the fact that individuals can and occasionally do freely diverge from cultural dictates or expectations. The history of the women's movement throughout the world is replete with examples of women doing just that. Fortunately, culturally sanctioned atrocities have always been challenged by individuals who act in accordance with conscience in opposition to cultural expectations or norms.

Assuming, then, that cultural values and practices are at least occasionally in conflict with the values and practices that individuals choose for themselves, we still need to ask what it means for them to make autonomous choices. The meaning of autonomy, as already suggested, is notoriously controversial and complex.[3] Minimally, it refers to the *capacity* of individuals to choose, which entails cognitive and volitional abilities that are not equally present or always present in all individuals. Maximally, autonomy also requires the ability to implement one's choices, which is often equated with freedom or liberty.[4] In other words, both internal and external resources are necessary to fulfill one's chosen goals.[5] To some extent, albeit paradoxically, the maximal meaning of autonomy involves dependence on those who provide or constitute such resources. Across the globe, as influenced by different cultural expectations and practices, this dependence varies considerably.

An egalitarian feminist standpoint subscribes to a prima facie rather than an absolute obligation to respect autonomy, acknowledging the importance of beneficence and nonmaleficence as additional prima facie obligations. Justice is the principle that mediates conflicts that arise in applications of the other principles. With regard to gender, as also with regard to race, class, sexual orientation, and ability, justice demands more than a minimal but less than a maximal conception of autonomy. In the fulfillment of obligations arising from beneficence and nonmaleficence, justice requires a distribution scheme that respects different needs and abilities, regardless of whether the recipients are autonomous.

Limitations to autonomy arise not only from differences in cognitive and volitional ability but also from different physical, educational, and economic abilities in potential decisionmakers, as well as in the information provided to them with regard to possible choices. While supporting the principle of respect for autonomy, gender justice goes farther than a minimal conception of autonomy because it requires attention to the limitations on autonomy that may be imposed on women both internally and externally.[6] The goal of gender justice is to reduce these limitations as much as possible, recognizing that discrepancies between the advantaged and the disadvantaged will remain. In most instances the gap between men and women or between other dominant and nondominant groups can only be narrowed by reducing the advantages of the dominant over the nondominant. In other words, men's advantages are inevitably lessened to the extent that women's are increased. This goal involves equality of respect for autonomy[7] as well as equality in the distribution of burdens and benefits. Conflicts between or among the principles of respect for autonomy, beneficence, and nonmaleficence are thus mediated through the principle of justice.

Although respect for cultural differences may be construed as respect for the autonomy of different cultures, that construal does not settle the question of whether the autonomy of an individual can or should be respected when it is at odds with the culture's "autonomy." At that point, it may be argued that the good defined by the culture is greater than the good defined by the individual whose decision is in conflict with a particular cultural value or practice. This argument is supportable on quantitative grounds, but it is hardly defensible on moral grounds. Unless we subscribe to a crude (and cruel) form of utilitarianism, few of us would support the notion that might makes right, even if might is defined by numbers alone.[8] The view that "cultural autonomy" supersedes individual autonomy is also defensible on grounds that the stability of a group is thereby maintained. Again, however, stability is not a good in its own right. Destabilization of a culture whose values or practices are morally questionable is in fact more desirable than maintaining its stability by overriding the autonomy of dissident members.

That said, the stability of a culture whose values and practices are generally moral and supportive of the majority of its members is probably a greater good than respect for the autonomy of an individual member of that culture. An egalitarian feminist standpoint concurs that the good of the majority may at times supersede the good of the few. Moreover, where contrary indications are absent, respect for individual autonomy is more likely than not to accord with respect for the culture to which the individual belongs. In situations where it is difficult if not impossible to determine the extent to which a given individual autonomously embraces the values embodied by her culture, respect for cultural differences should ordinarily prevail. However, a significant caveat to this prevalence arises from the fact that most if not all individuals belong to several overlapping, sometimes conflicting cultures. Women themselves compose a cultural group within and beyond the ethnic cultures to which they also belong. It follows that respect for the cultural differences that women as a group embody is part of what it means to respect their cultural differences. So, although an egalitarian feminist standpoint resists absolutizing the autonomy of individual women, it insists on the necessity of respect for the specific cultural milieu of women as women. That milieu is in fact broader than the ethnic cultures in which women find themselves, where values and practices have mainly been defined by men.

Specific cultural practices that are detrimental to women are surely questioned by most of the world's women and by many men. Consider, for example, female circumcision and suttee, the practice by which widows throw themselves on the funeral pyres of their husbands.[9] Given the pressures of socialization and fears of censure or exclusion, it is doubtful that women from cultures that encourage or demand these practices participate in them with genuine or full autonomy, even when they purport to do so. Only a very thin notion of autonomy, one which identifies it with whatever someone says or does that is not physically coerced, or with "choices" between extremely constraining options, would support the view that consent to genital mutilation or suttee is genuinely autonomous.

Another culturally sanctioned practice involving gender is sex selection. This may occur either before or after fertilization. As we will see in the next section, different cultures offer very different rationales in support of this practice.

Sex Selection from an Egalitarian Feminist Standpoint

When embryos are tested for specific anomalies, the test usually reveals the sex of the organism, regardless of whether such information is sought for medical reasons. Even when the information is not medically relevant, however, whether sex selection is sexist depends on the meaning of sexism and the rationale for the selection. Whether it is ethically justified depends also on the means by which it is undertaken. Sexism may refer to a preference for one sex, usually male, when there is no morally adequate reason for the preference. In particular cases, the preference may be morally justified if it is based on overriding moral reasons, such as avoidance of serious harm to another or others. In other cases, the preference may be based on morally neutral criteria, such as the desire to have children of both sexes. Typically, however, sexism refers to a preference for one sex for morally inadequate reasons. The inadequate reasons generally involve a gender bias.

According to the *Oxford English Dictionary*, sexism is "the assumption that one sex is superior to the other and the resultant discrimination practiced against members of the supposed inferior sex, especially by men against women."[10] By that definition sexism is wrong because it denies the essential equality between men and women. If sex selection has no impact on sex inequality, it is not sexist and may be morally neutral; if it reduces inequality, it is morally commendable. From an egalitarian feminist standpoint, selection of males is more problematic than selection of females because it reaffirms or reinforces male dominance. But selection of females is not necessarily commendable or even morally neutral; other factors may make it morally questionable or wrong.[11]

Sexism has been supported by many if not most cultures throughout history, just as racism, classism, heterosexism, and ableism have been supported.[12] In other words, women throughout the world have prevalently been viewed as inferior to men and treated as such.[13] Moreover, the cultural prevalence of sexism has coexisted in many instances with an underlying consciousness in members of both sexes that women are and should be treated as equal to men. Globally, people have been aware that sexism is wrong, even while practicing it.

The rationale for sex selection is not sexist, although it may be ableist if it is based solely on medical indications, such as the 50 percent risk that a male fetus will have hemophilia if a pregnant woman is a carrier for the condition.[14] It is sexist if the intent is to avoid the conception or birth of a child judged inferior because of sex. For either rationale, however, the means by which sex selection is undertaken raises further moral questions and controversy, depending on whether it occurs before or after conception. Except for its association with sexism, sex selection prior to conception is relatively uncontroversial. Following conception, it may be morally objectionable or acceptable solely on grounds of one's position on abortion. Except for its tie with abortion, however, sex selection is not really a morally different issue after conception than it is before conception. Cultural opposition to abortion is compatible with cultural encouragement of preconception sex selection, and cultural permissiveness of abortion is apparently compatible with opposition to sex selection, whether prenatal or postnatal.

Lest it be thought that a preference for males is limited to developing countries, data from the United States show that 84 percent of couples who request sex selection want boys.[15] A recent survey of Canadians shows a much weaker preference for sons.[16] Nonetheless, studies of sex preference for children across the globe illustrate a stronger bias in favor of male offspring. Until recently, the various methods available, such as timing of intercourse, ovulation induction medications, and artificial insemination, were generally unsuccessful.[17] A better success rate has been reported from in vitro separation of X-bearing sperm and Y-bearing sperm by gradient techniques, but these methods have not been validated by molecular techniques or controlled clinical trials. Two new techniques have proved much more reliable: preimplantation genetic diagnosis and sperm separation by flow cytometry. The latter method is less expensive and less invasive than the former because it involves artificial insemination rather than in vitro fertilization. According to Benjamin Reubinoff and Joseph Schenker, through the increased availability of sperm separation by flow cytometry, preconception sex selection "for social purposes" is likely to be sought, offered, and utilized more widely.[18]

Subsequent to implantation, the sex of the embryo is determinable through chorionic villus sampling, amniocentesis, or ultrasound. Fetuses of the undesired sex, usually female, may then be terminated. In developing countries, the practice is often explicit, with ultrasound increasingly used for sex determination.[19] In developed nations, people sometimes manipulate a system that is mainly opposed to prenatal testing for sex selection by requesting prenatal diagnosis for another reason, such as maternal age. When informed of their test results, they are also told the sex of the fetus if they wish to know. If the fetus is not the desired sex, they then ask for termination of the pregnancy, to which they have a legal right. Although most genetic counselors oppose prenatal testing for sex selection, the number of those who support the client's right to sex selection has been increasing.[20]

Christine Overall argues that "sexual similarity" and "sexual complementarity" are morally acceptable reasons for wanting a child of a certain sex. She bases her argument on the significance of sexuality, both heterosexuality or homosexuality, to interpersonal relationships. Sexual similarity, she says, "is a likeness, an affinity, of experience and capacities—the groundedness of being with one's own kind. The notion of sexual complementarity, on the other hand . . . is not merely a matter of dissimilarity . . . [but also] the desire for the new, for what will change and enlarge one's own experience."[21]

In arguing for the moral legitimacy of sex selection on this basis, Overall exhibits a sensitivity to the uniqueness of human relationships with which most feminists would agree. Neither for her nor for other feminists, however, does this imply support for sex selection policies.

Although Overall generally favors involving men in various aspects of child care, she stops short of advocating the same degree of involvement by heterosexual partners in the sex selection of their children.[22] Through its emphasis on attention to relevant differences, an egalitarian feminism would not only stop short but would insist that one partner, the woman, has a stronger claim in this regard. Since it is the woman who carries the main burden of bringing a child into the world, and usually also the main burden of child rearing, the woman's preference regarding the sex of her offspring is more compelling (but not necessarily adequate) when compared with such a preference on the part of her male partner. This reasoning would also apply to a lesbian couple when the partners have different preferences regarding the sex of a future child. If both women plan to share child rearing, the woman who would undergo insemination, gestation, and birth has the stronger claim regarding the sex of the child.

If the practice of sex selection led to numerical predominance of one sex over another, such a result would not necessarily be inegalitarian. It is at least possible for relationships between members of a numerical minority and majority to be fair and equal. It is also possible for a minority group to be politically stronger and to form an economic majority despite its numerical minority. So even if sex selection led to a majority of males in the population, as it has in parts of China, India, and Korea,[23] it does not necessarily follow that subjugation of women to men would thereby be supported or intensified. Nonetheless, the threat of increased sexism remains a matter of concern to those interested in promoting a feminist standpoint.

Ironically, another argument arises from the egalitarian feminist claims that women have historically been oppressed and such oppression is morally wrong. Both claims are relevant to the issue of sex determination. Consider, for example, the following rationale on the part of the potential mother, who wants what is best for her future child:

> I know that girls do not generally get a "fair shake" in society. Despite an egalitarian upbringing, a female child that I might bear is likely to have fewer advantages in life than a male child. Even with natural talents equal to a son, she probably would not reach the same income or prestige level. Marriage, parenthood, and gender stereotypes would reduce her chances of success, as they would not comparably affect a man. If I choose to have a daughter despite these drawbacks, I am choosing a future that is less than optimal for my child. Perhaps, therefore, I am morally bound to choose a son.[24]

Obviously, if every potential parent thought and acted in keeping with the preceding rationale, society would in time arrive at an overwhelming preponderance of males. Although such a situation is not necessarily sexist, it is likely to reinforce the sexism that already prevails even if the rationale for sex selection is the promotion of the future child's best interests. Accordingly, while the rationale is explicative of decisions by individual parents, it does not merit universalization or social approval.

Benefits of the availability of techniques for sex selection should be acknowledged. Among those cited are the virtual elimination of sex-linked diseases, reduced likelihood that children will be unwanted because of sex, reduction of the birthrate, and possibly a better balance of males and females in the elderly population.[25] The last result would occur because of the probability that the number of men in the general population would substantially increase. The greater longevity of women might be matched by the greater proportion of the larger population of men who survive to more advanced age.[26] Of course, achieving this end would also mean that the ratio of men to women would be greater earlier in life. So it is only in advanced age that numerical equality might be achieved, and it is even possible then that men would predominate. The anticipated numerical predominance of men is predicated on the well-supported preference of both men and women for sons, especially as firstborns.[27]

What are the potential harms of general availability of sex selection techniques? As already suggested, these have mainly to do with the reinforcement of sex-role stereotypes and sexist practices.[28] They may also intensify the burden, if the technique fails, of having or being an unwanted child. Regardless of their sex, firstborns are generally more ambitious and successful than second-born children, who are often more sociable than their older siblings. If firstborns are predominantly sons and second-born children are predominantly daughters, these differences parallel the sex-role stereotypes that already exist. With fewer women in the world, Amitai Etzioni maintains that the more venal traits of men, such as their tendency to violence and criminality, would prevail.[29] Women would more prevalently be treated as objects valued for their worth to men rather than for themselves, with their freedom suppressed to increase their availability. Men who least exemplify male stereotypes might also be exploited. Alternatively but improbably, women might dominate the mostly male world as supreme sovereigns. Neither scenario is acceptable from an egalitarian feminist standpoint.

It is hardly surprising that feminists as well as nonfeminists oppose sex selection for nonmedical reasons.[30] Nonetheless, many clinicians of both sexes support the practice. Interestingly, the rationale by which some genetic counselors support prenatal testing and termination of pregnancy for nonmedical sex selection may be considered feminist because it is based on respect for the pregnant woman's autonomy. In addition, this rationale suggests respect for the cultural attitudes and practices that may influence the request. The ethic of nondirectiveness that genetic counseling has long championed is inconsistent with opposition to sex selection for any reason, so long as the practice is uncoerced. Refusal of testing or termination for sex selection is effectively directive behavior.

A survey of nineteen nations conducted by Dorothy Wertz and John Fletcher found that the majority of geneticists in India and Hungary, as well as the United States, would offer sex selection for nonmedical reasons.[31] In the other nations surveyed, the majority would neither perform sex selection nor refer the couple to someone who would perform it. The case that elicited these responses involved a couple with four healthy daughters and no sons, requesting prenatal testing for sex determination in the absence of medical indications for the diagnosis. The couple tell the clinician that if the fetus is female they will abort it, and if their request is not honored "they will have an abortion rather than risk having a fifth girl."[32]

In the three countries that supported sex selection in this case, the reasons were very different. In Hungary, 60 percent of those surveyed would offer sex selection in order to prevent the otherwise certain abortion of a healthy fetus, which might be either male or female. In India, where 52 percent would offer sex selection during gestation, the principal rationale on both sides of the issue was concern about social implications. Those who opposed sex selection indicated concerns about exacerbating women's unequal position and furthering the already unbalanced sex ratio. Those who supported sex selection saw it as a means of practicing population control and reducing abuse toward women who do not bear sons and their unwanted daughters. In the United States, 62 percent of the clinicians surveyed would offer or perform sex selection on grounds of respect for the pregnant woman's or couple's autonomy. This rationale was generally framed in terms of rights: the right to this particular medical service, the right to decide, and the right to a referral.[33]

Data from a more recent survey by Wertz and her colleagues show an interesting contrast between the views of health professionals on sex selection and their views on other issues.[34] Throughout the world, women physicians were more directive than their male counterparts on most issues. On the issue of sex selection, however, U.S. women physicians were less directive than their male counterparts, genetic counselors, and non-U.S. physicians of either sex. Despite their overall emphasis on nondirectiveness, the U.S. genetic counselors were about as likely as non-U.S. physicians to refuse prenatal diagnosis for sex selection, even though they personally disagreed with the decision.[35] Wertz suggests that cultural differences and "professional locus" influence the disparate views of these groups more than gender influences them. Economic differences probably play a part as well.[36] Although some parts of the world were not included in the survey, the thirty-seven nations that participated represent a range of cultural differences not found among the U.S. respondents. Culture, class, and professional locus undoubtedly influence the different groups, but the interplay among the factors may be more influential still, and gender is another part of that interplay.

Philosophically, cultural support for sex selection well illustrates the problem of relativism. [37]In arguing against sex selection for nonmedical reasons, Wertz and Fletcher suggest a middle ground between ethical absolutism and ethical relativism. Although cultural diversity should generally be respected, they favor restrictions against culturally "intolerable" practices, one of which is sex selection.[38] Similarly, Susan Sherwin suggests a restricted form of relativism when she describes feminism as favoring respect for all differences except those that support gender injustice.[39] Presumably, sex selection is one of these differences. Neither view is actually supportive of relativism, however, because both entail the universal or absolute claim that sex selection for sexist reasons is never justifiable. Like it or not, then, Sherwin, Wertz, and Fletcher are not relativists but absolutists.

As with most issues, sex selection is not unalterably opposed on feminist or egalitarian grounds. Globally, selection of either males or females is justifiable for medical reasons such as avoidance of X-linked disease and is morally defensible in other situations as long as the intention and the consequences of the practice are not sexist. Sexist intentions are those based on the notion that one sex is inferior to the other; sexist consequences are those that disadvantage or advantage one sex vis-à-vis the other. Regardless of whether cultural attitudes condone or encourage it, sexism in either manifestation makes sex selection morally objectionable in any society.

Notes

Much of the discussion in this chapter, with some revision, is taken from chapter 6 of Mary Briody Mahowald, *Genes, Women, Equality* (New York: Oxford University Press, 2000). I wish to acknowledge with thanks permission from Oxford University Press to use this material in the current collection.

1. Tom L. Beauchamp and James F. Childress, *Principles of Biomedical Ethics*, 4th ed. (New York: Oxford University Press, 1994). The principles developed in this book, which has become a classic work in contemporary bioethics, are prevalently used in clinical ethics teaching and cited in articles on ethics topics in clinical journals.

2. Although few philosophers have analyzed the term, R. S. Downie and K. C. Calman have developed a very broad concept of "respect" in *Healthy Respect: Ethics in HealthCare* (London: Faber & Faber, 1987).

3. Etymologically, the term derives from the Greek *autos*, which means "self," and *nomos*, which means "rule" or "governance." According to Beauchamp and Childress (*Principles of Biomedical Ethics*), the term was first used to refer to the self-governance of the Hellenic city-states (p. 120). In the context of bioethics, however, autonomy generally means personal autonomy rather than political autonomy.

4. Beauchamp and Childress provide a societally less demanding or negative concept of liberty: "independence from controlling influences" (*Principles of Biomedical Ethics*, p. 121). Isaiah Berlin's famous distinction between "freedom to" (positive freedom) and "freedom from" (negative freedom) is consistent with their view. My egalitarian orientation finds this inadequate because it supports a system in which remediable and unjust inequalities are countenanced. See Isaiah Berlin, *Four Essays on Liberty* (New York: Oxford University Press, 1969).

5. Many years ago I distinguished between these concepts as intrinsic and extrinsic freedom. Cf. Mary B. Mahowald, "Beyond Skinner: A Chance to Be Moral," *Journal of Social Philosophy* 4 (1973): 1–4.

6. Susan Sherwin has developed the notion of "relational autonomy," which involves a critique of such limitations as particularly applicable to women in the health care setting. See Sherwin, "A Relational Approach to Autonomy in Health Care," in The Feminist Health Care Ethics Research Network, Susan Sherwin, coordinator, *The Politics of Women's Health: Exploring Agency and Autonomy* (Philadelphia: Temple University Press, 1998), pp. 19–44.

7. Because people are not equally autonomous, the term "equality" as used here refers to "respect" rather than "autonomy."

8. Although democratic government may take the form of rule by the majority, history offers some horrendous examples of corrupt decisions by the majority.

9. Literally, the term "suttee" (cf. *satti* in Hindi and *sati* in Sanskrit) refers to a "chaste and virtuous wife." Cf. *Webster's New World Dictionary*, 2d college ed. (1982), p. 1435. For an excellent account of female circumcision and its relation to ethical relativism, see Loretta M. Kopelman, "Female Circumcision/Genital Mutilation and Ethical Relativism," *Second Opinion* 20, no. 2 (1994): 55–71. For an account that reflects the ability of some U.S. physicians to respect the standpoint of African women on the issue, see Carol R. Horowitz and J. Carey Jackson, "Female Circumcision: African Women Confront American Medicine," *Journal of General Internal Medicine* 12 (August 1997): 491–499.

10. *The Compact OED New Edition*, p. 1727.

11. Selection of females to avoid the birth of a child affected with an X-linked disease may be viewed as commendable, but this is based on selection against the disease rather than selection of the sex. Morally questionable selection of females would occur if it were undertaken as a means of serving the interests of others (e.g., through their reproductive or domestic labor).

12. "Ableism" refers to a bias or prejudice against people with disabilities—a view that such individuals are inferior to those who are "able."

13. For documentation of philosophers from classical to contemporary times who viewed women as inferior to men, see Mary B. Mahowald, ed., *Philosophy of Woman* (Indianapolis: Hackett, 1994). With few exceptions, philosophers' concepts of woman are inconsistent with their concepts of "man" or human nature.

14. If selection of females is based on the desire to avoid suffering in an affected male, it is not sexist.

15. F. J. Beernink, W. P. Dmowski, and R. J. Ericsson, "Sex Preselection Through Albumin Separation of Sperm," *Fertility and Sterility* 59 (1993): 382–386. Although one recent American study of university students shows a fall in male preference over the past fifteen years, the preference for sons remains strong. Regarding the falling preference for sons, see J. B. Ullman and L. S. Fidell, "Gender Selection and Society," in J. Offerman-Zuckerburg, ed., *Gender in Transition: A New Frontier* (New York: Plenum, 1989), pp. 179–187. Regarding the strong preference for sons throughout the world, see T. M. Marteau, "Sex Selection," *British Medical Journal* 306 (1993): 1704–1705; G. Vines, "The Hidden Cost of Sex Selection," *New Scientist* 138 (1993): 12–13; V. Patel, "Sex Determination and Sex-Preselection Tests in In-

dia: Modern Techniques for Femicide, *Bulletin of Concerned Asian Scholars* 21 (1989): 1–11.

16. *Proceed with Care: Final Report of the Royal Commission on New Reproductive Technologies* (Ottowa: Canada Communications Group Publishing, 1993), 2:889–890.

17. Benjamin E. Reubinoff and Joseph G. Schenker, "New Advances in Sex Pre-selection," *Fertility and Sterility* 66, no. 3 (1996): 343–348.

18. Reubinoff and Schenker, "New Advances," p. 348. Note that blatantly sexist reasons may be included among "social purposes." Cf. Gina Kolata, "New Method Could Help Parents Choose a Baby's Sex," *International Herald Tribune,* September 10, 1998, pp. 1, 10.

19. The use of ultrasound for sex selection occurs despite governmental efforts to restrict its use for this purpose. Cf. Bob Herbert, "China's Missing Girls," *New York Times,* October 30, 1997, p. A23. In the United States as well, ultrasound for sex selection is available to individuals whose desire for sex selection is based on cultural values. Cf. Margie Slovan, "Some Go to Great Lengths to Avoid Having a Baby Girl," *Chicago Tribune,* August 3, 1997, sec. 13, pp. 1–2.

20. Dorothy C. Wertz, "Society and the Not-So-New Genetics: What Are We Afraid Of? Some Future Predictions from a Social Scientist," *Journal of Contemporary Health Law and Policy* 13 (1999): 315.

21. Christine Overall, *Ethics and Human Reproduction* (Boston: Allen & Unwin, 1987), p 27. The next few pages are slightly revised from my discussion of this issue in *Women and Children in Health Care: An Unequal Majority* (New York: Oxford University Press, 1993), pp. 84–86.

22. Personal communication with the author, September 25, 1989.

23. E.g., although the birthrate for girls is higher than that for boys worldwide, in Korea nearly 116 boys are born for every 100 girls, and in China 118.5 boys are born for every 100 girls. Cf. Sheryl WuDunn, "Korean Women Still Feel Demands to Bear a Son," *New York Times,* January 14, 1997, p. A3. Worse still is the incidence of female infants who "disappear" from the population because, in comparison with boys, they are neglected. Cf. Herbert, "China's Missing Girls," p. A23.

24. Mary Anne Warren suggests more compelling circumstances than I have here portrayed, for example, societies that are extremely oppressive toward women, where inheritance or other economic rights and privileges are limited to males. See Warren, *Gendercide* (Totowa, N.J.: Rowman & Allanheld, 1985), p. 85.

25. Warren, *Gendercide,* pp. 160–176; and Overall, *Ethics and Human Reproduction,* pp. 29–33.

26. Other ways of increasing the number of men in the population include more medical and social attention to the most frequent causes of death among men, for example, homicide and stress-related work roles.

27. William D. Althus, "Birth Order and Its Sequelae," *Science* 151 (January 1966): 44; and Overall, *Ethics and Human Reproduction,* p. 29.

28. Warren, *Gendercide,* pp. 108–158; and Overall, *Ethics and Human Reproduction,* pp. 29–33.

29. Amitai Etzioni, "Sex Control, Science, and Society," *Science* 161 (September 1968): 1109. I have long found this view both empirically and morally questionable.

30. Michael Bayles, for example, considered all cases of sex selection for non-medical reasons sexist. See his *Reproductive Ethics* (Englewood Cliffs, N.J.: Prentice-Hall, 1984), pp. 34–37. Even as she approves of sex selection for sex complementarity or sex similarity, Overall *(Ethics and Human Reproduction)* opposes institutional support for sex selection for nonmedical reasons.

31. Dorothy C. Wertz and John C. Fletcher, "Prenatal Diagnosis and Sex Selection in Nineteen Nations," *Social Science Medicine* 37, no. 11 (1993): 1359–1366. Moreover, according to Wertz and Fletcher, "more geneticists would perform prenatal diagnosis for sex selection in 1994 than in 1985. . . . Nevertheless, in most nations, with the exceptions of Russia, Hungary, Israel, and Portugal, fewer respondents would accede to such requests than they would in the United States." See Wertz, "Society and the Not-So-New Genetics," p. 316.

32. Wertz and Fletcher, "Prenatal Diagnosis," p. 1362.

33. Ibid.

34. Dorothy C. Wertz, "Is There a 'Women's Ethic' in Genetics: A 37-Nation Survey of Providers," *Journal of the American Medical Women's Association* 52, no. 1 (1997): 33–38.

35. This contrasts with the data obtained in Wertz and Fletcher's earlier study, which showed a significant difference between male and female geneticists: women were two times more likely than men to support sex selection. Cf. Wertz and Fletcher, "Prenatal Diagnosis," pp. 1359–1366.

36. According to Wertz, the average annual income of the U.S. physicians was greater than $100,000, whereas the average annual income of the non-U.S. physicians and of the U.S. genetic counselors was less than $50,000. See Wertz, "'Women's Ethic,'" p. 34. Of course, income is only one indicator of economic differences between groups. Moreover, as averages, these data do not reflect the wider range of income for U.S. physicians as compared with genetic counselors and non-U.S. physicians. Greater socioeconomic disparity often exists between individuals with similar cultural background, such as the Latino mayor of a major U.S. city as contrasted with his relatives in Cuba.

37. Ruth Macklin, *Against Relativism: Cultural Diversity and the Search for Ethical Universals in Medicine* (New York: Oxford University Press, 1999). Macklin provides a persuasive case against relativism while offering extensive documentation of cultural diversity.

38. Wertz and Fletcher, "Prenatal Diagnosis," p. 1364.

39. Susan Sherwin, *No Longer Patient* (Philadelphia: Temple University Press, 1992), p. 75.

12

Fatal Daughter Syndrome

WILLIAM M. ALEXANDER

True to animal behavior, humans act and react to survive within their ecosystem niche. The human niche of the Earth's biosphere includes thinking about twenty-first century sustainability. Humans seek to improve their well-being while living within the finite carrying capacities of the several ecosystems of the Earth's biosphere. Moving into this discourse, we shall consider how the inequitable provision of health care for females diminishes their capacity to create human well-being—well-being that can motivate and direct sustainable behavior. Provision of female health care in a universal context includes adequate food, clean water, education, and particularly the full utilization of female skills and strengths. Material sustenance and survival needs of humans reach farther into the ecosystems than the self-limited scope of professional health services in industrial nations.

Health care discrimination against females in high-consumption societies can be located in specific cases. However, the scope of such health care services is usually adequate to allow trickle down from males that is sufficient to avoid abnormal mortality rates among females. In order to clearly see the negative effects of female health care discrimination in real life, it is necessary to place this analysis within a low-consumption culture and society.

We find that India, with its large statistical base and wealth of health care studies, fits the low-consumption criteria. India has an additional analytical advantage as a social laboratory framing critical health care outcomes. One state in India, Kerala, uniquely contains both behaviors necessary for twenty-first-century human sustainability—modest consumption of the Earth's ecosystem services and the necessary corollary, small family sizes. Our analytical method may be simplified to a comparison of the measured well-being and fertility outcomes of India versus Kerala. In this analysis we first display sex-differentiated health care and then sex-differentiated contributions to the creation of a good life.

Within the future orientation of sustainability, we may view the low per capita Earth resource consumption in India throughout the twentieth century as analogous to the most likely condition (limited Earth resources per capita) in the human niche of the Earth's biosphere of the twenty-first century. As a sustainability problem, we see in twentieth-century India both sustainable and unsustainable behavior. Lessons learned about desirable human life within limited ecosystem services may be applied to the sustainability discourse concerning the whole Earth moving into the twenty-first century.

The U.N. Development Program *Report* for 1997 points to the excellent setting of this study.

> Many aspects of deprivation—from poor health to discrimination to domestic violence—have little to do with income. Haryana's [a North Indian state] per capita income is among the highest and fastest growing in India. Yet its infant mortality rate at 68 per 1000 live births, is four times Kerala's [a South Indian state]. Women in Haryana suffer systematic deprivation, reflected in one of the lowest female-to-male ratios in the country—865 to 1000. If all of India had Kerala's birth and child death rates, there would be 1.5 million fewer infant deaths in the country every year, and a dramatic reduction in population growth.[1]

In this chapter we shall focus on the abnormal death rates of female infants as the direct cause of the low female-to-male ratios. The causes of these female deaths, called fatal daughter syndrome, also impair the capacity of Indian women (excepting in Kerala) to create higher levels of well-being for their families.

Gender Differences

The common observation that women often fare better then men in social situations has been reconfirmed by recent genetic studies. Females (XX chromosomes) are less vulnerable to developmental disorders of language and social cognition than males (XY chromosomes).[2] Clear evidence of a male advantage in family, political, and commercial hierarchies during the last millennium might be explained first by larger body size and second by weak evidence of male advantage in abstract thinking. Males tend to think more about the control of ecosystems, including the control of large numbers of humans. The greater empathy of females, sharing and nurturing skills, may be learned in female relationships with others following their greater imprinted sociability and their biological experiences of child nurturing.

Both their more significant biological role in reproduction and their greater empathy draw the attention and focus of female thought to well-being. In contrast, the abstract thought advantage of males draws male focus and attention to the production of goods and services, economic growth. In day-to-day language we often say, "Dad brings home the bacon while Mom cares for the family." Generalizing men and women into analytical categories instead of viewing ourselves as individuals, we may carry our thinking beyond our personal experiences of gender relations into a useful twenty-first century scenario.

A practical gender question arises: Does an emphasis on male skills over females skills in the management of available ecosystem services produce some advantage? This question depends on an answer to another question: Are the available ecosystem services scarce or plenty? The closely related question we address here is, Can a large human population survive on Earth without utilizing female efficiency in the use of limited Earth resources to maintain high well-being?

Janet Jiggins makes our point:

> Women's increased sense of power typically does not lead to female dominance or to female hierarchies of power over men. It leads to an increased social capacity to determine common goals at the level of the family, the community, and the nation. It is profoundly democratic, enhancing the civil capacity to act in ways that satisfy societal goals. The call by women for an end to all forms of discrimination against women is not self-interested special pleading. The end of such discrimination is an essential condition for sustainable development.[3]

Well-Being and ZPG

Humans sometimes encourage and manage the survival of other life forms as necessary to their own well-being, a condition of more than survival for themselves. Humans seek well-being in a process that can make themselves sustainable. Measured aspects of desired well-being are long life expectancies, low infant mortality rates, high educational attainments, and low total fertility rates. These desired measurements are found together and are often used to explain one another in a circular fashion. In the specific questions addressed here, the natural unity of these well-being measures is maintained as an object and purpose of successful human behavior.

Well-being is also a qualitative characteristic of a society—happiness and contentment. A qualitative description of well-being has been documented with an appropriate emphasis on love and aesthetics.[4] Well-being has several positive measures with material connections, such as long life, low infant mortality, high literacy, and stable democratic systems, which will be featured here. We also know what well-being is not. Well-being is not welfare defined in dollars as income per capita. And well-being is not the charity of the wealthy, public or private.[5] One of the desired outcomes of high well-being, low fertility, provides a central linkage in this account. The low fertility of zero population growth may be located in any society where the total fertility rate has declined to two or less, that is, an average of two or fewer children in the lifetime of each female in a given society. Societal well-being necessary for the achievement of zero population growth provides a measurable benchmark for human sustainability.

Mixing Throughput with Knowledge

A material characteristic is integral to well-being, a modicum of matter and energy called throughput, that is, ecosystem services taken by humans. Throughput is a flow of matter and energy that humans withdraw from the Earth's biosphere each day for their use. Important parts of the throughput taken by humans are other life-forms, along with sunlight, air, water, and minerals. Throughput passes through the digestive tract of human civilization, often in a single day, usually within a year, while some recycling takes centuries, even millennia. All such matter and energy taken from the biosphere for human use is eventually returned in a degraded condition to be regenerated and reordered in the several ecosystems of the biosphere.[6]

Much, possibly most, human activity is the mixing of throughput with human knowledge, creating the desired end: well-being. Many human artifacts and most tools are huge repositories of knowledge. For example, keeping warm using little throughput in a cold climate is possible but requires a large input of knowledge. On the other hand, it is possible to keep warm using large amounts of throughput with little knowledge. The relative amounts of throughput and knowledge mixed to create well-being usually depends on which is easily available and which is in short supply.

Sustainability for humans means a limited amount of throughput taken from the finite ecosystem services of the Earth's biosphere. In simple arithmetic, a number of humans times human-taking per capita equals an amount of throughput that cannot be exceeded on a finite Earth. Either human numbers or per capita consumption may be maximized. If we wish to maximize human numbers, we may note that the application of more knowledge can increase well-being without increasing throughput. Searching for a value in increasing human numbers, we may find comfort in the reminder of an important pronatalist—more humans may create more knowledge.[7]

Zero population growth is most easily understood as a part of or as flowing from a condition of limited throughput growth. For life-forms other than humans, stabilized throughput for a particular species causes zero population growth. For humans the cause-and-effect relationships go both ways, that is, they are interactive. Limited throughput could also force zero population growth on humans, but human choice for zero population growth may lead humans to a sustainable throughput plateau. The human choice for zero population growth is mediated by the qualitative characteristic of a society: well-being. Well-being is defined by measures of several desired results—low infant mortality, long life, high education, and so on. In human behavior, high well-being measures correlate with total fertility rates of two or less.

Throughput Efficiency

As a positively defined qualitative characteristic of a society, well-being may be employed as a basic object and purpose of such society in an efficiency measure. Thus measured, efficiency is well-being divided by throughput per capita. In this efficiency formula, well-being would be set at one for any society that has a total fertility rate of two children or fewer. High well-being efficiency is thus the product of a society's low per capita throughput. Such efficiencies are the outcome of skilled application of knowledge.

These metaphors are drawn from our history and knowledge of biology in order to make this analysis intelligible to North Americans. Next, the usefulness of such metaphors in today's reality needs to be checked. Inasmuch as consumption (i.e., throughput per capita) in our industrial world is probably above sustainability, we must move our analysis into the developing world in search of a real-life society with a sustainable standard of living.

India and Kerala

Two criteria for this testing lead us to India. First, the standard of living—consumption per capita—in India seems likely to be on the scale of throughput per capita, which will be available worldwide during the twenty-first century. Second, India contains within its low consumption orbit a particular society in which the well-being is high enough to cause

TABLE 12.1   Death rates by Sex and Age groups for the population of eleven villages in Ludiana District of Punjab between July 1 and December 31, 1959, according to the Khanna Study

Age Groups	Male Death Rate	Female Death Rate	Male/Female Deaths Ratio
0–14	19.2	28.8	0.667
15–44	1.9	5.2	0.363
45+	30.7	31.9	0.962
All ages	14.6	19.1	0.764

SOURCE: Pravin, M. Visaria, "The Sex Ratio of the Population of India," *Census of India,* vol. 1, Monograph no. 10 (New Delhi: Office of the Registrar General, 1961).

TABLE 12.2   Death rates by Sex and Age groups for the population of the rural areas of Punjab, Himachal Pradesh, and Delhi between July 1958 and July 1959, according to the fourteenth round of the Indian National Sample Survey.

Age Groups	Male Death Rate	Female Death Rate	Male/Female Death Ratio
0–14	18.50	23.36	0.791
15–44	1.54	3.30	0.467
45+	22.61	17.94	1.261
All ages	12.39	14.15	0.876

SOURCE: Pravin, M. Visaria, "The Sex Ratio of the Population of India," *Census of India,* vol. 1, Monograph no. 10 (New Delhi: Office of the Registrar General, 1961).

moms and dads to voluntarily choose small families—Kerala. With a population greater than that of Canada, Kerala is an Indian state located between the Gnat mountain range and the Arabian Sea on the southern tip of India. In the following discussion twentieth-century India will be regarded as a case study foreshadowing twenty-first-century problems in human behavior and stresses in the Earth's biosphere. Within the evident cultural and lifestyle similarities of all Indians, the well-being contrasts between high-fertility India in general and low-fertility Kerala in particular are instructive.[8]

   In our search to explain why women live well in Kerala, we start by asking, Why are female death rates abnormally high in India? The basic data has long been known. The report of the 1961 Indian census displays the findings of the Khanna Study carried out by Harvard scientists, and places it within the larger context of the National Sample Survey carried out by the Indian government.

   In industrialized countries the ratio of male-to-female deaths in the right-hand column of Tables 12.1 and 12.2 would be one or more in every

TABLE 12.3 Three of India's Twenty-Five States with India and Four Asian
Neighbors

	Kerala	West Bengal	Uttar Pradesh	India	Bangla-desh	Paki-stan	Sri Lanka	China
Females per 100 males[a]	104	92	88	93	94	92	99	94
Infant mortality rate[b]	17	66	98	79	91	95	18	31
Female life expectancy[c]	74	62	55	59	56	59	74	71
Male life expectancy[d]	69	61	57	59	55	59	70	68
Female literacy rate[e]	86%	47%	25%	39%	23%	22%	74%	68%
Male literacy rate[f]	94%	68%	56%	64%	49%	49%	94%	87%
Economic growth[g]	0.3%	2.5%	2.2%	3.1%	1.9%	3.0%	2.6%	7.7%
Total fertility rate[h]	1.8	3.2	5.1	3.7	4.0	5.6	2.5	2.0
Population, millions[i]	29	68	139	884	114	119	17	1162

SOURCE: Jean Dre'ze and Amartya Sen, India: Economic Development and Social Opportunity (Delhi: Oxford University Press, 1996).
[a] Number of females per 100 males in the population.
[b] Infant mortality rate is the number of infants who die per 1000 live births. This is the best composite measure of well-being in a society. IMR is a sensitive indirect measure of the quality of the food and water, the quality of the housing and clothing, the quality of the health care, and the quality of the education in the whole society. By 1995 the IMR in Kerala had declined to thirteen.
[c] Life expectancy is the average number of years a child born into a given society may expect to live.
[d] Ibid.
[e] Literacy is the percentage of the female and male population over the age of seven who can read and write.
[f] Ibid.
[g] Economic growth is a ten year average of the annual growth of the economy of the state or nation.
[h] Total fertility rate is the average number of children of all females in their lifetime. In a population that has an equal amount of in- and out-migration, a TFR of less than two will create zero population growth within a generation or so. By 1995 the TFR in Kerala has dropped to 1.7.
[i] Population is the most recent census count given in millions.

age category. Comparison of these two tables shows that the abnormal death rates of females, or fatal daughter syndrome, was more intense in the Khanna Study area than in the larger area of the National Sample Survey.

As we proceed to real-life considerations, we must look at the comparative measures defining well-being. The high well-being measures found in Kerala will be considered normal, whereas the low well-being measures of India in general are abnormal. The data displayed in Table 12.3 is selected from the statistical appendix of Jean Dre'ze and Amartya Sen in their authoritative *Indian Economic and Social Opportunities* (1996). Additional data for the other Indian states and comparison nations may be found in this source.

First, we may need to confront our own mind-set, which may see economic growth as a necessary condition for fertility declines. Find the significant economic growth measured in India in Table 12.3 and note that the economic growth of Kerala is close to zero. In order to gain wider perspective, note also how economic growth plays out in the three states and four nations offered for comparison. Next note the consistency of the well-being measures displayed—infant mortality rate, life expectancy, and literacy. Kerala is not just the most desirable on each measure; critical well-being measures such as infant mortality are dramatically different between India and Kerala. It is difficult to believe we are looking at measures of similar populations. And before proceeding, consider the differences in the female-to-male ratios in Table 12.3, which will be referenced as a critical explanatory factor later in this chapter.

Looking further into Table 12.3, we may ask, Why is Indian fertility twice as high as that in Kerala? Since low fertility is encouraged by high well-being, we may restate our question. Why is well-being low in India and high in Kerala? We look at the levels of literacy, infant mortality, and length of life, and each begs a similar question. Why is literacy so much higher in Kerala than in all the rest, or any other part of India? Why is infant mortality in Kerala so low? Why do the men and women of Kerala live so much longer? Looking more particularly at these specialized questions, we see mirrored measurements integral to the well-being considered here as a unity, a human goal.

Popular Explanations

Much popular speculation has been offered to explain the causes of the desirable quality of life in Kerala. Let us note five differences: religion, caste demise, communist government, remittance income, and female education. The supporting relationship between increasing female literacy rates and declining infant mortality rates demonstrates two measures integral to well-being. This relationship is dramatically displayed in Figure 12.1. Increasing female literacy and declining infant mortality occurred together: the gender equity of the Kerala culture is the cause of both.

The religious profile of Kerala is somewhat different from the rest of India. The percentage of Muslims in the population of Kerala is higher than in all India—20 percent rather than 10 percent. And 20 percent of Kerala's population is Christian, compared to 2 percent for all of India. Looking at our linking measure, well-being to low fertility, we find that all three religious communities in Kerala have low fertility. The fertility rates for Hindus are lowest; Christian birthrates are a little higher, and Muslim rates only slightly higher than those of Christians.

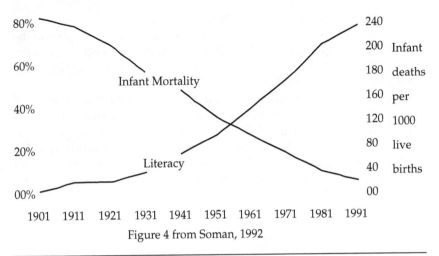

Figure 4 from Soman, 1992

FIGURE 12.1   Female Literacy Rises as Infant Mortality Rates Decline.

Source: CiR Soman, "Malnutrition, Mortality, and Child Development—Some Key Issues," in G.N. Menon, ed., *Epidemiology in Medicine* (Bangalore; Interline Publishing, 1942).

The social history of Kerala may offer a clue to the surprising ways in which Kerala differs from the rest of India. In 1900 Kerala was a madhouse of caste; its system the most rigid of all India. When Mahatma Gandhi returned from South Africa in 1912 to strike at India's great sin, caste, a religious, social, and political revolution was already under way in Kerala. Although slow and nonviolent, the far-reaching caste destruction in Kerala, when compared to all India, has been astounding. As early as 1960, the economic and political discrimination of caste had nearly disappeared.

Two further explanations have often been accorded much importance in the story of Kerala's successes. One is the election of a communist majority government in 1957. As the oppressed majority overthrew the oppressing minority, it endowed Kerala with vigorous, profoundly egalitarian democracy. That party labels are largely an election convenience is demonstrated by the failure of the communist parties to win a majority in any election since. The remaining argument claims that Kerala's higher well-being is financed by remittance income, particularly from the Persian Gulf. This money sent home is important and represents 12 percent of Kerala's income. However, this outside source of income only raises the spendable income per capita in Kerala to the low level of the Indian average. Much of this income is invested in private housing.[9]

As we review these popular explanations, we should not be diverted by them. They are of little help since they (1) are caused by the major explanatory factor, gender equity, (2) should have produced undesirable outcomes, (3) show a normal relationship between factors integral to the unity, well-being, or (4) are not differences between Kerala and India. Gender equity family structure is the only solid explanation of the different well-being outcomes.

Casual travelers and officials have long described the higher status of women in Kerala. An 1875 census report for a princely state later to become part of Kerala included the comment, "The partiality of parents in bestowing greater care on their female issues, will be hazarding an opinion based on insufficient data, though it is a fact that among [matrilineal] people a female child is prized more highly than a male one."[10] Looking back at India in 1999, data is no longer "insufficient."

Female-to-Male Ratio

Probing into the history of India and Kerala reveals hard data, helping to establish the gender equity explanation of caste demise, higher well-being, and lower fertility in Kerala. These significant measurements were revealed in the very first official enumeration of the Keralan population. For all India, typical of most nonindustrial countries of that time, the number of males exceeded the number of females. Yet in Kerala, as was expected only in industrialized countries, the number of females was greater than the number of males.

A century of census data shows female-to-male differences to be persistent and increasing. The favorable ratio of females-to-males in Kerala in 1901 was 101 to 100. As in the industrialized countries, this female share had increased to 104 by 1991. During this same century the female-to-male ratio began in India at 97 to 100 and by 1991 had declined to 92 per 100.[11] Impaired female survival is typical of developing countries, but the decline in female survival rates relative to males is abnormal.

A fundamental insight leading this analysis flows from the correlations between high fertility and low female-to-male ratios within the several Indian states. The fourteen major states of India are located in Figure 12.2 bisected by a trend line. The female-to-male ratios (number of females per 100 males) are shown as the increasing numbers from top to bottom. The increasing total fertility rates (births per female) related to the decline of female-to-male ratios are shown left to right. This figure clearly shows the critical relationship—as female-to-male ratios increase to normal levels, birth rates decline following improved well-being.

Figure 12.2, showing the significant impact of differential female-to-male ratios on human behavior (fertility rates) in Indian states, is based on 1991 census data. In a demographic transition a generation of delay is common between well-being improvements decreasing death rates,

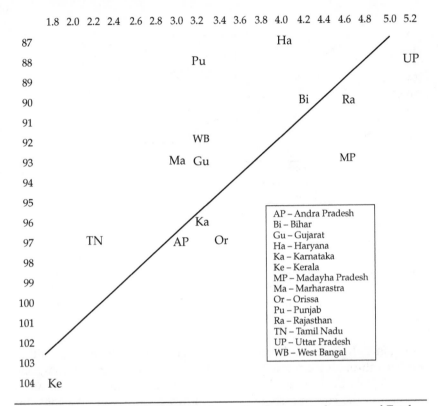

FIGURE 12.2   Female-to-Male Ratios increasing from top to bottom and Total Fertility Rates increasing from left to right in the 14 major Indian states.

SOURCE: Data from Jean Dre'ze and Amartya Sen, *India: Economic Development and Social Opportunity* (Delhi: Oxford University Press, 1996).

causing declines of birthrates. Therefore, to display the importance of female-to-male ratios through time, let us look at the abnormal decline in female-to-male ratios through the twentieth century in India.

Improvements in life conditions through time caused an increase in the female-to-male ratios in Kerala similar to the effect of such improvements throughout the Earth. However, in India, as these life improvements went forward, the female-to-male ratios regularly declined. We can see the extent of the Indian female-to-male ratio decline by calculating the size of the gap between the normal ratios in Kerala and the abnormal ratios in India. In Figure 12.3 the numbers of females that have been missing per 1,000 at each census is shown (left side) as a number increasing throughout the twentieth century.

A normal female numbers advantage, the four or more per hundred found in Kerala, may be called a gender balance. The abnormal condition

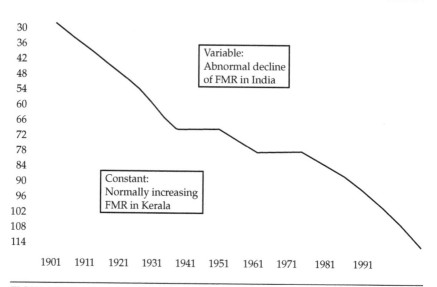

FIGURE 12.3   Female-to-Male Ratios Declining in Twentieth-Century India

SOURCE: Jean Dre'ze and Amartya Sen, *India: Economic Development and Social Opportunity* (Delhi: Oxford University Press, 1996).

found in all India is gender imbalance. Tracing the gender balance of Kerala back through the many centuries is difficult work for historians and archeologists. Such study shows gender balance predating the patriarchy integral to the Hindu caste system. Following the Aryan invasions, the development of commerce, and the caste division of labor, patriarchal family institutions spread and become dominant throughout India. But this powerful set of changes failed to overcome the female values and female valuation indigenous to Kerala. The persisting balance of gender in Kerala may explain Hindu toleration of Christians and Muslims, the early establishment of education for all, specifically including girls, and the overthrow of caste disabilities in Kerala.

Fatal Daughter Syndrome

Reports of female infanticide in twentieth-century India are rare. However, beginning in 1789 the officers of the British raj were reporting "almost wholesale female infanticide." Among 400 jadeja Rajput households, there was "not a single female child in any of them." The jadeja Rajputs were the highest-ranking subcaste of the wealthy land-owning caste. Family wealth was maintained by allowing sons to marry brides from lower subcastes paying dowries. For Muslims, the four-wives rule accommodated the surplus daughter problem at the top of social and wealth hierarchies. The monogamous Hindus of the highest-ranking families applied female infanticide.

Opium and other poisons were sometimes used, but the newborn infants were so vulnerable that the "refusal of the mother to feed the female infant or exposure to heat or cold were enough to finish them off." In 1856 census officials reported that castes practicing female infanticide were "resorting increasingly" to neglect of their female children to escape the accusation of killing their daughters.[12] Our current evidence shows that girl-child neglect, not infanticide, is the cause of the low female-to-male ratios in India. The devaluation of females by the highest castes has diffused into the practices of all lower castes and communities. We might expect the diffusion of excessive girl-child mortality to decline as we look down from the top to the bottom of the class/caste hierarchy. This is the case.

Traditional discrimination in health care that produces lower male than female mortality has been shown in eleven villages in the northern district of Ludhiana. These villages were the subject of intensive observation in the Khanna Study.[13] Similar methods were applied in the Mitlab project area in Bangladesh.[14] In both areas, female mortality was lower than male mortality in the early months after birth, consistent with the female physiological advantage in survivorship over the entire span of life. In the latter part of the first year and thereafter female death rates were higher than male death rates.

In the early interval after birth, when the source of nutrition is predominantly breast milk, the normal female advantage prevailed. After weaning, however, female death rates rose relative to male death rates. The more-sons incentive for the provision of better nutrition other than mother's milk for males is revealed in other studies. The higher female than male child mortality in the Khanna Study turned up particularly revealing evidence. The mortality of females under five who have no older sisters is little different from the male death rate, but the death rates of under-five females who have an older sister is about 50 percent higher than the rate for males.[15]

This set of evidence indicates that higher female mortality is caused by a lower regard for female infants—a lower regard that is less marked when a female child is the first daughter. Further evidence on the professional health care side is provided by an investigation of medical attendance during fatal illnesses in the Khanna Study area, 1957–1959. The overall death rate was 19.6 per 1,000 for females and 14.8 for males during these years. Fewer females than males had medical care during the fatal illness, and females were attended by personnel of lower competence.[16]

The most recent analysis of fatal daughter syndrome notes the slight numerical advantage of males at birth balanced by a slightly greater vulnerability of male infants, creating a parity between the sexes sometime after the age of five. We should expect the numbers of boys and girls aged five to nine to be about equal—as they are in Kerala. We may contrast Kerala with average girl-boy survivorship in the twenty-four adjoining districts in North India, parts of Haryana, Uttar Pradesh, Rajasthan, and Madhya Pradesh. The evidence of fatal daughter syndrome is extreme. Girl children have been reduced to 77 per 100 boy children.[17]

Family Structure in India

Indian census data allows us to identify districts with low and very low female-to-male ratios caused by fatal daughter syndrome. We may look within these districts to observe an all-pervasive class system marked by the ranking of the extended families that characterize the Hindu culture. That is, the extended families are the repositories of social power, economic power, and political power, a combination of powers rank ordered in the comprehensive hierarchical family systems of India.

These Indian class-ranked families are integral to the Hindu caste system. Muslims and Christians living in the same localities are accorded a kind of proportional class standing within the overall Hindu culture. Those districts with the lowest female sex ratios are clustered in the northern states adjacent to New Delhi, where the dominant caste is often the Rajputs. Although Rajputs are not the dominant caste in a majority of India census districts, naming a caste is important because marriages are not allowed (by hard-line religious and social traditions) across caste lines or into the Muslim or Christian communities.

The class hierarchy of the extended families among the Rajputs is replicated within the many castes and subcastes. That is, a highest-ranking (dominant) caste sets a pattern of family behavior that is emulated by other castes (also Muslims and Christians) in the locality or region. This commentary on the family class system is offered in a generalized form affording only a background for the relevant marriage and family life practices in India outside the special case, Kerala.

Among the Rajputs (and the customs established within other patriarchal castes) the purity of the male lineage, father to son, is the highest value and is consistently protected. Systematic suppression of female sexuality is the patriarchal method for maintaining male-lineage purity. The sexuality (physical beauty, demeanor, manners, and skills) of a female may be her means of self-expression (thus a part of her power relative to others, particularly males). This sexuality is suppressed by family institutions, disempowering females. Although more extreme in India, the struggles of females to circumvent such disempowerment in Western patriarchal families have been a familiar plot central to countless novels in the West. In India every opportunity for a female to express her sexuality, except in her husband's bed, is circumscribed or denied.

All marriages are arranged by family elders; girls are seldom allowed any role in these negotiations. Maintaining and improving the class status of the family is seen as the central goal of each marriage plan. A bride's opportunity to serve in the maintenance of her husband's family line is the secondary benefit. The arranged marriages among the royal and other high-ranking families of Europe often had this power-maintaining function.

The basic marriage rule is: outside of family and within caste. The critical problem in marriage arrangements flows from the need to maintain or improve the class standing of the extended family. If a daughter should be married into a family lower in the class ranking, the daughter's birth family loses status. On the other hand, a son may marry down, provided the bride's family can afford a large dowry. Inasmuch as class ranking is based on the somewhat interchangeable elements of wealth and social power, a significant infusion of wealth into the groom's extended family could maintain or even improve a family's class ranking.

As we compare the family structures in Kerala, it will become important to note that at marriage in North India the bride moves into the household of her husband. The daughter-in-law arrives as the least significant member of her new family, rather like a servant to her husband and his mother. She is cut off from her birth family by distance and restricted visiting customs. As an outsider in her new extended family, she may be denied female support and may exercise influence in family decisions only through the intervention of her husband speaking on her behalf. Even here she is disempowered. Husbands are discouraged from forming bonds of affection with their wives, since such attachments diminish the husband's allegiance to the family patriarch and the attention he pays to his first responsibility—his extended family.

Years may pass before the bride's status is established by the birth of sons bonded to her and speaking up on her behalf. Before puberty daughters are helpful to mothers, but at marriage their value to their mother's household disappears as they devote themselves to their husband's welfare, producing sons for the benefit of his family lineage and caring for his parents. Anthropologists have a word for this female-disempowering family structure—hypergamy—brides marrying upward within caste into richer and more esteemed extended families who require compensation for what would otherwise be a misalliance.

Family Structure in Kerala

Looking for census districts in India that display normal female-to-male ratios, we also discover different family structures and empowered females. None of districts in the Indian state of Kerala display the abnormally low female-to-male ratios characteristic of India in general, and the family structures are matrilineal and matrilocal, not patriarchal. At the same time, the extended families common to India as a whole (different from the nuclear families of Western societies) are common in Kerala.

The entire caste system of Kerala is quite different from the one in India in general. The Nayars, the dominant caste, originated in Kerala. Matrilineal and matrilocal family structures found in Kerala are unfamiliar in the experience and literature of Western societies. Lacking a patriarchal identity, the Nayar family structure is most easily explained in terms of its joint family residence, called a Taravad (also spelled Tharwad). A distinguished Indian jurist explains that a Taravad

> consists of a female ancestor, her children, and all such other descendants, however remote, in the female line. The male descendants themselves are its members but their children are not. A person belongs to the Tharwad of his or her mother only and the Tharwad membership arises by birth in the family. A female member of a Tharwad does not change her family by marriage unlike the other systems which follow the agnatic line of descent. . . . Each member of a Tharwad acquires an interest in Tharwad properties by reason of his or her birth alone, and when any member dies, the interest of that member devolves upon the other members of a Tharwad.[18]

Taravads were the female-lineage joint families (with female-owned properties and residences) of the high-ranking Nayar caste of historic Kerala. Advocates and jurists trained in English law brought the ownership of family property vested in females under concerted attack during the time of the British raj. In addition, a Christian attack on polyandry in the Taravads, joined by a low-caste attack on caste restrictions, generally moved with force in Kerala during the early twentieth century. Both the religious and the legal foundations of the Taravad institutions were severely undercut.[19]

From early times the gender equity found in Kerala appears to have grown out of the attitudes and beliefs of the indigenous Malayalee population later to become Nayars living in Taravads. These beliefs were secured by a special kind of marriages of Nayar women with the very small, ritually high, land-owning caste called Nambudiri Brahmins. Gender equity was diffused from the powerful Nayar households into the whole population of Kerala. The gender equity of the Taravads was and continues to be found in all parts of the Malayalam-speaking population—among lower-caste Hindus, Muslims, and Christians.

The experience of gender equity in the historic Taravads has been described by anthropologist Kathleen Gough.

> [In Cochin a] woman might have six or eight husbands of her own or a higher subcaste, and a man, any number of Nayar wives of his own or a lower subcaste. Residence was duo local: spouses lived separately in their

natal homes and a husband visited his wife in her home at night. Exact physiological paternity was, clearly, often unknown, and in any case a man had no rights in or nor obligations to his children. Among Nayars of this area [the male-lineage] family was not institutionalized as a legal, economic, or residential unit.[20]

Male support, discipline, and role models for each boy were provided by a mother's brother resident in the female-managed households.
In the hilly and sparsely populated areas, duo local residence was impracticable.

In most cases a man took his wife to live in his ancestral household in avunculocal residence and children were brought up until adolescence in the houses of their fathers. There was some polygyny, but polyandry was forbidden. Fathers had morally though not legally recognized rights in and obligations to their children and a strong affective bond with them. . . . Both in Kottayam and in Cochin, Nayar women were occasionally married to men of the highest, patrilineal caste of Nambudiri Brahmins. Children of such unions were Nayars, and rules of ritual pollution maintained distance between them and their higher caste fathers. The Nambudiri father might not eat with his wife and children, and might not touch them during the daytime while in a state of ritual purity. Only the eldest son of a Nambudiri house might marry a Nambudiri wife and beget children for his own family.[21]

Nambudiri daughters in excess of first sons were relegated to lifelong seclusion and denied the educational opportunities enjoyed by Nayar daughters. The numbers of Nambudiri Brahmins were small, less than 1 percent of the population, and remain numerically insignificant.
Jean Dre'ze summarizes the essence of the Nayar model of gender equity, the key to modern well-being in Kerala:

Nayar women had greater personal freedom than most women to take decisions regarding marital and sexual relations. Nayar women played a crucial role in making household decisions, the decision-making role being invested with great authority—inheritance was through them, and it was they who were the bearers of the family name. The birth of a girl in a Nayar household was welcomed; it was far from being considered a disaster as in other parts of India.[22]

Summary

Fatal daughter syndrome has been identified and described as a major cause of female mortality. The gravity of this bioethical problem has been highlighted by contrasting the abnormal female mortality rates that obtain throughout Indian in general with the normal female mortality rates that obtain in a particular Indian state: Kerala. Considering the increasing exploitation of ecosystem services by humans and the burgeoning human population, the amounts of material resources available per capita worldwide in the twenty-first century are likely to be similar to the limited resources available in India during the twentieth century. Thus, if the case of Kerala has any lessons to teach, it is that societies which value gender equity are much better at maximizing human well-being within conditions of relative scarcity than are societies which disvalue gender equality. Apparently, the world's long-term stability and viability will depend upon how well its peoples treat women.

Notes

1. UNDP [United Nations Development Program], *Human Development Report* (New York: Oxford University Press, 1997).

2. Peter M. McGuffin and Jane Scourfield, "A Father's Imprint on His Daughter's Thinking," *Nature* 387 (1997): 652–653.

3. Janice Jiggins, *Changing the Boundaries: Women-Centered Perspectives on Population and the Environment* (Washington, D.C.: Island, 1994), p. 15.

4. Guliz Ger, "Human Development and Humane Consumption: Well-Being Beyond the 'Good Life,'" *Journal of Public Policy and Marketing* 16, no. 1 (1997): 110–125.

5. Steve Dodds, "Towards a 'Science of Sustainability': Improving the Way Ecological Economics Understands Human Well-being," *Ecological Economics* 23, no. 2 (1997): 95–111.

6. Herman E. Daly, *Beyond Growth: The Economics of Sustainable Development* (Boston: Beacon, 1996).

7. Julian L. Simon, *Ultimate Resource* (Princeton: Princeton University Press, 1996).

8. William M. Alexander, "Exceptional Kerala, Efficient and Sustainable Human Behavior," in Valentine James, ed., *Capacity Building in Developing Nations* (New York: Praeger, 1997).

9. Thomas T. M. Isaac, "Economic Consequences of Gulf Migration," in K. C. Zachariah and S. Irudaya Rajan, eds., *Kerala's Demographic Transition* (New Delhi: Sage, 1997).

10. Nagam V. Aiya, *Report on the Census of Travancore, 1875* (Thiruvananthapuram, Travancore, India: Government Press, 1876).

11. Jean Dre'ze and Amartya Sen, *India Economic Development and Social Opportunity* (Delhi: Oxford University Press, 1996).

12. L. S. Vishwanath, "Efforts of the Colonial State to Suppress Female Infanticide: Use of Sacred Texts, Generation of Knowledge," *Economic and Political Weekly* 33, no. 19 (1998): 1104–1112

13. John B. Wyon and John E. Gordon, *The Khanna Study* (Cambridge: Harvard University Press, 1971).

14. Stan D'Souza and Lincoln C. Chen, "Sex Differences in Mortality in Rural Bangladesh," *Population and Development Review* 6, no. 2 (1980): 257–270.

15. Monica Das Gupta, "Selective Discrimination Against Female Children in Rural Punjab, India," *Population and Development Review* 13, no. 1 (1987): 77–100.

16. Sohan Singh, John E. Gordon, and John B. Wyon, "Medical Care in Fatal Illnesses of a Rural Punjab Population," *Indian Journal of Medical Research* 50, no. 6 (1962): 865–880.

17. Barbara Harriss-White, "Gender-Cleansing," in Rajeswari Sunder Rajan, ed., *Signposts: Gender Issues in Post-Independence India* (New Delhi: Kali for Women, 1999).

18. K. Sreedhara Variar, *Marumakkathayam and Allied Systems of Law in the Kerala State* (Ernaculam, India: K. Sreedhara Variar, 1969).

19. Robin Jeffrey, *Politics, Women, and Well-being: How Kerala Became a Model* (London: Cambridge University Press, 1992).

20. Kathleen E. Gough, "Cults of the Dead Among the Nayars," in Milton Singer, ed., *Traditional India: Structures and Change* (Austin: University of Texas Press, 1959).

21. Ibid.

22. Jean Dre'ze and Amartya Sen, *Indian Development: Selected Regional Perspectives* (Delhi: Oxford University Press, 1997).

13

Human Cloning and the Problem of Scarcity: A Sartrean Perspective

JULIEN S. MURPHY

Central to our humanity is a notion of freedom. What we prize most about ourselves is, if not our ability to master our destiny and shape the course of history, to make choices about some of the conditions of our daily lives. In a word, self-determination. What becomes of freedom in a society, in a world, in which human cloning is possible? At first glance, the choice to clone is a mark of our freedom, one of the many dazzling new possibilities of technoscience. But some fear that cloning will erode a basic sense of freedom by threatening our genetic uniqueness. What then becomes of individual identity and human dignity? These fears rest on certain assumptions about the role genes play in our psychological and moral well-being. We require a philosophical framework for assessing the larger implications of cloning. And as I see it, the later work of Jean-Paul Sartre, which feminists (among others) have found very useful,[1] promises to help us answer some of the questions that most distress us about cloning.

Cloning, Scarcity, and Immortality

Sartre, best known as the founder of French existentialism, is a transitional figure in the twentieth century. His play, *No Exit*, gave the world the famous line: "Hell is other people." (Will we someday say that hell is the clones of other people?) In his early writings on existentialism, Sartre emphasized human freedom. With the *Critique* (1960), his greatest political work, Sartre attempts to build an international philosophy of liberation for the second half of the century, reviving Marxism with an existential focus on individuals. Sartre analyzed oppression within the larger socioeconomic system that constitutes it, seeing it primarily in terms of scarcity.[2]

It is the perception of scarcity in reproduction that fuels, in part, the race to clone humans. For Sartre, scarcity is the basis of alienation in modern societies marked by competition over limited resources, and it characterizes all human relationships. Thrown together in a world of others, we find that there is never enough. From food to time, we struggle with scarcity. For Sartre, human needs stand in a dialectical relationship to scarcity. Hence our relationships to one another and the world are based on need. "The fact is that after thousands of years of History, three quarters of the world's population are undernourished. Thus, in spite of its contingency, scarcity is a very basic human relation, both to Nature and to men," Sartre wrote in the *Critique*. "In this sense, scarcity must be seen as that which makes us into *these* particular individuals producing *this* particular History and defining *ourselves* as men."[3] For many societies, technology is an important weapon in the struggle against scarcity. Throughout history, Sartre noted, tools, techniques, and technology were adapted precisely for this end. Biotechnology is a set of new techniques. We might say in our day that global food shortages demand bioengineered high-yield crops even though such innovations have yet to diminish hunger worldwide. The application of biotechnology to reproduction in animals and humans is now routine. Productivity concerns in agriculture have yielded reproductive techniques that were later modified and applied to treating infertility in humans. Cloning is the latest and most controversial of such techniques.

On a Sartrean view, then, cloning emerges as a praxis in response to scarcity. The scarcity it is meant to multiply is certainly not people, who are found in abundance on the planet. Nor is it meant to increase human genetic material, similarly abundant. Rather, cloning is meant to address the scarcity of specific DNA. Cloning favors our genetic specificity. We want to be able to reproduce using certain genes and not others; we need organs, bone marrow, or other replacement parts that are an exact match, not merely similar to ours. Although he wasn't thinking about genetic scarcity, Sartre wrote about the emphasis on uniqueness in relation to scarcity within capitalist economies:

Individualism is a form of interiorized scarcity belonging to bourgeois times. It can equally well mean family scarcity or class scarcity. You are what you have. Since the family's (or individual's) being is its possessions, to possess the scarce is to be scarce. At once, the scarce group's being is in danger in the world of the inert—for it is its goods, its property.[4]

Reproductive cloning presupposes a form of family scarcity—not enough or not any offspring from these particular parents becomes a problem for technology to address. Family scarcity is related to class scarcity insofar as technological solutions to infertility are largely financed privately and thus are inaccessible for many. Also, among those who could afford cloning, vanity and other motives could be present.

In confronting scarcity, some strategies, (e.g., industrialization) reshape the means of production. This too Sartre recognized. He claimed that "certain scarcities could condition a moment of History, if, in the context of changes of technique (which will themselves have to be explained), they take the form of abrupt changes in the standard of living. History is born from a sudden imbalance which disrupts all levels of society."[5] Cloning is one such strategy that would alter our modes of reproduction even if it were used for very few pregnancies. Who can say what all of the effects would be? The catalytic changes that cloning would cause might not change the standard of living abruptly but would raise the bar on what we might expect of reproduction. Therapeutic cloning would alter, in dramatic ways, our understanding of our bodily limits. Imagine one day being able to make our own replacement marrow, tissue, organs, and the like. While all the effects are not identifiable at this early stage in cloning research, we can speculate on some outcomes by exploring how cloning practices would become transformed into the practico-inert and would be affected by counterfinality.

Whereas Sartre claimed we use our freedom to act against scarcity, our praxes result in unintended consequences, overturned, as it were (Sartre calls this the practico-inert), and affected by the interplay of other praxes (which Sartre called counterfinality). His two famous examples of the practico-inert and related counterfinalities are the flooding produced by advancements in Chinese agriculture that deforested the land and the hoarding of gold from the New World by the Spanish that resulted in reduced value due to inflation. The Chinese peasants, in Sartre's example, intended to increase agricultural productivity but could not foresee the drastic countereffects of large-scale deforestation. Similarly, counterfinalities in animal cloning might not produce flooding but could have adverse environmental effects all the same. For instance, animal cloning, a developing science begun with a cloned South African frog in 1962 and continued with recent success in sheep (1997) and cows (1998), might save endangered species or might even reproduce a species after extinction, thereby preserving biodiversity. But to the extent that specific animal clones are preferred in great number, it could also reduce biodiversity in animals. These unintended and contradictory results illustrate a dialectical relationship between scarcity and overabundance.

In reproduction technology, counterfinality is easily seen when praxes to overcome scarcity result in overabundance and require reductive strategies. Consider cases of multiple pregnancies linked to the use of fertility drugs or multiple embryos for IVF. In the first case, in the interest of producing a live birth, women have had too many fetuses and thus, for the sake of viable fetuses and a healthy mother, fetal reduction may be recommended. In the second case, again to achieve one child, many embryos have been created. Once a successful pregnancy is achieved, reproductive couples are faced with the problem of what to do with their unneeded frozen embryos. Should they be disposed of, donated to others who wish to reproduce by IVF, used for research, or frozen indefinitely at a monthly cost? For couples using IVF I have known, this issue of abundance, more than the use of IVF itself, posed troubling religious and moral conflicts. In the case of cloning, overabundance is created by an attempt to address scarcity, since at present cloning is a highly inefficient mode of reproduction. In mammals, many embryos are produced to increase the chance of success. To clone Dolly, the first cloned sheep in the world, scientists used over 400 unfertilized eggs from donor ewes to then produce 277 reconstructed eggs, with very few developing embryos and only one healthy live birth. Some speculate that an even greater number of unfertilized eggs would be necessary to produce a single human clone.[6] The birth of a healthy child will no doubt require the production of many embryos that are unhealthy and unable to thrive, at least in the early years of cloning research. Whether children born by cloning techniques have a shortened life span, as some cloning scientists fear is likely, particularly if current mammalian techniques are applied to humans,[7] is a moral risk that will come with a heavy burden of responsibility.

The best-known counterfinality feared to accompany reproductive cloning would be the threat to our uniqueness. This is ironic given that, as noted earlier, cloning favors specificity, particular DNA. Unfortunately, when uniqueness is reproduced, it is destroyed. Cloning opponents frequently appeal to our human uniqueness, the way we differ one from another, to make their case. But their appeals to uniqueness are quite vague. Consider the following. One critic writes of human cloning that "no one has the right to jeopardize the precious uniqueness of all members of the human race in order to assuage individual heartbreak and gratify individual desires."[8] Ethicist Daniel Callahan repeats the uniqueness appeal when he writes that "engineering someone's entire genetic makeup would compromise his or her right to a unique identity."[9] The many appeals to uniqueness lead us to ask, What sort of uniqueness would be jeopardized by cloning? Our genetic uniqueness. Callahan's comment is particularly surprising because it follows his dismissal of the notion that we are our genes. ("True, we are not just our genes, environment, history and cultural context matter. That's why no two people, not even identical twins, are exactly the same.") Nevertheless, he goes on to link possession of a unique genetic makeup with the possibility of possessing a unique identity.[10] Callahan's emphasis on engineering the genetic endowment of a child builds the force of the argument not on the extent of cloning but on the fundamental role of genetics in making us specific individuals. Genetic determinism comes to mind in these appeals. Somehow a unique *genetic* makeup is necessary for a person's identity. Notice, no one says that large families jeopardize children's unique identities because they all share the same environment.

To trace personal identity to one's genes is an easy mark of genetic determinism, a move not uncommon among cloning opponents. These critics also ignore the implications of their views for issues of identity in identical twins. Callahan's point is echoed by Leon Kass, who similarly warns us that human clones would have serious identity problems,[11] and in the comments of science writer George Johnson: "If a cell can be taken from a human being and used to create a genetically identical double, then any of us could lose our uniqueness." Trouble enough, but then Johnson goes on to say, "One would no longer be a self."[12] Whether or not a self and personal identity are completely identical concepts depends on one's philosophical position. Again we find the assumption that it is one's genes, one's unique set of genes at that, that make a self possible. What can be said of these ill-founded appeals to uniqueness?

Within the framework of genetic determinism, freedom is understood as directly stemming from genetic uniqueness. But uniqueness, like scarcity, Sartre would remind us, is constituted within the socioeconomic system, a system in which genetic material of all types is seen as property, is patented, and is regulated by commerce. Indeed, the government has already sold the genetic information contained in the genome of the Icelandic people to a private biotechnology company for $200 million.[13] That our bodies, down to tiny parts of us, our genes, are products to market (will they soon be patented?) is a point graphically made by artist Rhee Sang with his exhibition, *Asexual Reproduction*, at a South Korean museum following claims that the world's first human cloning experiment had been conducted there. In one photo of a young boy from a poor country, Sang put prices on various parts of his body—his heart was priced at $91,000, his eyes at $900—and behind him in red paint, he wrote the words "HOW MUCH?"[14] This exhibit illustrates market forces at work in the commodification of the body.

The commodification of the body is one of the troubling counterfinalities of therapeutic cloning. The preservation of one's life may depend on the duplication and the termination of a genetic copy. It is unclear how developed an embryo would need to be in order for it to be useful as a source of replacement parts. Would it be unethical to create an embryo in vitro (or begin a pregnancy) exclusively for such ends and then terminate it when the parts have been supplied? This was suggested in a focus group investigating public sentiment in Britain on cloning. As one person exclaimed, "It could be psychologically disastrous if you created an embryo to create a part for yourself and then destroyed it."[15] There are many philosophical problems in determining the status of a human embryo, and therapeutic cloning complicates these matters by providing new pragmatic reasons to do research on early embryos. This is unfortunate. Although great benefit may come from early embryo research, bans against it that exist in many countries provide an important function: they set a limit on the extent of the permissible commodification of the body. Removing that limit will generate new dilemmas about the ontological status of the embryo and the human body, its limits and uses.[16] The Council for Responsible Genetics, a U.S. organization, fearing that cloning would contribute to the commodification of the body, likened cloning to other setbacks in history: involuntary servitude, slavery, torture, and the use of poison gas or biological weapons. In a position statement, the council draws an analogy between cloning and other practices of human exploitation claiming, "Just as the Thirteenth Amendment outlawed slavery, and other laws prohibited torture, child labor and other forms of human exploitation, the time has come to prohibit human cloning."[17] These are hard analogies to defend even if the council is right to worry about the proper uses of reproductive science.

For Sartre, freedom is marked not simply by our genetic makeup but by our ability to act in the world, to counter, or attempt to counter, scarcity. Like other projects in life, with reproduction there are advantages to involving others. To reproduce with someone else or with the genetic material of an anonymous donor introduces unpredictability that can offset the pervasiveness of one's own less-than-ideal traits and genetic propensities for disease. The wonder of life lies partly in the revelations of uncertainty. Is humanity about uncertainty or about control? Of course, it is about both—the need to feel at least partly in charge of the course of our life, the ability to marvel at the traits of our children that cannot be accounted for by shaking the family tree—the ways my son is not like me. Cloning may offer a way to take control over reproduction and disease. People differ in the degree of uncertainty and control they prefer. Meanwhile, the larger message of our interconnectedness, already becoming increasingly abstract and mediated by technology, is lost with cloning. Involving the genetic line of another person in reproduction can be a positive act, and when this is recognized, cloning would be the less desirable option. Although cloning might give us new choices over the genetic nature of our offspring, it also limits our freedom in many ways. For instance, it does not allow for the random variation in our own genetic patterns as they mingle biologically with those of others.

Cloning is about "introducing predictability and order into the wildly unpredictable crapshoot that is life," Barbara Katz Rothman reminds us.[18] It strikes us as the paramount act of control—the ability to delineate one's genetic offspring with nearly perfect specificity. Yet a clone is not an exact duplication. For one thing, it results from a different egg and a different pregnancy than that of the donor. Given the prospect of genetic mutations, our limited knowledge of the human genome, and the role of the environment (including the maternal environment), complete control of reproduction is illusory. Cloning seems to offer us a new form of immortality—it is as if we can live again if we clone ourselves. Yet here too we are cheated, for it is, after all, someone similar to us, but not us. But even if cloning were successful, it would not shield us from death, disease, failure, and historical calamity—the chaos of life. In fact, cloning can produce failure, disease, and frustration when we find certain traits not reproduced that we had hoped for, when we find it doesn't work or doesn't work well, that the clone is never the same, not as good or not good enough.

Cloning and Reproductive Technology

Must we clone humans? In addition to addressing scarcity, cloning is also about technological progress, the desire to transcend the realm of possibility by doing what we thought could not be done. Some say that human cloning is a sign of progress, a mark of living in a more developed time. Progress on this view means that some limitations of the past can be transcended in the future. It means that our strategies for overcoming needs identified in respect to scarcity have been successful. Sartre was critical of notions of progress. He did not believe there were any guarantees that things (civilization or science, for instance) would work out for the best. Moreover, he was critical of how we assess progress and at what point in time. His writing on the topic are found in his posthumously published notebooks on ethics and in an appendix to the unfinished second volume of the *Critique* (1961–1962). He traces the origin of progress to the end of the eighteenth century and describes it as a myth, not a reality.[19] "We can conceive of a fact of contemporary progress today," meaning something like the mechanization of the last century, "but that is because we have discovered progress. Progress is our myth."[20] The problem with progress has to do with its temporal quality. For Sartre, history is constituted by the multiple effects of coun-

terfinalities, ours and those of others. But counterfinalities make it difficult to assess progress in the short term because we really don't know
how things will turn out. A better assessment of progress lies in long-
term assessments. Even then, certain assumptions about human improvement and the end results are always at work. Hence progress
eludes us in the present moment, the moment when we are most eager
to declare its victories.

Progress promises to create something new. Cloning, however, does
not allow for anything radically new. Moreover, as it bypasses the genetic
lottery, it forecloses certain possibilities, such as the creation of a biological offspring of the opposite sex of the cell donor. There is an order or law
of progress that suggests things are always moving forward, conditions
are improving, human beings are happier now than they were in earlier
times. This assumption of change for the better is part of the myth of scientific progress as well. But Sartre warns us that so-called scientific
progress can be used as a means of oppression and offers expensive
weapons for warfare as an example. Sartre misjudges science in his claim
in the *Notebooks* that "science contains a call to democracy" because science "contains within itself the principle of equality in the face of knowledge."[21] With the increasing complexity and expense of technoscience,
including cloning research, such a call becomes more remote—a point to
which we will return. Finally, Sartre reminds us that we must always
evaluate progress within a political context by asking, Who is making
progress and who benefits from it?[22]

Given Sartre's remarks on progress, it would be premature to announce the outcomes of cloning for any society. Yet the myth of progress
is so pervasive that opponents seize critical ground by trying to show
negative outcomes for cloning in the near future. Some see their critiques
as a way of intercepting the powerful forward thrust of science. Kass, for
instance, believes that our freedom is at stake in how we regulate or
refuse to regulate cloning research. "The prospect of human cloning, so
repulsive to contemplate, is the occasion for deciding whether we shall
be *slaves of unregulated progress,* and ultimately its artifacts, or whether we
shall remain *free human beings* who guide our technique toward the enhancement of human dignity" (emphasis added).[23] Of course for Sartre,
our freedom is not so easily destroyed, even by the myth of progress.
And once again, we find a vague appeal, this one to the enhancement of
human dignity. Surely one could imagine something like cloning techniques in a society transformed by feminism. Perhaps cloning would be
used to counter high infertility rates created by environmental degradation. In such a case, cloning would not necessarily be at odds with human dignity. Still, Kass is right to wonder about the direction of science.
However, even if scientific progress appears to be largely unregulated, as

he suggests, particular values and interests are a driving force. Identifying who is controlling cloning research within a particular society and for what end is a worthy effort.

Critics try to evaluate the effects of cloning on the oppression of women around the world. Some now see human eggs, once thought of as plentiful, since most women possess at birth more eggs than they will ever need, as a scarce resource. If women seized control over human eggs that men needed for therapeutic cloning purposes, women could upset the power imbalance in sexist societies, or so one developmental biologist has claimed.[24] It is true that cloning research needs women's eggs or fetal material. South Korean scientists obtained permission from a woman who had successfully undergone IUF at the Kyung Hee University clinic to use her remaining six eggs for their human cloning experiment. The U.S. team that successfully isolated embryonic stem cells used aborted fetuses of Baltimore women.[25] As the suppliers of eggs and fetal material, women are also uniquely positioned to be their guardians and thus to have an investment in the ethics of cloning research.[26] Women have responded accordingly. A little noticed fact is that the alleged first human embryo created by cloning (and then quickly destroyed) was the clone of a woman egg donor. Two dozen protesters, among them many women, arrived at the front of Kyung Hee University on the day of the controversial cloning announcement. They called for government regulation of human cloning and denounced the cloning experiment as inhuman research.

Some critics worry that men's rights will suffer. In one study of public sentiment about human cloning in the United Kingdom, many people had "grave worries about a future society in which reproduction can occur without the need for men." In the words of one woman, "I was shocked to learn that babies can be conceived without a male being present."[27] Others see cloning as extending men's role as oppressors of women. Radical feminist Andrea Dworkin believes that men will control cloning decisions with the aim of reproducing subservient women. "The men who will clone the compliant women will control them both reproductively and sexually, and in the process, they will destroy all human meaning: The men will abandon change for absolute control, any chance of intimacy for absolute power."[28]

The same debate on whether cloning would liberate or further oppress people is found in discussions of the effects of cloning on gay men and lesbians. Cloning may offer possibilities for gay people to reproduce, but here too we find the practico-inert converted into counterfinality.[29] Cloning would free gay men and lesbians from a dependence on sperm and egg donors. However, since even one's own reproductive cells are the prior biological union of a male and female, cloning oneself does not displace but only reinscribes heterosexual reproduction. The ideal reproductive technology for many gay people would consist of techniques to achieve genetic fusion of reproductive cells from both partners, not the clone of one partner. Nor would cloning offer improved chances for pregnancy for lesbians (sperm banks would still be more affordable than cloning technology and insemination much easier than embryo transfer of an in vitro embryo produced by cloning) or for gay men (who would still rely on women as surrogates to carry their cloned offspring). It could be used for treating infertility in gay couples, but most likely the antigay prejudice already present in assisted reproduction practices will severely limit this particular application of cloning. At the same time, cloning can easily be used, as we have seen, to reinforce views of genetic determinism, and genetic determinism rarely favors gay liberation. Many believe that the cloning of a gay man or lesbian would once and for all decide whether or not there is a genetic basis for sexual orientation. The idea that cloning could decide the matter disallows for views that we have freedom to make sexual choices and underestimates the myriad of factors at work in shaping sexual desire.

Those who claim that cloning heralds progress for women cite treatment for infertility as a major women's issue. As the proliferation of IVF technology in urban areas in many countries indicates (there are reportedly thirty IVF centers in Seoul alone and eighty nationwide),[30] many infertile women want to become pregnant, even at high costs and even with donor eggs. The expanding field of infertility research is not without its opponents. As Callahan sees it, reproductive technology is an inappropriate use of technology. "It is as if infertility, once accepted as a fact of life, even if a sad one, is now thought to be some enormous menace to personal happiness, to be eradicated by every means possible." Some believe that reproductive rights ought to include medical research in infertility. Callahan disagrees: "The seemingly limitless aims of the reproductive right movement, and the obsession with scientific progress generally and the relief of infertility in particular, are nothing to be proud of."[31] One important feminist debate central to reproductive technology is whether infertility is a disease. Feminists can be found on both sides of the debate. Some believe that infertility research would give women greater control and hence greater freedom in reproductive choices. Others who claim it is not a disease worry that infertility research will increase social pressure for every woman to reproduce. No debate can be found on the benefits for women of therapeutic cloning. In fact, the examples of possible uses of therapeutic cloning are not gender marked, even though it would be easy to dream up some wonderful goals for this research. For instance, what if it were possible to replace reproductive organs lost to surgery with healthy ones? But this immediately raises the issue of how replacement parts would be generated. Presumably, embryonic stem cells would be required. Some women might become pregnant to produce embryos for replacement parts, radically altering women's relation to pregnancy.

Whether cloning will advance or impede women's liberation is a complex matter that is not discernable in the short term. There are some obvious implications that can be drawn nonetheless. To the extent that cloning is used to reinforce genetic determinism, it will serve to shore up current hegemonic power. Racial and ethnic groups marginalized within societies will most likely have diminished access to cloning, exacerbating social inequalities. Regulations may be placed on the sort of embryos that women bear, although even unregulated cloning confronts us with agonizing responsibilities, for example, how do we select a genetic endowment for our offspring? Cloning may reinforce a conservative view of the family by excluding gay men, lesbians, and single women from access, and by reemphasizing blood ties (over adoption, for example) even if it reverses so-called blood relationships in the family (e.g., is the clone of the mother her sister or her daughter?). Cloning also creates troubling moral dilemmas about the status of early embryos and extends the commodification of the body.

Cloning, when viewed from an international perspective, raises issues of social justice. The size of the health care industry, which accounts for 9 percent of the world's wealth, is matched only by remarkable inequalities in the distribution of its medical resources. Like other forms of medical technology, cloning could widen the gap in medical care between economic classes in most societies. The World Health Organization estimates that the poorer countries of the world bear 90 percent of the disease burden while having access to only 10 percent of the medical resources. Among diseases pervasive in poor countries, malaria, for instance, kills 3,000 children a day. Certain gene-linked diseases, avoidable by cloning specific genomes, may one day be diseases of the poor, not because they are linked to environmental degradation, civil unrest, or population displacement but because the privileged have used technology to benefit themselves, exacerbating social inequalities not only within societies but also on an international scale. Even as these new treatment options for infertility are being considered, the gap in maternal mortality between Western nations and poor countries is exceedingly large. One out of more than 4,000 women in the United States and Europe risk death from childbirth, compared to one out of sixteen women in the poorest countries. Because of globalization, as long as cloning is practiced somewhere, the affluent in any society will have access to it. Hence no country is free of cloning or its implications, though societies will differ in the meanings they attach to cloning and the uses, if any, they find for it. International consensus, when possible, on bioethics issues related to cloning and embryo research is increasingly important, as are global assessments of the distribution of medical resources.[32]

The hard questions of technoscience, its proper uses and limits, are clearly not getting easier. Perhaps it is not too late to remind ourselves that science is a collective project of the international community. Returning to Sartre's comment in the *Notebooks* that "science contains a call to democracy" is fitting here. Science, also a limited resource, must be used responsibly. If the international community will soon possess the tools to bring children into the world by cloning, an idea once relegated to mythology, fantasy, and science fiction, can we make the world a fitting port of arrival? The measure of human dignity, a concern prevalent in anticloning arguments, may lie not with the sanctity of the human embryo, as some religious groups believe, but in the possibilities societies make available for people, or as Sartre would say, in what we make of ourselves. Surely, human dignity requires that we direct our scientific efforts toward curing prevalent diseases and reducing high maternal mortality rates. It is not cloning per se that is at issue but specific cloning technology—what it demands of us, the values that drive the experimental work, the sorts of societies it is likely to produce. It is time to evaluate the end goal of technoscience, apart from the myth of progress, by examining not only what we might want science to do for us but what we might become in pursuit of it.

Notes

1. For instances of Sartrean feminist philosophy, see Linda Bell's Sartrean analysis of violence in her book, *Rethinking Ethics in the Midst of Violence: A Feminist Approach to Freedom* (Lanham, Md.: Rowman & Littlefield, 1993); and my edited anthology, *Feminist Interpretations of Jean-Paul Sartre* (University Park: Pennsylvania State University Press, 1999). Sartre did not address reproductive issues except in one instance of an unpublished manuscript. In the "Rome Lecture Notes," Sartre discusses the report of a group of Belgian women in the 1950s who chose to kill their infants, who had been seriously deformed by the use of thalidomide in pregnancy. For Sartre, the women chose death over subhumanity for their infants as a political act to pressure the government to work harder to ensure the safety of drugs for pregnant women. See Robert V. Stone and Elizabeth A. Bowman, "Dialectical Ethics: A First Look at Sartre's Unpublished 1964 Rome Lecture Notes," *Social Text: Theory/Culture/Ideology* 5 (1986): 195–515.

2. See Sartre's discussion of scarcity in Jean-Paul Sartre, *Critique of Dialectical Reason*, vol. 1, trans. Alan Sheridan-Smith (London: Verso, 1991); and Sartre, *Critique of Dialectical Reason*, vol. 2 [unfinished], ed. Arlette Elkaim-Sartre, trans. Quintin Hoare (London: Verso, 1991). See also Ronald Aronson, *Sartre's Second Critique* (Chicago: University of Chicago Press, 1987); and Ronald Aronson,

"Sartre on Progress," in Christina Howells, ed., *The Cambridge Companion to Sartre* (New York: Cambridge University Press, 1992), pp. 261–292.

3. Sartre, *Critique*, 1:123–124.

4. Sartre, *Critique*, 2:423.

5. Sartre, *Critique*, 1:126, 138.

6. Harry Griffin, "Cloning and Nuclear Transfer—On Proposals to Clone Humans," paper, October 25, 1998; on-line http://www2.ri.bbsrc.ac.uk.library/research/cloning/humans.html Accessed March 21, 1999.

7. Mammalian research suggests that cloning adult cells can lead to a number of cell mutations in the cloned mammal, which could result in a shortened life span or increased cancer risk. These mutations result from changes in the donor cells that may be caused by aging and exposure to ultraviolet radiation. See Paul G. Shiels et al., "Analysis to Telomere Lengths in Cloned Sheep," *Nature*, May 27, 1999, pp. 318–319.

8. Susan Jacoby, "Entitled to the Embryo?" *New York Times*, November 1, 1993, p. A19.

9. Daniel Callahan, "A Step Too Far," *New York Times*, February 26, 1997, p. A23. Callahan is the former director of the Hastings Center.

10. Ibid.

11. Leon Kass, in Leon Kass and James Q. Wilson, eds., *The Ethics of Human Cloning* (Washington, D.C.: American Enterprise Institute, 1998). Kass is a humanities professor at the University of Chicago.

12. George Johnson, "Soul Searching," in Martha C. Nussbaum and Cass R. Sunstein, eds., *Clones and Clones: Facts and Fantasies About Human Cloning* (New York: Norton, 1998), p. 67.

13. See Simon Mawer, "Iceland, the Nation of Clones," *New York Times*, January 23, 1999, p. A29; and R. C. Landon, "People Are Not Commodities," *New York Times*, January 23, 1999, p. A29.

14. Edward Kim, "Art Exhibition Condemns Human Cloning," *Korean Herald*, February 8, 1999; on-line http://164.124.96.164/kh0208/m0208c01.html Accessed March 20, 1999.

15. "Public Express Concern over Cloning," BBC News, Science and Technology report, December 3, 1998; on-line http://news2.thdobbc.co.uk.hi/english/sci/tech/newsid_227000/227129.stm. Accessed April 27, 1999. The research was done by the Wellcome Trust, the world's largest medical charity.

16. The moral aspect of conceiving a child in order to obtain bone marrow has already seen public discussion. See Lance Morrow, "When One Body Can Save Another," *Time*, June 17, 1991, pp. 54–58. In one study, the majority (71 percent) of people polled answered no to the question, Is it morally acceptable to conceive and intentionally abort a fetus so the tissue can be used to save another life?

17. Position statement on genetic discrimination by the Council for Responsible Genetics; on-line http://www.gene-watch.org/cloning.html Accessed April 27, 1999.

18. Barbara Katz Rothman, "On Order," in *Clones and Clones*, p. 280.

19. Jean-Paul Sartre, *Notebooks for an Ethics*, trans. David Pellauer (Chicago: University of Chicago Press, 1992), p. 41.

20. Sartre, *Critique*, 2:412.

21. Sartre, *Notebooks*, p. 43.

22. Sartre, *Critique*, 2:416.

23. Leon R. Kass, "The Wisdom of Repugnance," in John D. Arras and Bonnie Steinbock, eds., *Ethical Issues in Modern Medicine* (Utah: Mayfield, 1998), p. 510.

24. Gina Kolata, "In the Game of Cloning, Women Hold All the Cards," *New York Times,* February 22, 1998, pp. 6–7. The reference is to a statement made by Dr. Davor Solter, director of developmental biology at the Max Planck Institute of Immunobiology in Freiburg, Germany.

25. Gregg Easterbrook, "Will Homo Sapiens Become Obsolete?" *New Republic,* March 1, 1998, p. 20. See also Nicholas Wade, "Panel Told of Vast Benefit of Embryo Cells," *New York Times,* December 3, 1998, p. A24.

26. See Julien S. Murphy, "Egg-Farming and Women's Future," in Rita Renata Duelli Klein and Shelly Minden, eds., *Test-Tube Women: What Future for Motherhood?* (Boston: Pandora, 1984), pp. 68–75; and Murphy, *The Constricted Body: AIDS, Reproductive Technology, and Ethics* (Albany: State University of New York Press, 1995).

27. "Public Express Concern over Cloning."

28. Andrea Dworkin, "Sasha," in *Clones and Clones,* p. 77.

29. See William N. Eskridge and Edward Stein, "Queen Clones," in *Clones and Clones,* pp. 95–113; and Timothy F. Murphy, "Our Children, Ourselves: The Meaning of Cloning for Gay People," in *Flesh of My Flesh,* pp. 141–149. See also Julien S. Murphy, "Should Lesbians Count As Infertile Couples? Antilesbian Discrimination in Assisted Reproduction," in Anne Donchin and Laura H. Purdy, eds., *Embodying Bioethics: Recent Feminist Advances* (Lanham, Md.: Rowman & Littlefield, 1999), pp. 103–120.

30. Michael Baker, "Korean Report Sparks Anger and Inquiry," *Science,* January 1, 1999, p. 17.

31. Daniel Callahan, "Cloning: Then and Now," *Cambridge Quarterly of Healthcare Ethics* 7 (1998): 141–144.

32. Meredith Wadman, "Ethicists Urge Funding for Extraction of Embryo Cells," *Nature* 399 (1999): 292; Declan Butler, "Breakthrough Stirs U.S. Embryo Debate," *Nature* 398 (1999): 10; Meredith Wadman, "Embryonic Stem-Cell Research Exempt from Ban, NIH Is Told," *Nature* 397 (1999): 185–186; "Time to Lift Embryo Research Ban," *Nature* 396 (1998): 97; Nicholas Wade, "Presidential Commission Expected to Endorse One Form of Research Using Embryos," *New York Times,* May 24, 1999, p. A1; Susan Mayor, "UK Authorities Recommend Human Cloning for Therapeutic Research," *British Medical Journal,* December 12, 1998, 1613.

14

Maria's Desire: Considerations About a Moment of "Genetic Counseling" for Breast Cancer

FERNANDA CARNEIRO
ROBERTO DOS SANTOS BARTHOLO JÚNIOR

Martin Buber, Women, and Bioethics

Ethics, as it is applied to the biological or medical sciences, should never be disconnected from real life, in our estimation. The attempt to theorize at the moral level is always an exercise in existential thinking—of looking reality in the face and then, if necessary, transforming that reality for people's good. Here we narrate a moment of great importance in a particular woman's life—the dialogue, or the attempted dialogue, between a woman and a geneticist as he communicates to her the results from a genetic test that will indicate either the presence or absence of BRCA1 or BRCA2 (genetic factors to which 5 percent of breast cancer cases are attributed).

Institutionally, we call this moment "genetic counseling."[1] But what should we call this moment at the personal level, and how should geneticists help their clients withstand its emotional intensity? In this chapter we address these and other questions about genetic counseling, sketching a theory that we believe has the power to root this practice in existence as ordinary people experience it.

As we see it, Martin Buber's relational ontology provides the theoretical framework within which geneticists can learn how to counsel their clients in a morally appropriate way.[2] Buber's entire philosophy rests on the pri-

macy of human relationships in the construction of a life truly worth living. His fundamental insight is the notion that there is a basic difference
between relating to a thing, or "It," which I observe on the one hand, and
to a person, or "Thou," who addresses me and requires a response from
me on the other hand. This difference is the difference between relating to
objects like rocks and to people like us. To be sure, says Buber, there are
times when one person will view another person "objectively," as a thing.
When a person does this to someone, that other person becomes a mere
"It," a thing like any other thing. This state of affairs will change, however, if the "It" refuses to remain a thing and personally addresses the person who tried to reduce him or her to a thing. Suddenly, the "objectifier"
will have the opportunity to recognize the essential "I-ness" of the "objectified," to recognize instead his or her unique individuality.

According to Buber, one of the most significant differences between an
I-It relationship and an I-Thou relationship is that we invest only a part
of ourselves in an I-It relationship. There is always a part of us that remains outside an I-It relationship. In contrast, there is no holding back in
an I-Thou relationship. Our whole being must be involved. Otherwise
we will become observers of the relationship rather than participants in
it. Clearly, I-Thou relationships are much more risky than I-It relationships. In an I-It relationship the part of the self that remains outside the
relationship cannot be hurt by the other person because that other person cannot reach it. In contrast, in an I-Thou relationship the whole of
one's self is exposed to the other person. We are both living entirely in
the present moment of our encounter, not knowing for certain where our
communication will take us. In this present moment, we must both be
prepared for any and every address and response. It is this readiness
that constitutes genuine listening. The purpose of genuine listening is to
really hear what the other is saying, constantly being aware that the
other is revealing something unique about himself or herself that the
hearer did not already know.

As we see it, genetic counselors are always confronted with the Buber-
ian duality: I-Thou or I-It. These two relationships determine the possibilities of the relationship between a geneticist and the patient before him
or her, in this case, the woman in our story. The desire to engage in an authentic dialogue with patients enables the geneticist to create an environment in which patients can express themselves freely and reveal themselves as "Thous" rather than "Its." Unless patients feel they are being
met as persons, they will tend not to act as persons, that is, as men and
women who, on account of their freedom, are capable of assuming responsibility for their decisions and actions. Thus, in our estimation, autonomy or freedom is a value in genetic counseling precisely because it is
the necessary condition for responsibility.

The human being is the only creature known to us, capable of assuming responsibility. This property must be understood as something more than just a mere empiric statement. It is a distinct and decisive characteristic of the essence of the human being and its existential equipment. We recognize therefore the essential character of this human property and also recognize, instinctively, its value, but not as one more value in a scenery already replete of living things, but as a value that exceeds everything existent until now by means of something that generically transcends it and before which we are responsible.[3]

Another paramount value in genetic counseling is beneficence. The purpose of the dialogue between geneticists and patients is, after all, the patient's good. The geneticist must search with each patient for that patient's good, never imposing his or her own good on the patient.[4]

Conditions for Freely Given Consent

As we understand it, genetic diagnosis and counseling is a procedure that deals with the most intimate and singular identity and destiny of a person: "Who am I?"[5] The contact between a geneticist, who is usually a man in Brazil, and a patient who wants to know whether she is at risk for genetic breast cancer, for example, is an asymmetric relationship, marked not only by the experience of gender but also by other circumstances involving power. The geneticist is armed with the official authority of expertise, whereas his patient has only the unofficial voice of experience. Obtaining authentic consent from a person with less official power than oneself requires a pedagogical dialogue based on subjective as well as objective knowledge of that person. For the geneticist, this asymmetric relationship requires taking responsibility for the patient's psychological and spiritual state of being as well as her physical state of being. But the geneticist is not the only one with responsibilities in the geneticist-patient relationship. The patient as well as the geneticist is a person in search of the truth. They are exposed to each other in all their vulnerability, facing each other as free and responsible persons capable of connecting to each other.[6] In order for the truth to emerge between them, however, the geneticist must, because of his official position, be sure that the patient is able to hear and understand the information that will be provided to her. Only then will the stage be set for a true dialogue.

Maria's Desire

In the case at hand, we must ask what Maria desired when she came to the Public Health Institution. No doubt, she desired one simple thing—

good news—news that her body was not marked by BRCA1 or BRCA2. But was her desire to be fulfilled? To find out, we must enter a room in which a team consisting of the geneticist, a trainee and me, Fernanda, an observer, assembled to meet Maria. She seemed to be about fifty (but she could have been forty) and she wore the uniform of a bus conductor. Maria apologized for her appearance, stating that although she was not employed by the bus company, she wore the uniform to avoid paying for the bus ticket. No one could call Maria a beautiful woman. Her hair was a mess, and her smile was marred by missing teeth. But there was something about her eyes, fixated on the geneticist and oblivious to me. They were curious and attentive; from time to time Maria cast them down, revealing her discomfort with the situation.

The geneticist seemed unconcerned about their encounter, confident that he had the situation under control. He started the conversation in an informal tone without excessive seriousness. "Maria, all the information given or received here is confidential and will only be used with your consent," he calmly stated. "For me that is no problem," said Maria, almost interrupting the end of the geneticist's sentence in order to push him toward revealing the "truth" in his possession.

Maria had already lost one breast. It had been removed after a standard diagnosis of cancer when it was too late to proceed in any other fashion. She wanted to get to the punch line. "Where did you find out about the National DNA Bank?" he asked.

"In the newspapers," she said matter of factly.

The geneticist started making side comments to the trainee, murmuring technical phrases like "difficult prognosis," "predictive exam," and so on. It was clear to me, the observer, that Maria understood none of these phrases, a lack of understanding that would, of course, impede her ability to understand and act on the information she was on the verge of receiving.

Referring to the removal of her breast, the geneticist asked, "When did you have your first 'diagnosis' of breast cancer?" Her eyes, squinting slightly because of her effort to hear, opened with the despair of someone who does not understand something that is fundamental. "What 'osis'?" Maria asked.

In that moment, Maria's otherness penetrated and altered us. She did not understand the geneticist, although the trainee and I did. It was clear to us that Maria, who had presumably had a "pedagogical session" about "informed and free consent" with another health care team at the time of her first surgery, had never fully understood what they tried to communicate to her. Maria must simply have to guess what words like "diagnosis" mean. What words can we use to help her understand her situation?, I thought.

The "technical dialogue" with Maria continued, but there was a para-dox in the air.[7] The team wondered whether they could understand Maria's silence any more than she could understand their words. They began to doubt whether authentic dialogue was possible. "Tell me a bit about your history. How many brothers and sisters do you have? Who has had cancer in your family?," probed the geneticist.

"My great-grandmother and my grandmother had cancer. It started in their skin. My mother, who is sixty years old now, had her breast re-moved six years ago. My aunt lost her uterus to cancer; my brother lost his brain to cancer; and, oh, my sister . . . her breast was removed just a while back," answered Maria.

The geneticist, taking care with his words, tried to explain that certain families are genetically predisposed to getting certain kinds of breast can-cer. He explained the characteristics that mark such families. He talked slowly. It seemed that he wanted to hide from himself the explanatory chasm between Maria and himself, a chasm in which his words con-tained no significance whatsoever, a gap in which diagnoses became "osis." The revelation of the inaccessibility of his scientific terms had clearly disconcerted the geneticist as well as the rest of the team. His technical words lost their communicative strength; they burst like soap bubbles before us. Still, Maria was attentive. She was waiting for her mo-ment of truth. Was *she* a "victim" of her family's genetic destiny?

Finally, the geneticist spoke. "Maria, your diagnosis is negative," he said.

"Negative? What do you mean?" she asked.

The "house of language" opened a door.[8] In its normal usage, the term "negative" is associated with something that is not good. But Maria wanted good news; she did not think a "negative" result was good news.

The geneticist sensed Maria's "Thou-ness." "'Negative' means that you will not get a genetic cancer in your other good breast. Whatever kind of cancer took your first, bad breast, it was not genetic cancer," he said.

Had Maria understood that "negative" was good? The team was not sure, for Maria asked no questions at this point and continued to stare. What was going on inside her? What uncertainties did her heart shelter? Probing, the geneticist asked, "Maria, do you have any other questions?"

This time, the "house of language" opened one of its intimate chambers. Maria seemed to glow. She brightened up. She began to look like someone who expects happiness. The dialogical moment swelled and Maria ap-peared in all her personhood. She exclaimed, "Yes, I do, doctor. I want to know when I shall receive my 'prosthesis' for my missing breast."

How surprising! She knew very well how to pronounce this piece of medical jargon without stuttering. Until that moment she had been too frightened to express anything in a straightforward manner, but now she was not afraid of making a demand. The word "prosthesis" signaled something that was part of her intimacy, her personal dignity. Maria was not that interested in learning about BRCA1 and BRCA2—about her susceptibility to it. Rather, she was interested in her appearance and in the ability of the geneticist and his team to restore her corporeal integrity.

Turning her question into a declaration of her personhood, Maria said to the team, "My breasts are my beauty. They are the beauty of all women!" Maria's words touched the team. She had exposed to everyone her desire to be beautiful, to be in possession of her body and to feel like a whole woman. For Maria, cancer was a threat to her femininity; what she wanted from the team was not a diagnosis but a prosthesis. She wanted us to see her as someone who used to be beautiful and could again be beautiful with a prosthesis.[9]

Reflections on Maria's Desire

Although this narrative opens many paths for theoretical reflection, we will look back only at the moment in which the geneticist says to Maria, "All the information given or received here is confidential and will only be used with your consent." She answers, "For me that is no problem." The unexpectedness of Maria's response permits us to consider the complex responsibilities of geneticists who deal with biological information of great import. If Maria does not seem to understand how important it is for her to safeguard genetic information about herself and how important it is for her to understand her biological destiny, chances are that many people lack the same kind of understanding. If Maria's understanding is limited, no matter how many papers she is given to sign or how many discussions she is asked to attend, her ability to give full informed consent will remain limited. Thus it is the responsibility of geneticists and other health care professionals to make sure that Maria's best interests are not jeopardized and that, whenever possible, her desires be fulfilled. What Maria, a poor woman, wants is what an affluent woman could get easily: a prosthesis or, better yet, reconstructive surgery for her breast. What is just and good for Maria is that she have her "beauty" back. Although geneticists may wish to limit their assistance to Maria, providing her only with scientific information about her cancer genes, if they are true healers, they must try to see if there is any way that they can make her a whole woman again.

Maria is not an It. She is a Thou, and as a Thou she demands that we recognize her person and her desires. By recognizing her and entering her world, we come closer to healing ourselves as well as Maria. Our fates become intertwined.

Notes

1. Linked to the Breast Cancer and Genetics project of the National DNA-BNDA Bank of the Fernandes Figueira Institute, Oswaldo Cruz Foundation.

2. The works of Buber express his deep commitment to life. For Buber, to philosophize is to explain the lived concreteness of human existence. Buber is rather skeptical with regard to the great concepts established by different philosophical movements. He shows affinity with the position of the Lebensfilosophie (philosophy of life) widely diffused in Central Europe at the time he wrote his masterpiece, I and Thou.

3. Hans Jonas, "La fundamentación ontologica de uma etica caro ao futoro," in Herder, ed., Pensar in Dios e otros essayas (Barcelona, 1998).

4. The term "freely given and informed consent" represents in Brazil one of the most rigorous ethical standards acknowledged by the respective Committees on Ethics in Research on Human-Subjects. According to resolution CNS 196/96-IL 10, there must be consent of the research subject and/or his/her legal guardian without deception, incompetency, subordination, or intimidation, and after complete and detailed explanation of the investigation, its objectives, methods, foreseen benefits, potential risks, and discomforts.

5. Roberto dos Santos Bartholo Jr., "Da vida provisoria," in A Dor de fausto (Rio de Janeiro: Revan, 1992).

6. Martin Buber, Do diálogo e do dialógico, trans. Marta Ekstein de Souza Queiroz and Regina Weinberg (Sao Paulo: Editora Perspectiva, 1982).

7. Ibid.

8. Ibid.

9. On March 2, 1999, the Brazilian House of Representatives initially approved a bill permitting hospitals in the public health system to perform reconstructive surgery in cases of mutilations caused by breast cancer. This fact reflects the social relevance of physical integrity, which is of great cultural value to the Brazilian feminine community. At the time of this study the bill has not received final approval. As a result, reconstructive surgery is still not available for all Brazilian breast cancer survivors.

15

Female Genital Circumcision and Conventionalist Ethical Relativism

LORETTA M. KOPELMAN

Traditionally Masai girls from Kenya are circumcised at seven or eight in order to be eligible for marriage at fourteen or fifteen. Their fathers, however, are now arranging marriages for them at increasingly early ages, sometimes when they are only nine years old. A Kenya news account offers an economic explanation for this social change, saying that "fathers are motivated by greed and the desire to get their hands on the dowries they receive in exchange for their daughters as early as possible." They seek a top bride price, such as "two cows, several crates of beer and some money" before the girls are old enough to resist.[1] Masai girls want to go to school and escape marriages to men often as old as their fathers. Sometimes they run away and find sanctuary at a boarding school about an hour south of Nairobi, headed by Priscilla Nankurrai. She helps them get schooling, avoid arranged marriages, and obtain medical attention for their all-too-frequent emotional and physical scars. The girls' mothers may help them escape, although they risk beatings if discovered. A developmental consultant who is herself Masai, Naomi Kipury, says conservatives fiercely oppose schooling for girls because they believe "the girls will reject the traditions of Masai culture if they are allowed to go to school. I think some parents are trying to get their children out of school to marry them quickly and regain control. Education opens up a whole other world and they fear the girls will get lost from the community."[2]

This news account reminds us that what some of us view as child abuse, neglect, or exploitation is viewed by others as traditional family and cultural values. In many parts of the world female genital cutting, child marriages, and denying girls the same opportunities for schooling that boys receive are regarded as violations of the law. Female genital cutting, the subject of this chapter, is viewed as mutilation and abuse in many parts of the world, including the United Kingdom, France, Canada, and the United States.[3] National medical societies such as the American Medical Association and influential international agencies including UNICEF, the International Federation of Gynecology and Obstetrics, and the World Health Organization (WHO) openly condemn and try to stop these practices. Around the world, women's groups protest the practice of female genital cutting and infibulation, denying that it is just a cultural issue and arguing that these rites should be treated with the same vigor as other human rights violations.[4]

These procedures involve the removal of some, or all, of the external female genitalia, denying women orgasms and causing disease, disability, and death in women, girls, and infants in these regions. These surgical rites, usually performed on girls between infancy and puberty, are intended to promote chastity, religion, group identity, cleanliness, health, family values, and marriage. Most of the people practicing this ritual are Muslim, but it is neither required by the Koran nor practiced in the spiritual center of Islam, Saudi Arabia.[5] These rites predate the introduction of Islam into these regions.

At least 80 million living women have had some form of this mutilation, and each year 4–5 million girls have it done.[6] It is hard to collect data, however, since these rites are technically illegal in many of these countries, the unenforced remnants of colonial days. The United Nations has a special ambassador on female genital mutilation, fashion model Waris Dirie, who, like some of the little Masai girls, ran away from her home in Somalia after undergoing a form of ritual circumcision making it impossible for her to have orgasms. She believes that these practices are wrong and should be stopped but warns that well-meaning Westerners may do more harm than good by attacking African practices. She urges them to use their energies to stop these rites in their own countries.[7] The Center for Disease Control estimates that around 48,000 girls currently living in the United States are likely to undergo these rites, over half of them living in the New York City area. Parents sometimes believe it is especially important to have these procedures done in the United States, since they view it as a sex-obsessed society where it is especially necessary to control female sexuality. Like the Masai fathers, these parents fear they will lose control of their daughters if they go uncircumcised. Immigrants generally get around laws prohibiting these rites by taking their girls back home or going to practitioners within their communities.

The U.S. federal laws are relatively new, however, and immigrants may not even know about them. Senator Pat Schroeder helped frame and pass the federal law upon hearing of the plight of Fauziy Kasinga.[8] In 1994, with the help of her female relatives, she fled Togo after learning she was about to be mutilated. She was imprisoned in the United States for illegal immigration but ultimately was allowed to stay. Her case set a precedent that female genital mutilation is a form of persecution.[9] In what follows, I argue against tolerating these rites as having cultural approval in these communities. I begin by defining some terms and clarifying the problem, since "female circumcision" and "relativism" have many different meanings.

Defining Terms and Setting the Problem

Female genital cutting or circumcision is commonly classified according to three types. Type 1 circumcision is the removal of the clitoral hood or prepuce (skin around the clitoris). Type 2, or intermediary circumcision, is the removal of the entire clitoris and most or all of the labia minora. Type 3, or pharaonic circumcision, is the removal of the clitoris, labia minora, and parts of the labia majora. Infibulation refers to stitching shut the wound to the vulva from genital cutting, leaving a tiny opening so that the woman can pass urine and menstrual flow.

People who want to continue these practices resent crosscultural criticisms, seeing them as assaults on their social traditions and identity. A version of ethical relativism supports their judgment, holding that people from other cultures have no legitimate basis for such condemnation. Anthony Flew defines ethical relativism as follows: "To be a relativist about values is to maintain that there are no universal standards of good and bad, right and wrong."[10] To avoid confusion with other definitions of "ethical relativism," I will, following Louis P. Pojam,[11] call this position *conventionalist ethical relativism*. It denies the existence of any underlying universal moral principles among cultures, asserting that moral principles depend entirely on cultural notions and acceptances. It rejects all forms of objectivism (a view that social differences can have underlying similarities with universal validity).[12] David Hume disavowed conventionalist ethical relativism when he wrote, "Many of the forms of breeding are arbitrary and casual; but the thing expressed by them is still the same. A Spaniard goes out of his own house before his guest, to signify that he leaves him master of all. In other countries, the landlord walks out last, as a common mark of deference and regard."[13]

Conventionalist ethical relativism is different from, although sometimes confused with, certain noncontroversial views.[14] For example, descriptive relativism holds that notions of moral right and wrong vary among cultures (sometimes called the diversity thesis). Conventionalist ethical relativism, however, goes beyond this to claim that no crosscultural moral judgments have moral force, since something is wrong or right only by the standards of some cultural group.[15] Conventionalist ethical relativism does not stop at asserting that different rankings and interpretations of moral values or rules by different groups exist but goes on to maintain that we have no basis for saying that one is better than another. Anthropologists sometimes use the locution "ethical relativism" differently, to mean what philosophers would call "descriptive relativism." Some simply use "ethical relativism" to signal that we should be very careful about making crosscultural judgments or that it is very hard to discern underlying similarities. To add to the confusion, both philosophers and anthropologists have used the locution "cultural relativism" to refer to normative as well as descriptive views.[16]

In addition, some philosophers and anthropologists seem to advocate a weaker version of "ethical relativism," especially those attracted to postmodern views. They hold that some crosscultural judgments have moral force but show disdain for substantive and fully articulated moral theories clothed as purely rational, abstract, and universal. For example, Susan Sherwin maintains that traditional moral theorists generally support the subservience of women and concludes, "Feminist moral relativism remains absolutist on the question of the moral wrong of oppression but is relativist on other moral matters."[17] She argues that female circumcision is wrong. By maintaining that some judgments have crosscultural moral authority, however, Sherwin is not defending conventionalist ethical relativism in the sense defined.

Female genital cutting and infibulation serve as a test case for conventionalist ethical relativism because these rites have widespread approval within the cultures that practice them and thus on this theory are right. Yet they have widespread disapproval outside their cultures for reasons that seem compelling but on this theory lack any moral authority. Thus many discussions in ethics about female genital mutilation examine which forms of ethical relativism entail that genital cutting is a justifiable practice in societies that approve it.[18]

Despite its popularity, there is a substantial logical problem with conventionalist ethical relativism.[19] From the fact that different cultures have different moral codes or norms, it does not follow that there is no objective moral truth or standards *of any sort* underlying our different behavior. The relativists' conclusion about what is the case (there are no universal moral codes or standards or any sort) does not follow from premises about what people believe is true.[20]

In response to this logical problem the conventionalist ethical relativists might argue that our different social lives and codes offer the best evidence that there are no objective moral standards and that what is right or good is determined by social approval. Therefore, I propose to consider the evidence and argue that it does not support the plausibility of conventionalist ethical relativism or a justification for tolerance of female genital circumcision or infibulation.

Morbidity and Mortality of Female Genital Circumcision

Of the three forms of female genital mutilation, Type 1 is the least mutilating and, unlike the other types, may not preclude orgasm. Type 1 circumcision, however, is very difficult to perform without removing additional tissue.[21] Types 2 and 3 are the most popular forms of circumcision and preclude orgasms. These rituals are so widespread that they probably contribute to the belief of men and woman in these regions that sex cannot be pleasurable for women, other than knowing that they bring pleasure to their husbands.[22] More than three-quarters of the girls in the Sudan, Somalia, Ethiopia, Egypt, and other north African and southern Arabian countries undergo type 2 or type 3 circumcision, with many of the others circumcised by type 1.[23] One survey by El Dareer shows that over 98 percent of Sudanese women have had this ritual surgery, 12 percent with type 2 and 83 percent with type 3.

A series of pioneering studies conducted in the Sudan by El Dareer, in Sierra Leone by Koso-Thomas, and in Somalia by Abdalla document that female genital cutting harms girls and women in many ways, having both short- and long-term complications. Later studies confirmed their findings.[24] The operation causes immediate problems that can even be fatal. They find initial problems are pain, bleeding, infection, tetanus, and shock. The degree of harm correlates with the type of circumcision. El Dareer found that bleeding occurred in all forms of circumcision, accounting for 21.3 percent of the immediate medical problems; infections are frequent because the surgical conditions are often unhygienic. She also found that the inability to pass urine was common, constituting 21.7 percent of the immediate complications. Finally, she found that these rites cause many long-term medical complications, including difficulty in the consummation of marriage and hazardous labor and delivery. Of the women surveyed, 24.5 percent estimated that these rites cause long-term complications from urinary tract infections and 23.8 percent recognized that the rituals has caused chronic pelvic infection.[25]

As high as the rate of these reported complications are, investigator El Dareer believes that the actual rates are probably even higher for several reasons. First, there are unenforced laws against female genital cutting. Although it is nonetheless widely practiced, people are reluctant to discuss illegal activities. Second, people may be ashamed to admit that they have had complications, fearing they are to blame. Third, some women believe that female circumcision or infibulation is necessary for their health and well-being and may not fully associate these problems with the surgery. They assume that their problems would have been worse without it. Of course, many other women, as these studies show, are well aware of the complications from these rituals.[26]

Reasons for Female Genital Cutting

Investigators have identified five primary reasons for these rites: (1) religious requirement, (2) group identity, (3) cleanliness and health, (4) virginity, family honor, and morality, and (5) marriage goals, including greater sexual pleasure for men.[27] These investigators, who are members of cultures practicing female genital mutilation, report many factual errors and inconsistent beliefs about the procedure and the goals they believe these rites serve.[28] They therefore argue that the real reasons for continuing this practice in their respective countries rest on ignorance about reproduction and sexuality and, furthermore, that these rites fail as means to fulfill established community goals.

Meets a Religious Requirement

According to these studies, the main reason given for performing female genital cutting and infibulation is that it is a religious requirement. Most of the people practicing this ritual are Muslims, but it is not a practice required by the Koran.[29] El Dareer writes that "there is nothing in the Koran to suggest that the Prophet [Mohammed] commanded that women be circumcised."[30] Female genital cutting and infibulation, moreover, is not practiced in the spiritual center of Islam, Saudi Arabia. Another reason for questioning this as a Muslim practice is that clitoridectomy and infibulation predate Islam, going back to the time of the pharaohs.[31]

Preserves Group Identity

According to the anthropologist Scheper-Hughes,[32] when Christian colonialists in Kenya introduced laws opposing the practice of female circumcision in the 1930s, African leader Kenyatta expressed a view still popular today:

> This operation is still regarded as the very essence of an institution which has enormous educational, social, moral, and religious implications, quite apart from the operation itself. For the present, it is impossible for a member of the [Kikuyu] tribe to imagine an initiation without clitoridectomy. . . . the abolition of *IRUA* [the ritual operation] will destroy the tribal symbol which identifies the age group and prevents the Kikuyu from perpetuating that

spirit of collectivism and national solidarity which they have been able to maintain from time immemorial.[33]

In addition, the practice is of social and economic importance to many women who are paid for performing the rituals.[34]

Investigators Koso-Thomas, El Dareer, and Abdalla agree that people in these countries support female circumcision as a good practice, but only because they do not understand that it is a leading cause of sickness, or even death, for girls, mothers, and infants, and a major cause of infertility, infection, and maternal-fetal complications. They conclude that these facts are not confronted because these societies do not speak openly of such matters. Abdalla writes, "There is no longer any reason, given the present state of progress in science, to tolerate confusion and ignorance about reproduction and women's sexuality."[35] Female circumcision is intended in these cultures to honor women as male circumcision honors men, and members of cultures that practice the surgery are shocked when clitoridectomy is likened to removal of the penis.[36]

Helps to Maintain Cleanliness and Health

The belief that the practice advances health and hygiene is incompatible with stable data from surveys done in these cultures, where female genital mutilation has been linked to mortality or morbidity such as shock, infertility, infections, incontinence, maternal-fetal complications, and protracted labor. The tiny hole generally left to allow for the passage of blood and urine is a constant source of infection.[37] Koso-Thomas writes, "As for cleanliness, the presence of these scars prevents urine and menstrual flow from escaping by the normal channels. This may lead to acute retention of urine and menstrual flow, and to a condition known as *hematocolpos*, which is highly detrimental to the health of the girl or woman concerned and causes odors more offensive than any that can occur through the natural secretions."[38] Investigators Dirie and Lindmark, completing a recent study, wrote that "the risk of medical complications after female circumcision is very high as revealed by the present study [conducted in the capital of Mogadishu]. Complications which cause the death of the young girls must be a common occurrence especially in the rural areas. . . . Dribbling urine incontinence, painful menstruations, hematocolpos, and painful intercourse are facts that Somali women have to live with—facts that strongly motivate attempts to change the practice of female circumcision.[39]

Although promoting health is given as a reason for female genital mutilation, many parents seem aware of its risks and try to reduce the morbidity and mortality by seeking good medical facilities. Some doctors and nurses perform the procedures for high fees or because they are concerned about the unhygienic techniques that traditional practitioners may use. In many parts of the world, however, these practices are illegal, and medical societies prohibit doctors and nurses from engaging in them even if it might reduce morbidity and mortality.[40]

Preserves Virginity and Family Honor and Prevents Immorality

Type 3 circumcision and infibulation is used to control women's sexual behavior by trying to keep women from having sexual intercourse before marriage or conceiving illegitimate children. In addition, many believe that types 2 and 3 circumcision are essential because uncircumcised women have excessive or even uncontrollable sexual drives. El Dareer, however, believes that this view is not consistently held in her culture, the Sudan, where women are respected and men would be shocked to apply this cultural view to members of their own families.

Beliefs that uncircumcised women have uncontrollable sexual drives, moreover, seem incompatible with the general view that sex cannot be pleasant for women, which investigators El Dareer, Koso-Thomas, and Abdalla found was held by both men and women in these cultures. Investigators also found that female circumcision and infibulation did not represent a foolproof way to promote chastity. These procedures can actually lead to promiscuity because they do not diminish desire or libido, even though they make orgasms impossible.[41] Some women continually seek experiences with new sexual partners because they are left unsatisfied in their sexual encounters.[42] Some even pretend to be virgins by getting stitched up tightly again.[43]

Furthers Marriage Goals, Including Greater Beauty for Women and Sexual Pleasure for Men

Those practicing female genital cutting not only believe that it promotes marriage goals, including greater sexual pleasure for men, but that it deprives women of nothing important, according to investigator Koso-Thomas. El Dareer and Abdalla also found widespread misconceptions that women cannot have orgasms and that sex cannot be directly pleasing to women coexisting with beliefs that these rites are needed to control women's libido and keep them from becoming "man-crazy."[44]

To survive economically, women in these cultures must marry, and they will not be acceptable marriage partners unless they have undergone this ritual surgery.[45] It is a curse, for example, to say that someone is the child of an uncircumcised woman.[46] The widely held belief that infibulation enhances women's beauty and men's sexual pleasure makes it difficult for women who wish to marry to resist this practice.[47] They view uncut female genitals as ugly.[48]

For those outside these cultures, beliefs that these rites make women more beautiful are difficult to understand, especially when surveys show that many women in these cultures attribute keloid scars, urine retention, pelvic infections, puerperal sepsis, and obstetrical problems to infibulation.[49] Even some people from within these cultures, such as Koso-Thomas, have difficulty understanding this view:

> None of the reasons put forward in favor of circumcision have any real scientific or logical basis. It is surprising that aesthetics and the maintenance of cleanliness are advanced as grounds for female circumcision. The scars could hardly be thought of as contributing to beauty. The hardened scar and stump usually seen where the clitoris should be, or in the case of the infibulated vulva, taut skin with an ugly long scar down the middle, present a horrifying picture.[50]

The investigators who conducted these studies believe that education about these misconceptions may be the most important means to stop these practices. Some activists in these cultures such as Toubia[51] and Abdalla want an immediate ban. Others encourage type 1 circumcision (removal of the clitoral hood) in order to "wean" people away from types 2 and 3 by substitution. Type 1 has the lowest association with morbidity or mortality and, barring complications, does not preclude orgasm in later life. The chance of success through this tactic is more promising and realistic, they hold, than what an outright ban would achieve; people could continue many of their traditions and rituals of welcome without causing so much harm.[52] Other activists in these countries, such as Raquiya Abdalla, object to equating type 1 circumcision in the female with male circumcision: "To me and to many others, the aim and results of any form of circumcision of women are quite different from those applying to the circumcision of men."[53] Nahid Toubia also objects because type I circumcision causes considerable, albeit unintended, harm to the clitoris.[54]

Debates over Conventionalist Ethical Relativism

Do moral judgments made by outsiders concerning these rites simply reflect their own moral codes, which carry no moral authority in another culture? For example, when international agencies such as UNICEF or WHO condemn female genital mutilation, do they just express a cluster of particular societal opinions having no moral standing in other cultures? Consider some key points of this debate over how to answer these questions.

How Do You Count Cultures?

Debates over female genital cutting and infibulation illustrate a difficulty for defenders of conventionalist ethical relativism concerning the problem of differentiating cultures. People who take the practice of female circumcision with them when they move to another nation claim that they continue to make up a distinct cultural group. Some who moved to Canada, the United States, France, and Britain, for example, resent laws that condemn the practice as child abuse, claiming interference in their culture. If ethical relativists are to appeal to cultural approval in making the final determination of what is good or bad and right or wrong, they must tell us how to distinguish one culture from another.

How exactly do we count or separate cultures? A society is not a nation-state because some social groups have distinctive identities within nations. If we do not define societies as nations, however, how do we distinguish among cultural groups, for example, well enough to say that an action is child abuse in one culture but not in another? Subcultures in nations typically overlap and have many variations. Even if we could count cultural groups well enough to say exactly how to distinguish one culture from another, how and when would this be relevant? How big or old or vital must a culture, subculture, or cult be in order to be recognized as a society whose moral distinctions are self-contained and self-justifying?

A related problem is that there can be passionate disagreement, ambivalence, or rapid changes within a culture or group over what is approved or disapproved, as illustrated in the Masai people of Kenya. According to conventionalist ethical relativism, where there is significant disagreement within a culture there is no way to determine what is right or wrong. But what disagreement is significant? As we saw, some people in these cultures, often those with higher education, strongly disapprove of female genital cutting and infibulation and work to stop it.[55] Are they in the same culture as their friends and relatives who approve of these rituals?

It seems more accurate to say that people may belong to distinct groups that overlap and have many variations. Members of the same family may belong to different professional groups and religions, or marry into families of different racial or ethnic origins. To say that we belong to overlapping cultures, however, makes it difficult to see conventionalist ethical relativism as a helpful theory for determining what is right or wrong. To say that something is right when it has cultural approval is useless if we cannot identify distinct cultures.

Do We Share Any Methods of Assessing False Beliefs and Inconsistencies in Moral Judgments?

Critics of conventionalist ethical relativism argue that a culture's moral and religious views are often intertwined with beliefs that are open to rational and empirical evaluation, and this can be a basis of crosscultural examination and intercultural moral criticism. Defenders of female genital cutting and infibulation do not claim that this practice is a moral or religious requirement and end the discussion; they are willing to give and defend reasons for their views. For example, advocates of female genital cutting and infibulation claim that it is a means of enhancing women's health and well-being. Such claims are open to crosscultural examination because facts can be weighed to determine whether these practices promote the ends of health or really cause morbidity or mortality. Beliefs that the practice enhances fertility and promotes health, that women cannot have orgasms, and that allowing the baby's head to touch the clitoris during delivery causes death to the baby are incompatible with stable medical data.[56] Thus shared medical information and values offer an opening for genuine crosscultural discussion or criticism of the practice.

As we saw in the section discussing the morbidity and mortality associated with these rites, some moral claims can be evaluated in terms of their consistency with one another or as means to goals. These rituals are incompatible with goals to promote maternal-fetal health because they imperil mothers and infants. We need not rank values similarly with people in another culture (or our own) to have coherent discussions about casual relationships, such as what means are useful to promote the ends of maternal-fetal safety. Even if some moral or ethical (I use these terms interchangeably) judgments express unique cultural norms, then critics argue they may still be morally evaluated by another culture on the basis of their logical consistency and their coherence with stable and crossculturally accepted empirical information.

Defenders of conventionalist ethical relativism could respond that we do not *really understand* their views at all, and certainly not well enough to pick them apart. The alleged inconsistencies and mistaken beliefs we find do not have the same meaning to people raised in the culture in question. In short, some defenders of conventionalist ethical relativism argue that we cannot know enough about another culture to make any crosscultural moral judgments. We cannot really understand another society well enough to criticize it, they claim, because our feelings, concepts, or ways of reasoning are too different; our so-called ordinary moral views about what is permissible are determined by our upbringing and environments to such a degree that they cannot be transferred to other cultures.

Philosophers point out that there are two ways to understand this objection.[57] The first is that nothing counts as understanding another culture except being raised in it. If that is what is meant, then the objection is valid in a trivial way. But it does not address the important issue of whether we can comprehend well enough to make relevant moral distinctions or engage in critical ethical discussions about the universal human right to be free of oppression.

The second, and nontrivial, way to view this objection is that we cannot understand another society well enough to justify claiming to know what is right or wrong in that society or even to raise moral questions about what enhances or diminishes life, promotes opportunities, and so on. Yet we think we can do this very well. We ordinarily view international criticism and international responses concerning human rights violations, aggression, torture, and exploitation as important ways to show that we care about the rights and welfare of other people and, in some cases, think these responses have moral authority. Travelers to other countries, moreover, quickly understand that approved practices in their own country are widely condemned elsewhere, sometimes for good reasons.

People who deny the possibility of genuine crosscultural moral judgments must account for why we think we can and should make them, or why we sometimes agree more with people from other cultures than with our own neighbors about the moral assessments of aggression, oppression, capital punishment, abortion, euthanasia, rights to health care, and so on. International meetings also seem to employ genuinely crosscultural moral judgments when they seek to distinguish good from bad uses of technology and promote better environmental safety, health policies, and so on.

Do We Share Any Goals or Values?

Although we may implement them differently, *some* common goals are shared by people from different parts of the world, for example, the desirability of promoting people's health, happiness, opportunities, and cooperation, and the wisdom of stopping war, pollution, disease, oppression, torture, and exploitation. These common values help to make us a world community. By using shared methods of reasoning and evaluation, critics argue we can discuss how these goals should be implemented. We use these shared goals, critics argue, to assess whether genital cutting is more like respect or oppression, more like enhancement or diminishment of opportunities, or more like pleasure or torture. Genuine differences among citizens of the world exist, but arguably we could not pick them out except against a background of similarities. Highlighting our differences presupposes that we share ways to do this.

Defenders of conventionalist ethical relativism argue that crosscultural moral judgments lack genuine moral authority and perpetuate the evils of absolutism, dogmatism, and cultural imperialism. People rarely admit to such transgressions, often enlisting medicine, religion, or science to arrive at an allegedly impartial, disinterested, and justified conclusion that they should "enlighten" and "educate" the "natives," "savages," or "infidels." Anthropologist Scheper-Hughes[58] and others assume that if we claim we can make moral judgments across cultures, we thereby claim that a particular culture knows best and has the right to impose its allegedly superior knowledge on other cultures.

This presupposition is incorrect because being able on some occasions to judge aspects of other cultures in a way that has moral force does not entail that one culture is always right, absolutism is legitimate, or we can impose our beliefs on others. Relativists sometimes respond that even if this is not a strict logical consequence, it is a practical result. Philosopher Susan Sherwin writes, "Many social scientists have endorsed versions of relativism precisely out of their sense that the alternative promotes cultural dominance. They may be making a philosophical error in drawing that conclusion, but I do not think that they are making an empirical one."[59] I find even this more modest conclusion problematic, as I explain in the next section.

Does Conventionalist Ethical Relativism Promote or Avoid Oppression or Cultural Imperialism?

Defenders of ethical relativism such as Scheper-Hughes often argue that their theoretical stance is an important way to avoid cultural imperialism. I argue, in contrast, that it causes rather than avoids oppression and cultural imperialism. Conventionalist ethical relativism entails not only the affirmation that female genital cutting is right in cultures that approve it but that anything with wide social approval is right, including slavery, war, discrimination, oppression, racism, and torture. That is, if saying that an act is right means that it has cultural approval, then it follows that culturally endorsed acts of war, oppression, enslavement, aggression, exploitation, racism, or torture are right. The disapproval of other cultures, on this view, is irrelevant in determining whether acts are right or wrong. Accordingly, the disapproval of people in other cultures, even victims of war, oppression, enslavement, aggression, exploitation, racism, or torture, does not count in deciding what is right or wrong except in their own culture.

Consequently, conventionalist ethical relativism instructs us to regard as morally irrelevant the approval or objections by people in other cultures; the approval and complaints are merely an expression of their own cultural preferences and have no moral standing whatsoever in the society that is engaging in the acts in question. I have argued that this leads to abhorrent conclusions.[60] If this theoretical stance is consistently held, it leads to the conclusion that we cannot make intercultural judgments with moral force about *any* socially approved form of oppression, including wars, torture, or exploitation of other groups. As long as these activities are approved in the society that does them, they are right. Yet the world community believed that it was making important crosscultural judgments with moral force when it criticized the Communist Chinese government for crushing prodemocracy student protest rallies, apartheid in South Africa, the Soviets for using psychiatry to suppress dissent, and the slaughter of ethnic groups in the former Yugoslavia and Rwanda. In each case, representatives from the criticized society usually said something like, "You don't understand why this is morally justified in our culture even if it would not be in your society." If conventionalist ethical relativism is plausible, these responses should be as well.

Defenders of conventionalist ethical relativism may respond that cultures sometimes overlap and hence the victims' protests within or between cultures ought to count. But this response raises two further difficulties. If it means that the views of people in other cultures have moral standing and oppressors *ought* to consider the views of victims, such judgments are incompatible with conventionalist ethical relativism. They are inconsistent with this theory because they are crosscultural judgments with moral authority. Second, as we noted, unless cultures are distinct, conventionalist ethical relativism is not a useful theory for establishing what is right or wrong.

Conventionalist ethical relativists who want to defend sound social, crosscultural, and moral judgments about the value of freedom, equality of opportunity, or human rights in other cultures seem to have two choices. On the one hand, if they agree that some crosscultural norms have moral authority, they should also agree that some intercultural judgments about female genital cutting and infibulation also may have moral authority. Sherwin is a relativist taking this route, thereby rejecting the conventionalist ethical relativism being criticized here.[61] On the other hand, if they defend this version of conventionalist ethical relativism yet make crosscultural moral judgments about the importance of values like tolerance, group benefits, and the survival of cultures, they will have to admit to an inconsistency in their arguments. For example, Scheper-Hughes advocates tolerance of other cultural value systems but fails to see that claim as being inconsistent.[62] She is saying that tolerance between cultures is *right*, yet this is a crosscultural moral judgment using a moral norm (tolerance). Similarly, relativists who say it is *wrong* to eliminate rituals that give meaning to other cultures are also inconsistent in making a judgment that presumes to have genuine crosscultural moral authority. Even the sayings sometimes used by defenders of ethical relativism (e.g., "When in Rome do as the Romans") mean that it is *morally permissible* to adopt all the cultural norms of whatever culture one finds oneself in.[63] Thus it is not consistent for defenders of conventionalist ethical relativism to make intercultural moral judgments about tolerance, group benefit, intersocietal respect, or cultural diversity.

I have argued that, given these difficulties, the burden of proof is on defenders of conventionalist ethical relativism. They must show why we cannot do something we think we sometimes ought to do and can do very well, namely, engage in intercultural moral discussion, cooperation, or criticism and give support to people whose welfare or rights are in jeopardy in other cultures. Defenders of conventionalist ethical relativism need to account for what seems to be the genuine moral authority of international professional societies that take moral stands, for example, about fighting pandemics, stopping wars, halting oppression, promoting health education, or eliminating poverty. Responses that our professional groups are themselves cultures of a sort seem plausible but are incompatible with conventionalist ethical relativism, as already discussed.

Some defenders of conventionalist ethical relativism object that eliminating important rituals from a culture risks destroying the society. Scheper-Hughes insists that these cultures cannot survive if they change such a central practice as female circumcision. This counterargument, however, is not decisive. Slavery, oppression, and exploitation are also necessary to some ways of life, yet few would defend these actions in order to preserve a society. El Dareer responds to this objection, moreover, by questioning the assumption that these cultures can survive only by continuing clitoridectomy or infibulation. These cultures, she argues, are more likely to be transformed by war, famine, disease, urbanization, and industrialization than by the cessation of this ancient ritual surgery. Further, if slavery, oppression, and exploitation are wrong, whether or not there are group benefits, then a decision to eliminate female genital mutilation should not depend on a process of weighing its benefits to the group.

It is also inconsistent to hold that group benefit is so important that other cultures should not interfere with local practices. This view elevates group benefit as an overriding crosscultural value, something that these ethical relativists claim cannot be justified. If there are no crosscultural values about what is wrong or right, a defender of conventionalist ethical relativism cannot consistently make statements such as,

one culture ought not interfere with others,
we ought to be tolerant of other social views,
every culture is equally valuable, or
it is wrong to interfere with another culture.

Each claim is an intercultural moral judgement presupposing authority based on something other than a particular culture's approval.

Conclusion

Female genital cutting and infibulation cause disability, death, and disease among mothers, infants, and children. It leads to difficulty in con-
summating marriage, infertility, prolonged and obstructed labor, and
increased morbidity and mortality. It strains the overburdened health
care systems in developing countries where it is practiced with im-
punity. Investigators who have documented these health hazards come
from these cultures but draw upon interculturally shared methods of
discovery, evaluation, and explanation in concluding that female genital mutilation fails as a means to fulfill many of the cultural goals for
which it is intended, other than control of female sexuality. Although
many values are culturally determined and we should not impose
moral judgments across cultures hastily, we sometimes seem to know
enough to condemn practices such as female genital mutilation, war,
pollution, oppression, injustice, and aggression. Conventionalist ethical
relativism challenges this view, but a substantial burden of proof falls
on upholders of this moral theory to show why criticisms of other cultures *always* lack moral authority. Because of the hazards of even type 1
circumcision, especially on children, many groups, including WHO and
the AMA, want to stop all forms of ritual genital surgery on women.
Unenforced bans have proven ineffective, however, since this still popular practice has been illegal in most countries for many decades.[64]
Other proposals by activists in these regions focus on fines and enforcement of meaningful legislation, but education of the harms of genital
cutting and infibulation may be the most important route to stop these
practices.[65] Thus an effective means to stopping these practices may be
to promote education.

Notes

1. Rosalind Russel, "Child Brides Rescued by Shoestring School: Masai Fathers
Sell Daughters for Cows, Beer, Money," *Saturday Argus,* January 30–31, 1999, p.
13.
    2. Ibid.

3. June Thompson, "Torture by Tradition," *Nursing Times* 85, no. 15 (1989): 17–18; Patricia Schroeder, "Female Genital Mutilation—A Form of Child Abuse," *New England Journal of Medicine* 331 (1994): 739–740.

4. Nah Toubia, "Female Circumcision As a Public Health Issue," *New England Journal of Medicine* 331 (1994): 712–716.

5. Asthma El Dareer, *Woman, Why Do You Weep? Circumcision and Its Consequences* (London: Zed, 1982); Daphne Williams Ntiri, "Circumcision and Health Among Rural Women of Southern Somalia as Part of a Family Life Survey," *Health Care for Women International* 14, no. 3 (1993): 215–216.

6. Ntiri, "Circumcision and Health," pp. 215–216.

7. Amy Finnerty, "The Body Politic," *New York Times Magazine*, May 9, 1999, p. 22.

8. Schroeder, "Female Genital Mutilation" pp. 739–740.

9. Sharon Lerner, "Rite or Wrong: As the U.S. Law Against Female Genital Mutilation Goes into Effect, African Immigrants Debate an Ancient Custom," *Village Voice Worldwide*; on-line http://www/ village voice.com./ inl/lerner.html Accessed March 3, 1997.

10. Anthony Flew, "Relativism," *Dictionary of Philosophy* (New York: St. Martin's, 1979), p. 281.

11. Louis P. Pojman, "Relativism," in Robert Audi, ed., *The Cambridge Dictionary of Philosophy* (Cambridge: Cambridge University Press, 1995), pp. 690–691.

12. Edward Craig, "Relativism," in Edward Craig, ed., *Routledge Encyclopedia of Philosophy* (London: Routledge, 1998), 8:189–190.

13. David Hume, *An Enquiry Concerning the Principles of Morals*, 1777. References are to section and paragraph 8:2.

14. The definition of ethical relativism used here is similar to that found in the most recent and important encyclopedias of philosophy (Craig) and two influential dictionaries of philosophy (Flew and Pojman).

15. To add to the confusion, some call ethical relativism "cultural relativism."

16. Richard Shweder, "Ethical Relativism: Is There a Defensible Version?" *Ethos* 18 (1990): 205–218.

17. Susan Sherwin, *No Longer Patient: Feminist Ethics and Health Care* (Philadelphia: Temple University Press, 1992), pp. 58, 75.

18. Sherwin, *No Longer Patient*; Loretta M. Kopelman, "Female Circumcision and Genital Mutilation," in *Encyclopedia of Applied Ethics* (1998), 2:249–259. Portions of this article were used or adapted in writing this chapter.

19. Craig, "Relativism," pp. 189–190; Flew, "Relativism," p. 281; James Rachels, *The Elements of Moral Philosophy*, 2d ed. (New York: McGraw-Hill, 1993).

20. Rachels, *Elements of Moral Philosophy*.

21. Toubia, "Female Circumcision," p. 713.

22. Ibid.; Koso-Thomas, *The Circumcision of Women* (London: Zed, 1987); Ruquiya H.D. Abdalla, *Sisters in Affliction: Circumcision and Infibulation of Women in Africa* (London: Zed, 1982).

23. El Dareer, *Woman*; Ntiri, "Circumcision and Health," pp. 215–216; Koso-Thomas, *Circumcision of Women*.

24. Loretta M. Kopelman, "Medicine's Challenge to Relativism: The Case of Female Genital Mutilation," in Ronald A. Carson and Chester R. Burns, eds., *Philosophy of Medicine and Bioethics: A Twenty-Year Retrospective and Critical Appraisal* (Dordrecht: Kluwer, 1997), pp. 221–238; Kopelman, "Female Circumcision," pp. 249–259.

25. El Dareer, *Woman*; Koso-Thomas, *Circumcision of Women*; Abdalla, *Sisters in Affliction*; June Thompson, "Torture by Tradition," *Nursing Times* 85, no. 15 (1991): 17–18.

26. Ibid.

27. El Dareer conducted her studies in the Sudan, Koso-Thomas in and around Sierra Leone, and Abdalla in Somalia.

28. El Dareer, *Woman*; Koso-Thomas, *Circumcision of Women*; Abdalla, *Sisters in Affliction*; Ntiri, "Circumcision and Health," pp. 215–216.

29. El Dareer, *Woman*; Ntiri, "Circumcision and Health," pp. 215–216.

30. El Dareer, *Woman*.

31. Ibid.; Abdalla, *Sisters in Affliction*.

32. Nancy Scheper-Hughes, "Virgin Territory: The Male Discovery of the Clitoris," *Medical Anthropology Quarterly* 5, no. 1 (1991): 25–28.

33. Ibid.

34. El Dareer, *Woman*; Koso-Thomas, *Circumcision of Women*; Abdalla, *Sisters in Affliction*; Faye Ginsberg, "What Do Women Want? Feminist Anthropology Confronts Clitoridectomy," *Medical Anthropology Quarterly* 5, no. 1 (1991): 17–19.

35. Abdalla, *Sisters in Affliction*.

36. El Dareer, *Woman*.

37. Ibid.; Koso-Thomas, *Circumcision of Women*; Abdalla, *Sisters in Affliction*; Ntiri, "Circumcision and Health," pp. 215–216.

38. Koso-Thomas, *Circumcision of Women*, p. 10.

39. M. A. Dirie and G. Lindmark, "The Risk of Medical Complication After Female Circumcision," *East African Medical Journal* 69, no. 9 (1992): 479–482.

40. Thompson, "Torture by Tradition," pp. 17–18.

41. El Dareer, *Woman*.

42. Koso-Thomas, *Circumcision of Women*.

43. El Dareer, *Woman*.

44. Lerner, "Rite or Wrong."

45. Abdalla, *Sisters in Affliction*.

46. Koso-Thomas, *Circumcision of Women*.

47. Ibid.; El Dareer, *Woman*.

48. Lerner, "Rite or Wrong."

49. Ntiri, "Circumcision and Health," pp. 215–216; Abdalla, *Sisters in Affliction*.

50. Koso-Thomas, *Circumcision of Women*.

51. Toubia, "Female Circumcision," pp. 712–716.

52. El Dareer, *Woman*.

53. Abdalla, *Sisters in Affliction*.

54. Toubia, "Female Circumcision," pp. 712–716.

55. El Dareer, *Woman*; Koso-Thomas, *Circumcision of Women*; Abdalla, *Sisters in Affliction*.

56. Koso-Thomas, *Circumcision of Women*.

57. Elliott Sober, *Core Questions in Philosophy* (New York: Macmillan, 1991); Kopelman, "Medicine's Challenge to Relativism," pp. 221–238; Kopelman, "Female Circumcision," pp. 249–259.

58. Scheper-Hughes, "Virgin Territory," pp. 25–28.

59. Sherwin, *No Longer Patient*, pp. 63–64.

60. Kopelman, "Medicine's Challenge to Relativism," pp. 221–238; Kopelman, "Female Circumcision," pp. 249–259.

61. Sherwin, *No Longer Patient*.

62. Scheper-Hughes, "Virgin Territory," pp. 25–28.

63. Ibid.

64. El Dareer, *Woman*.

65. Ibid.; Abdalla, *Sisters in Affliction*; Dirie and Lindmark, "The Risk of Medical Complication" pp. 479–482; Toubia, "Female Circumcision," pp. 712–716.

16

HIV/AIDS and
Prostitution in Mainland China:
A Feminist Perspective

WANG JIN-LING

Mainland China has been affected by the spread of HIV/AIDS over the past several years. Many Chinese, including policymakers, believe that the commercial sex trade is a major means of spreading HIV/AIDS. This view, which is typical transglobally, can be traced back to traditional Chinese moral standards which teach that "seeking sexual pleasure tops the list of all evils" and "chastity for women weighs more than life." Such negative teachings about sexuality help explain why, in mainland China, the majority of policies and regulations that aim to curb the spread of HIV/AIDS are targeted against female sex workers and prostitutes. This is unfortunate because, first, such a state of affairs demonizes an already oppressed group of women and, second, as I argue in this chapter, the commercial sex trade is not the *primary* cause of the rapid spread of HIV/AIDS throughout mainland China.

Spread of HIV/AIDS in Mainland China

The first reported case of HIV in mainland China occurred in 1985. By 1994, the total number of reported HIV cases was 1,774, a number that rose to 3,341 by 1995.[1] As of 1998, there were 9,970 reported cases of HIV/AIDS in mainland China. Of these cases, a total of 173 patients with AIDS died. Specialists believe, however, that there are many unreported cases of HIV/AIDS in mainland China. They estimate that there are probably 200,000 to 250,000 Chinese with HIV/AIDS[2] and that the number is increasing.

TABLE 16.1   1995–1996 Results from HIV / AIDS Monitoring Posts

| Year | People with STDs | | Prostitutes | | IV-Drug Users | | Long-Distance Automobile Drivers | |
	Total	*HIV/AIDS Patients*	Total	*HIV/AIDS Patients*	Total	*HIV/AIDS Patients*	Total	*HIV/AIDS Patients*
1995*a	9916	2	6454	1	5245	1	1174	—
1996*b	9546	1	5611	1	5395	105	800	—
Total	19462	3	12065	2	10640	106	1974	—

*a Department of Disease Control, Ministry of Health, et al, *"Establishment of HIV Sentinel Surveillance System in China and Report of Surveillance in 1995," Chinese Journal of Prevention and Control of STD/AIDS,* (May 1996): 193–197.

*b Qu Shu-quan, *"The Report of HIV Sentinel Surveillance in China, 1996," Chinese Journal of Prevention and Control of STD/AIDS,* (May 1997): 193–197.

That there is a close relationship between the spread of the commercial sex trade and the spread of HIV/AIDS in mainland China is undeniable. According to a report issued by the Ministry of Public Security, the number of prostitutes and clients arrested in 1984 was 12,281, rising to 115,289 in 1989, 287,995 in 1994,[3] and 418,000 in 1996.[4] Moreover, estimates indicate that those arrested account for only about 25–30 percent of the persons actually involved in the commercial sex trade.[5] This means that at the end of the 1990s, there were more than 1 million persons working in the commercial sex industry.

Given that the Chinese public is well aware that persons in the commercial sex trade do not practice safe sex, it is not surprising that they attribute the rapid spread of the HIV virus in mainland China to prostitutes in particular. What is not always known by the Chinese public, however, is that intravenous drug use and contaminated blood transfusions are two other important ways of spreading the HIV virus. In order to study the spread of HIV/AIDS effectively, forty-two posts were set up in 1995 to monitor the HIV/AIDS status of four groups of Chinese: persons seeking treatment at STD clinics, prostitutes, drug addicts, and long-distance automobile drivers. The 1996 results of this monitoring effort indicated that IV-drug use is the leading cause of the spread of HIV/AIDS in mainland China, where approximately 70 percent of all HIV/AIDS patients are IV-drug users.[6] See Table 16.1.

Another important source of HIV/AIDS in mainland China is contaminated blood. In fact, the first mainland Chinese to contract HIV/AIDS were all infected by "bad" blood from abroad. When some of this "bad" blood got into the bodies of people who routinely sell their blood for money, the HIV virus found a home in mainland Chinese blood banks, which sadly became the locus of transfer of the HIV virus to unsuspecting members of the population. Consider a typical case. There were 134 patients with HIV and one patient with AIDS in ShanXi Province. The patient with AIDS was a male blood donor. He had sold his own blood more than forty times (400cc each time). Of the 134 patients with HIV, 132 became infected with HIV through transfusions of blood obtained from the site where the patient with AIDS had sold his blood.[7] Specialists pointed out that because there are so many donor bloodmobiles in China, few of them equipped with adequate blood screening technologies, infected blood is routinely collected and accepted.

Despite the fact that IV-drug users and contaminated blood account for most of the cases of HIV/AIDS in mainland China, neither the drug trade nor commercial blood banks but the commercial sex trade is the primary target of policymakers. Moreover, although the clients of prostitutes as well as prostitutes themselves are penalized by government laws, prostitutes are penalized more frequently and more severely. For example, far more prostitutes than clients are arrested and sent to reform schools. In fact there are women's reform schools in each of mainland China's provinces, municipalities, and autonomous regions for female prostitutes, whereas men's reform schools for clients are few and far between.

As I see it, viewing those who work in the commercial sex trade, but particularly prostitutes, as the *main* transmitters of HIV/AIDS is the result of a cultural bias against women, according to which women are sexual seductresses preying on weak men. It is, therefore, unjust as well as counterproductive for policymakers to concentrate their efforts on controlling prostitutes' behavior in order to stop the spread of HIV/AIDS, when they should be focusing their efforts instead on the main causes of this state of affairs: drug addicts and blood donors.[8] Since one of my main interests as a feminist is improving the lives of Chinese women, particularly women who work as prostitutes, the main focus of my chapter is on developing public policies that not only help slow the spread of HIV/AIDS but also improve the lives of Chinese prostitutes.

Commercial Sex, the Spread of HIV/AIDS in Mainland China, and Bias Against Women

Worldwide, studies show that preventive measures, such as condom use, effectively reduce HIV/AIDS transmission.[9] Not sex per se, but unsafe sex contributes to the escalating rate of HIV/AIDS in mainland China. Regrettably, condom use is relatively rare in the commercial sex trade. A 1995–1996 surveillance report on HIV/AIDS transmission in mainland China revealed that the clients of prostitutes rarely or never use condoms, even when the prostitutes request them to so (see Table 16.2).

TABLE 16.2   Condom Use by Prostitutes in Mainland China: 1995–1996
HIV/AIDS Surveillance Report

Year	Every Time (%)	Often (%)	Rare (%)	Never (%)	Unclear (%)	Total Number (N)
1995 (1)						
(April-June)	13.0	6.7	14.6	65.6	0.1	3297
1995 (2)*a						
(October-December)	12.9	4.2	14.1	68.3	0.6	3160
1996 (1)						
(April-June)	8.6	5.2	17.8	68.1	0.3	2635
1996 (2)*b						
(October-December)	8.8	9.1	23.6	58.4	0.1	2736

*a Department of Disease Control, Ministry of Health, et al, *"Establishment of HIV Sentinel Surveillance System in China and Report of Surveillance in 1995," Chinese Journal of Prevention and Control of STD/AIDS,* (May 1996): 193–197.

*b Qu Shu-quan, *"The Report of HIV Sentinel Surveillance in China, 1996," Chinese Journal of Prevention and Control of STD/AIDS,* (May 1997): 193–197.

A 1997 surveillance report revealed that although the overall rate of prostitutes who never ask their clients to use condoms had decreased to 50 percent, in some rural provinces the proportion of prostitutes who engage in unprotected, unsafe sex had reached 92 percent.[10]

It is a fact that infected female prostitutes transmit HIV to their healthy male clients. But it is also a fact that healthy prostitutes are infected with HIV by unhealthy male clients. Many of these HIV-infected clients are foreigners on business in mainland China, but others are native-born mainland Chinese men. Even women who are not involved in the commercial sex trade are sometimes the victims of unsafe sex. For example, among the twenty-one patients reportedly infected with the HIV virus between 1988 and 1996 in Wenzhou, East China Zhejiang Province, two were native-born Chinese women with foreign, HIV-infected husbands.[11] In South China Yunnan Province, where IV-drug use is the chief source HIV transmission and where the majority of IV-drug users are men, the numbers of wives infected with HIV by their husbands keeps rising.[12]

On the whole, the citizens of mainland China are very unsympathetic to victims of HIV/AIDS, especially sexually active ones. HIV/AIDS is generally viewed as punishment for immoral and/or illegal acts and not simply as a tragic human disease. As a result, HIV/AIDS victims are viewed as morally corrupt persons rather than as suffering patients who need help. They are condemned as people who brought their disease upon themselves and deserve to be punished for their promiscuous sexual conduct. Although all people with HIV/AIDS are severely criticized, the harshest words and punishments are reserved for sexually active women, a state of affairs that accounts for the fact that HIV-infected prostitutes rather than their HIV-infected clients are more likely to be viewed as the people responsible for the spread of HIV/AIDS throughout mainland China.

From a humanitarian point of view, AIDS should be viewed simply as a disease that can infect both men and women, and not as a reflection on the infected person's moral character (especially females). Because people with AIDS are viewed as sinners or criminals rather than as patients and because HIV-infected females are considered somehow morally worse than HIV-infected males, mainland China provides poor health care to all AIDS patients, but particularly to female HIV/AIDS patients who work in the commercial sex trade. This is a blatantly unfair state of affairs for several reasons. First, women's lives are just as valuable as men's lives; second, female sex workers and prostitutes often have no other way to support themselves and their families other than selling their bodies to men; and third, women with HIV/AIDS are entitled to the same health care that men with HIV/AIDS receive. Therefore, gender inequities in HIV/AIDS prevention and control must be recognized and challenged by the people of mainland China so that equitable and effective HIV/AIDS policies can be instituted.

Because of the large amount of money generated by the commercial sex trade and the increasing number of Chinese women who see sex work as a viable job option, mainland China is turning its attention to this issue. Based on research findings and analyses, I recommend a new assumption to ground future HIV/AIDS public policies: HIV transmission within the commercial sex trade must be conceptualized and treated as an occupational disease, just like all other occupational diseases. Furthermore, women in the commercial sex trade who become infected with HIV must be treated with respect and dignity, just like any other patient in the health care system. Sympathy, not condemnation, is what these women need—a sense that they are worthy human beings who deserve to be cared for in their hour of need.

For the most part, prostitutes in mainland China do not know how to say no to male clients who pose a very real threat and danger to them. In need of money to support themselves and, in many instances, their families, prostitutes often say yes to unsafe sex with their male clients. For example, in a survey of fifty prostitutes in a women's reform school in Qingdao, Shangdong Province, forty-six responded to the question, "What direct cause led you not to use a condom?" See Table 16.3.

TABLE 16.3   Reasons for Not Using Condoms

Causes	Male Visitors Refuse to Use It	Not Necessary	Policemen Will Find It	It Is Difficult to Buy It	Total
Number	28	10	7	1	46
Percentage	60.9	21.7	15.2	2.2	100

SOURCE: Liou Jin-zhen, et al, *"A Survey on Situation and Cause of Condom Use by Prostitutes,"* *Chinese Journal of Prevention and Control of STD/AIDS.* (May 1997): 215–217.

In another survey of 200 prostitutes, a majority of them said that they would agree to sex without a condom if a male client said, "I will look for another woman if you ask me to use a condom" or "I will pay more money for sex without a condom."[13]

When a prostitute says yes to sex without a condom, she may or may not know how HIV is transmitted. Many prostitutes in mainland China have no knowledge about sexually transmitted diseases except the information they get from vulgar pornographic publications and from persons already engaged in the commercial sex trade. Under such conditions, it is not surprising that many prostitutes have no idea about what constitutes so-called safe sex. In large measure, prostitutes lack this kind of information because of the high rate of female illiteracy in mainland China, especially among its poorest women, who drop out of school at a very young age.[14]

Clearly, prostitutes are not born; they are made by a society that values women less than men and drives women to sell the only "commodity" they have at their disposal: their bodies.[15] As a group, women in mainland China are discriminated against in the distribution of social and familial resources. Burdened by heavy family responsibilities that require them to continually sacrifice themselves for the good of their children in particular, some women are drawn into prostitution because they erroneously think they can make more money and thus escape the heavy duties of being a wife and mother with no money to spend on themselves. There are, of course, reasons other than lack of money that push women into prostitution. For example, in a 1990 study of 389 prostitutes in Zhejiang Province, I discovered that women became involved in the commercial sex trade for the following sorts of reasons:

16 percent   "disappointment with love or love failure"
13 percent   "lure and temptation from somebody"
13 percent   "lack of care or excessive care from their parents"
12 percent   "retaliation against men"

12 percent	"domestic economic difficulty"
9.8 percent	"despair"
9.5 percent	"quarrel with husband"
5.7 percent	"pleasure seeking"
4 percent	"curiosity"
2.8 percent	"need for protection and care"
1.3 percent	"need for sexual satisfaction"
1.3 percent	other reasons

A few claimed to have become prostitutes in order to secure funds for a new home or to pay off their husband's gambling debts.[16]

Concluding Reflections

Among the points I wish to stress in conclusion are the following. First, compared with IV-drug use and contaminated blood transfusions, the spread of HIV/AIDS by sex workers and prostitutes is of only secondary importance in mainland China.

Second, it is primarily the lack of adequate safety precautions that accounts for the major role the commercial sex trade plays in the spread of HIV/AIDS. Were those who buy sex and those who sell sex better protected (through condom use, for example), far fewer sexually active people would become infected with HIV/AIDS.

Third, male clients' refusal to use condoms and prostitutes' lack of information about STDs, including HIV/AIDS, largely account for the lack of general safety precautions in the commercial sex trade. Because so many prostitutes are poor and illiterate, they are at the mercy of their clients.

Fourth, it is unfair to blame female prostitutes as the persons most responsible for the transmission of HIV/AIDS. Their male clients are just as responsible for the spread of this disease. Most prostitutes are not prostitutes because they want to be. If they were better educated and had a fair share in society's social goods and services, these women would most probably choose another occupation.

Clearly, faulty logic and sexist assumptions about immoral, worthless women drive mainland China's current public policy on prostitution. If society truly cares about all its members—female and male—and if it wishes to stop the spread of HIV/AIDS among its populace, then society must make some major changes in its treatment of women, including prostitutes.

Among the steps society can take now are the following: (1) correctly evaluating the situation in the commercial sex trade and its effect on the spread of HIV/AIDS; (2) withdrawing its condemnation of prostitutes as "bad" women; (3) educating prostitutes about HIV/AIDS prevention, helping them whenever possible to change their high-risk lifestyle and teaching them how to say no to male clients who refuse to practice safe sex; (4) educating male clients about HIV/AIDS prevention and punishing them if they abuse prostitutes; (5) educating the entire population about sex, including safe sex; and (6) convincing the entire population that HIV/AIDS is an awful disease and that the people afflicted with it are not to be viewed as criminals and sinners but as patients who deserve compassionate treatment.

Reform of laws, rules, and public policies in regard to the commercial sex trade will not be easy but must be done, not only to help stop the spread of HIV/AIDS in mainland China but also to improve the lives of mainland Chinese prostitutes and women. I urge Chinese policymakers, in accomplishing this task, to base their efforts on three principles: (1) respect for the human dignity of all people, irrespective of their chosen occupation; (2) promotion of distributive justice in families and society; and (3) encouragement of education, including sex education, as the best means to increase people's opportunities for freedom and well-being.

Notes

1. Chen Cun-ming, "The Trend of HIV/AIDS Spread in Mainland China," in *The Collected Works of Clinical Diagnosis and Treatment of HIV/AIDS in Mainland China* (Beijing: Restricted Publication, 1996), p. 7.

2. Zhang Qing, "AIDS Spreads Rapidly," *Chinese Women Daily*, May 6, 1998.

3. Zhang Ping, ed., *Social Problems in China* (Japan: YAJI Bookhouse, 1997), p. 150.

4. Li Li-zhen, "Wipe Out Prostitution Continuously and Firmly," *Chinese Women Daily*, September 1, 1997.

5. Ping, ed., *Social Problems*, p. 4.

6. Wu Juan, "Keep the Lives from Drugs," *Wenhui*, June 6, 1998.

7. Ren Jun-bing, "A Man with HIV Has Sold His Own Blood Forty Times," *Wenhui*, January 1, 1998.

8. Zhang Qing, "Sound the Alarm About HIV in Our Country Again," *Chinese Women Daily*, October 17, 1996.

9. For example, there is an introduction in the abstracts of the Fourth International Congress on AIDS in Asia and the Pacific.

10. Zhang Qing, "Let Us Say 'No' to HIV," *Chinese Women Daily*, November 11, 1997.

11. Chen Da-jin, "The Trend of HIV/AIDS Spread in Wenzou," in *The Collected Works of the Reference on Control of HIV/AIDS* (Zhijiang: Restricted Publication, 1996), p. 49.

12. Che He-he, "Control of HIV/AIDS in Yunnan Province," in *Collected Works of Clinical Diagnosis*, p. 91.

13. Wang Jin-ling et al., "A Gender Analysis of Prostitutes and Clients in Mainland China," *Zhejiang Academic Journal* 110 (March 1998): 53–59; Wang Jin-ling, *Analysis of Prostitutes in Mainland China* (Jian Shu: Publishing House, 1998).

14. Research Institute of All China Women's Federation and Department of Social Science and Technology Statistics, State Statistics Bureau, *Gender Statistics in China (1990–1995)* (China Statistical Publishing House), p. 235.

15. Wang Jin-ling et al., "The New Prostitution: Their Construction, Features, and Causes," *Research on Sociology* 44 (February 1993): 111–123.

16. Ibid.

PART THREE

Medical Research and Treatment

17

Ways to Approach the Problem of Including Women in Clinical Drug Trials

NADINE TAUB

As more countries are developed and industrialized, we can expect the use of sophisticated chemical and biological medications now being produced and distributed in one part of the world to assume an important role worldwide. Thus there will be a need globally for solutions to problems that now are of relevance only in the industrialized nations.

The problem of illness caused by "correctly" prescribed medication has attracted a fair amount of attention recently.[1] In this chapter I look at a somewhat different but related problem, one connected with deciding what is a "correct drug" and what is an appropriate dosage for women. Thus I am concerned with the problem of ensuring the inclusion of women in the clinical testing of drugs required to determine their safety and efficacy. The assumption that men can serve as proxies for women, so that women need not be included in testing, is simply wrong. Certain drugs may be neither safe nor effective for women. Others may require different doses for the two sexes. Thus the inclusion of women in tests that now are often done with men only would seem crucial.

The questions I consider in this chapter involve government bodies that decide whether drugs and devices will be licensed for distribution and, in that sense, regulate the release of medical drugs and devices. I consider positions taken by the U.S. Federal Drug Administration (FDA), which regulates medical drugs and devices in the United States, in some detail. Seeking insight into the conflicting perspectives, I look briefly at the European Agency for the Evaluation of Medicinal Products (EMEA), which regulates medical drugs and devices manufactured by members of the European Union, and at the International Conference on Harmonisation (ICH), which is an ongoing attempt to coordinate the regulation of medical drugs and devices in the European Union, the United States, and Japan. I look overall at the role women play in agency-required testing of these products. More specifically, I ask whether these agencies require women to be subjects in testing the products, to what extent, and whether such rules are desirable.

In the United States

In the United States, the history of the FDA reflects two competing concerns: (1) the need for inclusiveness in testing to ensure the accuracy of results for many and (2) the need to protect potentially vulnerable subjects. The relative importance of these two concerns has varied over time. It is now recognized, for example, that "emphasis on the need to protect research subjects burgeoned in the 1950s and 1960s."[2] Indeed, during this period, the protective concern far outweighed testing concern, particularly with respect to the reproductive function.

In 1977, the FDA excluded women with the potential for becoming pregnant, in addition to those who were actually pregnant, from participating in testing.[3] The rule's prohibition extended beyond those who actually conceived during the trial period to anyone who might conceive. To a large extent, this avoidance of deformity creation (in an anti-abortion world) reflected the post-Nuremberg concern for human life and a reaction to tragedies related to thalidomide, DES, and the like.

In the 1980s and 1990s, however, other concerns came to the fore. One major argument was that without women as subjects in the clinical trials, there was no assurance that the trial results would actually apply to women. In this view, biomedical research had "not given the same attention to the health problems of women that it ha[d] given to those of men, and that women may not have benefited from advances in medical diagnosis and therapy because of their lower rates of participation in clinical studies."[4]

Moreover, with the appearance of HIV and AIDS, as well as other very serious, often life-threatening conditions that did not respond to known medications, there was a real interest in being able to obtain medicines that were still at the experimental stage. If, however, women were not included in the experiments, there was no real hope of access.

In 1993, the FDA issued a new guideline concerning persons to be included in clinical trials that replaced the 1977 provision.[5] Reflecting the growing concern about the effects of drugs on women, the new guideline claimed to increase the number of women involved in clinical trials—without sacrificing their safety. The 1993 guidelines permitted women of childbearing potential to participate in early clinical trials, but not pregnant women. The revisions were thus intended to gain needed information about women's exposure. Female participants can now make decisions about fetal risk and try to forestall pregnancy.

The 1993 change did not, however, satisfy all those who were unhappy with the 1977 guideline. Critical response to the 1993 FDA guideline came particularly from groups involved with HIV/AIDS sufferers. Women who needed new medications were displeased with having to wait. Such restrictions were particularly difficult for women with AIDS or HIV, as medications to treat their conditions were not otherwise available.[6]

The FDA kept the 1993 guideline intact while it gathered a new committee of "experts" to consider the problem of obtaining access to experimental drugs for AIDS infection and the like where medication was only available on an experimental basis.[7] Following their work, a new regulation was issued in 1997.[8] Pursuant to this regulation, those faced with life-threatening diseases, such as AIDS, are permitted to take drugs that have not yet been approved for licensing and distribution. No distinction is made between males and females. This FDA action remains in effect to this day.

How should the compromise represented by the 1993 and 1997 developments be evaluated? It is, of course, a definite move toward greater inclusiveness, although falling short of *total* inclusion. Is it enough that the regulation proposed in 1997 specifically addressed the need for persons with life-threatening diseases to participate in the early stages of clinical drug trials? When this provision went into effect, the basis for criticizing the 1993 guideline was much reduced. Thus the United States resolved the seemingly conflicting needs of pregnant or potentially pregnant women for access to drugs in the early stages of testing and the needs of fetuses to avoid the danger of exposure during this period by allowing pregnant or potentially pregnant women to expose themselves to drugs in the period of unknown risk, but only when the disease they face is life threatening. This gives a woman with AIDS access to new medication being tried on men when nothing else has seemed to work.

In the United States, at least, we speak of adults being able to make decisions, to have the right—the power and the opportunity—to decide for themselves whether to take certain medicines and whether to participate in experiments to test them. This supposes that they have both the ability to obtain and the ability to evaluate available information about the drugs being tested. Are these assumptions close enough to the truth that we want to honor them?

The life-threatening case seems to be the easy one. The fetus in most situations will die if the woman does. Is the resolution completely satisfactory? Obviously, yes, for women facing life-threatening diseases who thus have access to new possibilities for cures (even if some find existing medication worth using). What about fertile women facing incapacitating illness that does not threaten their lives? Does the threat of incapacity outweigh risks to the fetus? Who should decide? Are these cases in which the mother (or the parents together) should decide what's best for the future child? Or do the potentially conflicting interests suggest that someone else should decide whether a prospective mother may take a medicine still under investigation? Or should the state, in barring all, some, or no one access to the investigational drug, substitute some other party? By barring women access in early stages of investigation, both the United States and, as we shall see, the European Union have made the state the decisionmaker in this context.

Usually, giving people the right to decide whether they will take medicine that is still experimental assumes that they are making decisions about risks and benefits for themselves. Those decisions may well have consequences for both themselves and their offspring, as embryos or, ultimately, as children. In the United States, at least, the embryo is considered part of the mother. Given that unity and the near unity of interest, it would seem that the mother-to-be is generally able and should be permitted to make decisions concerning their mutual body and how to maximize its well-being. The situation seems quite different from the drug or alcohol-inclined mother-to-be. In substance abuse cases, the woman is acting in accordance with her own interest and not her future child's, if she is even aware of what she is doing.

What does this mean for the father-to-be? We might just assume that his situation is different and his interests are distinct from the future child's interests, since there is no bodily unity between them. But this is an assumption to question. The future father's choices also affect the future child. For example, certain conditions—and diseases—may be passed on to a later-born child through paternal exposures or ingestion. As a bottom line, then, does that mean the future father should not be allowed to take certain products? Should he be prohibited from engaging in certain work for fear of harming the child-to-be? Does our reluctance to impose limits on the man suggest anything about the limits imposed on the woman?

In short, participation in the testing of medicines, particularly early in the process, is both like and unlike other types of exposures common in the United States. A number of situations—one thinks of drug and alcohol consumption—would seem to involve a greater conflict between parental and fetal interest than the medicine-testing situation. In the case of yet unlicensed medicines, the parent-to-be is undertaking a possibly high-risk treatment in order to help both herself and her fetus. (With regard to the fetus, the drug may have potential for "helping the future child" in two respects—helping the fetus reach birth and enhancing its life after birth.) By contrast, in the drug and alcohol situation, it is clearly the behavior of the mother-to-be, apparently seeking to satisfy a craving or habit of her own, in disregard of the fetus's interest, that is at issue. The medical products testing thus seems to be a different situation, even when a fetus is involved.

The European Union and
the International Conference on Harmonisation

By contrast, the regulations governing drug trials in the European Union make no specific reference to gender. Instead, the later phases[9] of the clinical trials require the tests to be performed on a proper sample of the population affected by the disease. But the sample need not depend on the frequency/type of the disease/type and population. It seems clear that if women (or men) are particularly subject to the disease, they will require medication, presumably of the sort tested. Thus they are to be included in the clinical trials—even if not in exact proportion to their share in the affected population. This is true even of phase 1 trials testing for safety and efficacy, which is ultimately subject to the ICH.

The ICH, as already noted, includes the United States and Japan in addition to the European Union. Thus different approaches between and among the treaty parties regarding the necessity *vel non* of explicitly requiring women to be included in testing are to be expected. As already noted, the United States, in keeping with its own analysis and history, would have the ICH require women's inclusion in the first phase of clinical trials, whereas the European Union is only willing to specify their inclusion in the latter phases, when safety and efficacy tests have been performed.[10]

The European resistance to specifying gender at the outset of testing is probably due to experiences akin to those of the United States following the imposition of the 1977 approach and has the same flaws. On the other hand, the United States has found that an approach that eschews sex specifics totally is not completely satisfactory either (whether to scientist or advocate); hence the U.S. call for specificity, at least to some degree. Given these differences, one possible ICH solution is simply to tolerate difference in the parties' systems and regulations, but this approach seems contrary to the very purpose of the ICH.

What course should the ICH take, then, with respect to the pregnant and potentially pregnant? To try to answer that question in context, we must ask who should have the power to decide whether a prospective mother's judgment—about her own conduct—should be superseded by another's, namely, the state's. In most situations, of course, parents and prospective parents are regarded as able to make decisions in the best interest of their offspring. Are there situations, besides those involving possible conflict of interests, in which the mother-to-be should be deprived of her decisionmaking power? One variation on this circumstance that comes readily to mind involves questions about a future parent's behavior and her or his right to endanger future offspring by behavior in connection with work-related risks, such as chemical exposures (mentioned before).

Concluding Discussion

Whether a procedure for testing a medical product is a good one is obviously a question that could be answered from a number of perspectives. In this chapter we have focused on the woman's point of view. Does including women in the first phase of clinical trials help or hurt them? The histories of thalidomide, DES, Depo-Provera, and the like are well-known examples of medication harming women (and their offspring). What conclusion is to be drawn from these unfortunate experiences? Is it that women, for their own protection, should not be exposed to such drugs unless and until they are determined to be safe for humans? Perhaps, if "humans" includes females. However, since the basic tests conducted to determine safety and efficacy occur in phase 1 of the trials, it would seem necessary to include women at that point.

It is, of course, extremely difficult to determine what's "right" on an individual, state, national, or international basis. But failure to come to terms with the difficult questions may result in both the failure to recognize and protect the needs of women and the unborn and the failure to facilitate the functioning of collective bodies.

Notes

1. See, e.g., "Danger at the Drugstore: Those Fatal Side Effects," *International Herald Tribune*, April 16, 1998, p. 1.
2. "General Considerations for the Clinical Evaluation of Drugs," U.S. HEW Publication no. (FDA) 77–3040, 1997.
3. Ibid.
4. Anna C. Mastroianni, Ruth Faden, and Daniel Federman, *Women and Health Research: Ethical and Legal Issues of Including Women in Clinical Studies* (Washington, D.C.: National Academy Press, 1994), p. 1.
5. 58 Federal Register 39406 (1993).
6. Terry McGovern, then director of the HIV Law Project and part-time instructor at the Women's Rights Litigation Clinic at Rutgers School of Law in Newark, New Jersey, USA, played a leading role in cocoordinating the comments of AIDS groups on the guideline.
7. Terry McGovern was a member of one of the new committees.
8. "General Considerations for the Clinical Evaluation of Drugs," U.S. HEW Publication no. (FDA) 77–3040, 1997.
9. These restrictions apply to phases 3 and 4 of the clinical trials described in earlier guidelines.
10. Martin Harvey of EMEA, telephone conversation with author, winter 1999.

18

Globalization, Gender, and Research

FLORENCIA LUNA

In 1997 and 1998 there was a heated debate about the use of placebo-controlled AZT drug trials on HIV-infected pregnant women in developing countries. As I see it, this debate is most instructive for the project of shaping a global bioethics. First, it deals with the relation between developed and developing countries and the ethical standards or values that should be respected throughout the world. Are all moral issues global, or are some of them peculiar to developing countries? Should we maintain unitary or different moral standards for developing countries and developed countries? How do we respect the particularity of different countries and cultures? When, if ever, is it justified to apply different standards of health care to different individuals and/or groups? When do people deserve the same treatment and when do they deserve different treatment?

Second, since the primary aim of giving AZT to HIV-infected pregnant women is to benefit their fetuses, this debate invites us to strike an appropriate moral balance between the interests of fetuses and the interests of HIV-infected pregnant women. In all nations, but especially in nations that still view women's interests as less important than their fetuses' interests, a feminist perspective must be applied. Only then can we be sure that women are being treated justly.

In this chapter I propose a way to handle debates such as the one I just described. I argue that supporting universal ethical standards for human research, such as the ones proposed in the Helsinki Declaration ("assuring the best proven treatment") does not necessarily mean lack of sensibility for local problems.[1] On the contrary, the best way to honor the rights of persons, made diverse by their race, class, gender, and nation of origin, may be to treat them all with the same respect and consideration.

Setting the Stage for Global Justice

Before offering my analysis on the ways in which AZT research was conducted on HIV-infected women in sub-Saharan Africa, I think it is important to focus on the phenomenon of globalization in general. Globalizing is an all-pervasive, complex phenomenon that manifests itself in positive as well as negative forms, depending on the context in which it appears. Although peoples in developing nations resist globalization insofar as it undermines their unique cultural heritages, they tend to embrace it insofar as it accords them the same moral, legal, and economic status as peoples in developed nations.

Among the gifts of globalization to all peoples is an increased recognition of human rights as the moral property of one and all. That the world is less and less willing to tolerate abuses in human rights seems clear in global authorities' recent condemnation of Chile's former president and dictator, Augusto Pinochet. When Pinochet went to London in October 1998 for surgery, a Spanish judge presented an extradition order for him to British authorities. The order accused Pinochet of violating the human rights of Spanish citizens living in Chile during his dictatorship. Pinochet pleaded diplomatic immunity, but his plea was not accepted by the British House of Lords, which agreed to hear the extradition petition. Although Pinochet appealed the House of Lords' decision, he was prevented from leaving England pending resolution of the extradition debate, which lasted for about two years. Regrettably, Britain's ultimate resolution of the case suggested that all its talk about human rights had been a fake.* But at least the affair refocused international attention on the issue of human rights—an issue that always seems in danger of being forgotten. Given England's resolution of the Pinochet case, it is no wonder that some critics in developing countries suspect that the entire pursuit of human rights abuses by powerful nations is a sham. Powerful nations like England are willing to challenge human rights violations only if they occur in small, relatively powerless countries like Chile, and even then they, like England, cave in under pressure. These same powerful nations would, however, never challenge human rights violations in countries equally or more powerful than

---

*When this article was originally written, Pinochet's case was still pending resolution. Then the presumption was that England was prepared to grant the extradition. Unfortunately, this presumption proved wrong. Noting Pinochet's poor health and age, England invoked humanitarian reasons for its ultimate decision not to extradite Pinochet. In point of fact, Pinochet was not as bad off as England claimed. After a twenty-four-hour flight back to Chile, Pinochet threw away his cane and strode off the plane. What a mockery! However, the final joke may be on Pinochet. As this book goes to press, Chile has decided that Pinochet may, afterall, be put on trial.

they are. In other words, powerful nations .invoke "global standards" only when they want to control powerless nations in harmful ways.

To be fair, the critics seem to have a point. Why, we must ask, did the United States, for instance, vote against the creation of an international criminal court? In June 1998 there was a World Conference in Rome to debate the creation of such a court. The United States insisted that it would vote in favor of such a court only if the five permanent members of the U.N. Security Council had veto power over the cases to be judged. Apparently, the United States did not want its soldiers to be judged for war crimes in other countries.[2] However, despite strong U.S. opposition and pressure,[3] on July 17, 1998, the World Conference in Rome voted to create a permanent International Criminal Court to judge the perpetrators of war crimes and crimes against humanity. The significance of this vote cannot be overemphasized. It is the victory of an idea of justice born in the Nuremberg trials, postponed by the Cold War, and renewed because of the ethnic crimes in Rwanda and ex-Yugoslavia.

What does this example as well as the Pinochet case show? To me it shows that just because a country uses the term "human rights" to bolster its own agenda does not mean that the ideas served by the term "human rights" are not of great value. To be sure, powerful countries will be more eager to punish war criminals in countries that they disfavor and/or in countries that are less powerful than themselves, but this does not mean that less powerful countries will be unable to convince the world community that war criminals should be punished wherever they are found: be they found in developing countries such as Chile, Argentina, Rwanda, or Yugoslavia, or in developed countries such as the United States, England, and Russia. Even if all the nations in the world can never agree on every aspect signaled by the term "human rights," their willingness to embrace minimum standards of what counts as a human rights violation is an extremely important starting point. It is never right to torture and kill innocent human beings.

In addition to highlighting the importance of human rights, globalization focuses its lenses on women's rights, especially in those countries in which women are routinely oppressed. In the same way that appeals to human rights helped women in developed countries attain rough parity with men earlier this century, they are now helping women in developing countries to do the same. A globalized view of women as men's equals provides women everywhere with the ideas they need to fight against their oppression. No matter where a woman lives she deserves the same economic, political, cultural, religious, and health care rights that a man has.

The positive aspects of globalization invite all people to recognize and insist on their basic human rights. All individuals are entitled to the same respect and consideration irrespective of their race, class, gender, or country of origin. Before we can take into account the particulars of a culture's moral code, we have to be certain that it is not systematically oppressing any of its minority populations or its women. A somewhat similar rule applies to medical research. Only after we are certain that the basic human rights of research subjects have been taken into account, should we consider whether there are factors that permit us to do research somewhat differently in developing countries than in developed countries.

Global Justice and Medical Research on Women

Although my focus is on placebo-controlled AZT drug trials on HIV-infected pregnant women in sub-Saharan Africa, my analysis applies to similar research in other developing countries. In general the purpose of the sub-Saharan drug trials was to identify effective yet affordable drug treatments for HIV-infected pregnant women. However, there was a major problem with the design of these drug trials, which provided AZT to HIV-infected women only during the last four weeks of their pregnancy. In the United States AZT had already been proved effective in blocking approximately two-thirds of maternal transmission of HIV to the fetus. In the AIDS Clinical Trials Group (ACTG) study 076, women were given AZT five times daily, starting in the second trimester of pregnancy. In addition to these women being given intravenous AZT during labor, their infants were given AZT syrup for the first six weeks of their lives.[4] As soon as it became apparent how effective this kind of treatment was, the study was terminated so that all the women in the study could receive the proper treatment for their fetuses. After the results of this study were published in 1994, the U.S. Public Health Service concluded that the ACTG 076 regimen should be recommended as the standard of care for all HIV-infected pregnant women without substantial prior exposure to zidovudine.[5]

When the U.S. Public Citizen's Research Group—a private nongovernmental health watchdog organization—became aware that some pregnant HIV-infected women in developing countries were not being given the standard of care, it protested. Peter Lurie and Sidney Wolfe, members of this group, published an article in the *New England Journal of Medicine* in which they claimed that the AZT trials being conducted in sub-Saharan Africa violated the Helsinki Declaration's provision that every patient enrolled in a clinical trial must be assured the "best proven treatment."[6] Lurie and Wolfe were not impressed by arguments that the "means" of providing HIV-infected pregnant women in the control group with a worse-than-best treatment justified the "end" of answering the question, Is the shorter regime better than nothing?[7]

Defenders of the AZT trials in sub-Saharan Africa stressed that in countries such as this one it is morally acceptable to provide women with less than the best proven therapy because some treatment is better than no treatment. Other defenders of the AZT trials, equally convinced of the standard practice argument, argued that placebo-controlled trials were justified because such trials are the "gold standard" in clinical trials. What's more, they produce results quickly and are very cost-effective. Finally, still other defenders of the AZT trials claimed that these trials had proven to be beneficial, since they demonstrated that a short AZT treatment is far better than no AZT treatment and, in some instances, was comparable to long AZT treatment. Although I think that there are some good arguments in favor of placebo designs—for example, those based on socioeconmic difficulties such as rural deliveries or the risks of breast-feeding in countries where water may expose newborns to multiple life-threatening diseases—most of the arguments in defense of the AZT trials strike me as overly reliant on the need to keep science "pure" and on the need to save money.[8] Why, then, do U.S. researchers and researchers from other developed countries think that as long as they do not leave research subjects in developing countries worse off than "nature" has already left them, they may view research practices considered harmful in their own nations as harmless here?[9]

I do not think that researchers should treat people in developing countries differently than they treat people in developed countries. Research subjects everywhere assume certain burdens on their time, resources, and energies. Such burdens are particularly heavy for poor people in developing countries, especially women. In the AZT trials under discussion women had to take time off from work; they had to find someone to take care of their children; they had to travel by public transportation to get to the hospital; and they had to medicalize and make "public" their pregnancy in ways that alienated them from their own bodies. Instead of treating these women as the "lucky" recipients of what amounts to substandard care, researchers should treat them as persons willing to make major personal sacrifices in order to possibly help their fetuses.

In addition, I do not think that lack of infrastructure, poverty, or lack of available treatment should condition the level of research and type of treatment provided. In many developing countries following the standard "ordinary" practice will mean jeopardizing the health and even lives of the women participating in a research study. To be sure, researchers might have to modify the design of a research study because of certain socioeconomic problems, but such modifications must always respect the women or other persons participating in such research. What is considered the standard treatment in developed countries should not be viewed as "too much" for developing countries. Research subjects deserve equal treatment. One's geography should not negatively affect one's moral worth.

Other Conditions in Developing Countries
That Should Be Considered in the Debate

Some bioethicists might reject a universal standard of care as an unrealistic policy that fails to acknowledge the differences among countries. But as I see it, embracing a universal standard of care does not entail blindness to local conditions. On the contrary, embracing such a standard is often the best way to protect vulnerable research subjects whose "local conditions" are ones of poverty, illiteracy, and the like.

In order to establish the truth of the assertion I have just made, I plan to focus not on the African situation but on the situation in my own country, Argentina. To be sure, Argentina's economy is better than the economies of most African countries. It has a large middle class and a relatively good system of public education. But it is still a developing country which shares the kinds of problems that plague developing countries throughout the world. First, there are the pressures that impinge on Argentinian physicians and researchers. In Argentina, physicians and researchers in public institutions are not well paid. Argentinian physicians generally supplement their paltry public salaries by accepting simultaneous positions in several hospitals or by accepting private patients in addition to their public patients. In addition, researchers routinely accept money from pharmaceutical companies eager to win approval for their drugs. They provide money to researchers to pay each research subject they enroll in a study (which may raise doubts as to the adequate selection of certain research subjects). These and other moneys are not paid directly to the institutions for which the researchers work. Rather, they are paid on the sly to the researchers, who pocket a large percentage of the money for their personal use. In addition to these cash payments, researchers are tempted with other kinds of "incentives," like trips to conferences and family vacations. To be sure, many physicians and researchers refuse to be seduced by these incentives; but it is undeniable that money tempts many researchers and physicians.

Second, there are Argentinean women who agree to be research subjects for reasons that do not always serve their best interests. Since most research is done in public hospitals and not in private clinics, the available patient population for research is typically the most vulnerable: illiterate men and women with scarce resources and with no other access to health care. In general, this population is grateful for anything that is offered to them and is disinclined to challenge or question authorities about any aspect of their health care. Behavior toward them is paternalistic, particularly if they are women.[10] Pregnant women, most especially if they are poor, are subjected to additional pressures. Argentina is a Catholic country in which some of the Church's precepts are followed in the public as well as the private domain. Research done with the goal of benefiting the fetus must be accepted because fetuses are considered persons. Hence poor pregnant women in a public hospital with nowhere else to go find it extremely difficult not to participate in research studies that aim to benefit fetuses. Told that they have a duty to their fetuses, vulnerable pregnant women feel they have no other choice than to serve as research subjects.

Third, the Argentinean political environment does not encourage respect for persons. In countries where killings are common (Argentina has a long history of dictatorships, murders, and violations of human rights), there is a general tendency not to respect persons.[11] To compound this problem, in Argentina the patient-physician relationship remains relatively paternalistic and quite authoritarian, particularly in those instances in which physicians' patients are female, poor, and illiterate. In addition, in Argentina "informed consent" is a legal instrument used to protect physicians and their institutions from liability. As long as patients sign on the dotted line, there is little effort to ensure that they really understand the risks to which they have consented. Ethics committees are of little help here, for there is a tendency to use these committees to justify whatever physicians and researchers wish to do.

To be sure, none of these three variables is unique to developing countries. Some of them are present in developed countries. However, these variables are more pronounced in developing countries where there are, in general, *very poor mechanisms to control or punish wrongdoing such as systemic corruption.*[12] Hence, the cumulative effect of all these elements together should be carefully considered in assessing appropriate safeguards for research subjects, particularly in developing countries.

Concluding Reflections on Women's Interests in Medical Experimentation

Just because the research environment in developing countries requires careful scrutiny does not mean that any research study conducted within them is invalid or not worth doing. To deprive people in the developing world of the benefits of appropriate clinical research is to make a bad situation worse. All men and women, but especially women, who wish to participate in research should be permitted to do so.

Traditionally, women were excluded from clinical trials. Drugs and therapies were not tested on them, and differences in male-female body functions and hormone alterations were not considered.[13] American biologist Sue Rosser points out two studies that dramatically demonstrate the research community's failure to consider important sex differences in research: (1) a study in which the effects of cholesterol-lowering drugs were tested on 3,806 men and no women[14] and (2) a similar study in which the effects of aspirin on cardiovascular disease were tested on an all-male sample.[15] Rosser claims that researchers' justifications for excluding women from their studies (cleaner data due to lack of interference from estrus or menstrual cycles, fear of inducing fetal deformities on pregnant subjects, and higher incidence of some diseases in males) might be "practical when viewed from a financial standpoint."[16] Nevertheless, observes Rosser, excluding women from research studies in order to keep the costs of these studies as low as possible "results in drugs that have not been adequately tested in women subjects before being marketed and lack of information about the etiology of some diseases in women."[17]

Moreover, as Rosser correctly points out, using only male research subjects not only ignores the fact that females may respond differently to the variables tested but also leads to less accurate models in the male.[18] Clearly, it is in the best interests of men as well as women that women, including pregnant women, be proportionately represented in clinical research studies. But is it in the best interests of fetuses, whose moral status remains debatable (are they actual persons, potential persons, or nonpersons), that women, including pregnant women, be represented in such studies? As it stands, it seems that many researchers are particularly loath to endanger fetuses, although the same rule does not apply to women.

Although fetus-oriented researchers claim that they exclude pregnant women from their research studies in order to protect them, in point of fact they are trying to protect not these women but their fetuses. Comments bioethicist Loretta Kopelman, "Barring women from participating in trials just because they are or might become pregnant denies them the same access to new and promising therapies as men. It assumes that there will be a conflict of interest between the mother and the fetus, and that the welfare of the fetus should come first as a matter of policy."[19]

It is not that it is wrong to exclude women from clinical research studies because fetuses have *no* rights. Rather, it is wrong to do so because women's rights are no less important than fetuses' or men's rights. Realizing this, the U.S. government, for example, has refused to provide federal funds to researchers unless they include women as well as men in their studies if at all possible.

Increasingly, it is becoming clear that when the drugs being tested promise significant benefits—in some instances life-saving benefits—the morally appropriate way to proceed is to provide as many people as possible with an opportunity to gain access to experimental drugs. Nowhere is this more evident than in AIDS research. Initially, researchers set unrealistically high criteria for inclusion in their AIDS-related clinical drug trials. When it became apparent that the drugs being tested were indeed therapeutic, AIDS activists persuaded researchers to devise ways to make these drugs available to people not included in their studies. As a result, "the parallel track" strategy was devised. It permits HIV-infected patients who aren't in a clinical research trial to gain access to experimental drugs if there are no therapeutic alternatives to the drugs being tested, there is some evidence of their efficacy, there are no unreasonable risks for the patients, and the patients cannot participate in the clinical trials for some reason or another.[20]

Perhaps the greatest humanitarian contribution to clinical research trials consists in searching for endpoints other than death for calling a halt to a clinical trial and measuring the therapeutic effect of a new drug. For example, when the drug AZT was shown to help some AIDS patients, a double blind, placebo-controlled, randomized clinical trial was begun. Some patients received AZT, others a mere placebo. After several months of testing the AZT against the placebo, 16 of 137 patients on the placebo arm died, whereas only 1 of 145 patients receiving AZT died. At this point the trial was ended and all the patients were switched to AZT.[21] Critics complained, however, that this trial should have ended before the sixteen people on the placebo had died. Responding to the critics' complaints, the research community agreed that in the future endpoints research should shift from mortality of research subjects to CD 4 level of lymphocytes or the appearance of opportunistic infections.[22]

Although the research community is sometimes reluctant to modify its research protocols and bend the rules of scientific studies, it increasingly recognizes that humanitarian considerations sometimes require making exceptions to the rules.[23]

For instance, AIDS vaccine trials will have to test different manifestations of the virus in different parts of the world, since the HIV virus presents itself differently in different environments. Research done in the United States or France will not be usefully applied all over the world, nor can it be tested only in developing countries. But this justification of variations in vaccine trials is quite different from one that aims to justify, for example, the use of research subjects in developing nations, where antiretroviral drugs are not readily available, as "guinea pigs" to test if vaccine-infected individuals can survive infection without antiretroviral therapy. This procedure is by no means accepted in developed countries, where antiretroviral drugs are available.

Thus it worries me when researchers urge their colleagues to do their research in developing countries for the kind of wrong reasons that Barry Bloom among others has suggested:

> In developed countries, it will be ethically required that individuals in vaccine trials who are found to have acquired HIV infection will be offered antiretroviral therapy, which usually dramatically reduces virus levels. If vaccines can-

not achieve protection against infection, however, treatment with antiretrovirals will compromise the ability of the trial to measure the efficacy of the vaccine in preventing disease. It may also obscure possible secondary end-points of vaccine efficacy, such as reduction in viral loads (a promising correlate of disease progression) or immunological correlates of protection. Because of these complications, determination of the protective efficacy of HIV vaccine *candidates may only be possible in trials in developing countries where the resources are not available to provide antiretroviral drugs*. It is that circumstance, plus the fact that development of successful vaccines will be an incremental process requiring multiple trials, that presents the most challenging ethical issues.[24] (emphasis added)

Because of all the challenges AIDS vaccines present, UNAIDS organized a series of regional "community consultations" to gather the views of relevant groups in the nations targeted for AIDS studies. These workshops were conducted in April 1998 in Brazil, Thailand, and Uganda. The views about the treatment to be provided varied among the different countries. Brazil's group argued that it would be unethical to deprive participants of antiretroviral treatment solely for the purpose of making a vaccine trial more valid or statistically powerful. They insisted that any Brazilian who became infected with HIV as the result of participating in a clinical trial should be provided the standard of care treatment offered to HIV-infected patients in the nation sponsoring the clinical trial. In contrast to Brazil, Thailand and Uganda agreed to a lower standard of care.[25] So desperate are these countries to stop the spread of AIDS among their populations that they seemed willing to deprive some of their own citizens of needed therapy. We have to be very careful in accepting such a double standard. It may imply treating people from developing countries as mere guinea pigs, opening the possibility of doing cheap research at their expense.

Clearly, AIDS is a major problem in much of the developing world, and developing nations need the help of developed nations in order to save their populations from decimation and enormous suffering. However, the best way for developed nations to help developing nations overcome AIDS is not the way that tramples the rights of men and women who are poor, illiterate, and perhaps very frightened. Rather, it is up to researchers to use some of their intellectual talents to devise ethically sound as well as scientifically rigorous research protocols. They should take the lead in respecting human rights, striving to maintain universal ethical standards.

Notes

A longer version of some of the ideas presented in this chapter is contained in *Bioethics and Research in Argentina,* in press for the series *Philosophy in Latin America*, RODOPI.

1. "In any medical study, every patient—including those of a control group, if any—should be assured of the best proven diagnostic and therapeutic method." Declaration of Helsinki, II, 1989, p. 3.

2. Aryeh Neier, "Los EE.UU. Y el poder de veto," *La Nación*, July 8, 1998, p. 19.

3. "Aprobaron la creación de la Corte Criminal Internacional," *La Nación*, July 18, 1998, p. 3. The statute can be signed any time before December 31, 2000. It will function sixty days after it is ratified by sixty countries and will not be retroactive thereafter.

4. James Mc Intyre, "AZT Trials to Reduce Perinatal HIV Transmission: A Debate About Science, Ethics, and Resources," *Reproductive Health Matters* 6, no. 11 (1998): 129–130.

5. Paul Lurie and Sidney M. Wolfe, "Unethical Trials of Interventions to Reduce Perinatal Transmission of the Human Immunodeficiency Virus in Developing Countries," *New England Journal of Medicine* 337, no. 12 (1997): 853. At the time of the controversy some of these trials had been stopped. See E. Marshall, "Controversial Trial Offers Hopeful Result," *Science*, February 27, 1998, p. 1299.

6. Lurie and Wolfe, "Unethical Trials," p. 853.

7. Ibid., p. 854.

8. See Florencia Luna, *Bioethics: Latin American Perspective,* Value Inquiry Book Series (Amsterdam: Rodopi Publishing House, forthcoming).

9. Deborah Zion, criticizing this argument, points out its disturbing implications: "it is ethically acceptable to exploit the suffering of vulnerable populations even though the means to alleviate it are known, because if no trial at all were offered the women in question would have passed on the infection to their children anyway." "Ethical Considerations of Clinical Trials to Prevent Vertical Transmission of HIV in Developing Countries," *Nature Medicine* 4, no. 1 (1998): 11.

10. Florencia Luna, "Paternalism and the Argument from Illiteracy," *Bioethics* 9, no. 3–4 (1995): 283–290.

11. Ibid.

12. See Florencia Luna, "Corruption and Research," *Bioethics* 13, no. 3–4 (1999): 262–271.

13. Sue Rosser, "Re-visioning Clinical Research: Gender and the Ethics of Experimental Design," *Hypatia* 4, no. 2 (1989): 127.

14. Jean Hamilton, "Avoiding Methodological Biases in Gender-Related Research," in *Women's Health Report of the Public Health Service Task Force on Women's Health Issues* (Washington, D.C.: U.S. Department of Health and Human Services).

15. Steering Committee of the Physician's Health Study Research Group, *Science and Government Report*, Washington, D.C., March 1, 1988, p. 1. Special report of findings from the aspirin component of the ongoing physician's health study, *New England Journal of Medicine* 318, no. 4 (1998): 262–264.

16. Ibid.

17. Ibid.

18. Rosser, "Re-visioning Clinical Research," p. 129.

19. Loretta Kopelman, "How AIDS Activists Are Changing Research," in J. Monagle and David Thomasma, eds., *Health Care Ethics: Critical Issues* (Gaithersburg: Aspen, 1994), p. 206.

20. Ibid., p. 201.

21. Ibid., p. 207.

22. T. C. Merrigan, "You Can Teach an Old Dog New Tricks: How AIDS Trials Are Pioneering New Strategies," *New England Journal of Medicine* 323 (1990): 1341–1343.

23. I do not endorse a merely "consumerist" view of research. Research in the case of illness may put women and men in a very vulnerable situation and this should be acknowledged. See Florencia Luna, "Sida e investigación: ¿Fin de un paradigma en investigación?" *Análisis Filosófico* 17 (1997): 2. I do favor the idea of a cooperative venture, particularly Loretta Kopelman's proposition. However, because of possible corruption in developing countries, I would carefully monitor such a process.

24. Ibid., p. 196.

25. Ruth Macklin, "International Collaborative Research: Recent Developments" (manuscript presented at PAHO meeting, May 1999).

19

Realizing Justice in Health Research for Women: Reflections on Democratizing Decisionmaking

LISA A. ECKENWILER

Advocates for women's health worldwide are pressing the importance of incorporating democratic ethical and political ideals in scientific projects. Appealing to ideals of social equality and self-determination, they agree on the quite general notion that women who bear the consequences of decisions should be integrally involved in the process of making them. Yet the meaning of the word "democratic" and accounts of how such a concept will work in specific contexts are issues that demand further attention. Such attention is, of course, vital, given accounts of injustice against certain groups, women chief among them.

My aim in this chapter is to contribute to this endeavor, which joins philosophical theory with practice, by exploring different models of democratic decisionmaking, specifically for the purposes of setting health research agendas, allocating funds for such research, and reviewing ethical concerns raised by programs of research and the particular protocols that compose them. This is a project of global significance, since women all over the world are involved (to varying degrees, of course) as participants in health research, and virtually all are affected by its results. In my estimation, although others have made efforts to develop models of democratic decisionmaking in the women's health research arena, so far neither the communitarian model of democratization proposed in the United States nor the strategies deployed in some developing countries adequately promotes ideals of equality and liberty. Although these models have promising elements, I believe there are better alternatives, alternatives conceived from some of the insights of feminist thought.

Communitarian Models for
Democratic Research in the United States

The Theory Explained

The fundamental notion at work in the social ontology of much of liberal moral and political theory is that persons are appropriately regarded as radically individualized, that is, as atomistic, self-sufficient entities which, because they are abstracted from social contexts, share the same moral rights and capacities for reason and action and for formulating a conception of the good.[1] Challenging this notion, communitarians insist that the self is essentially social, that is, embodied, constituted, and defined by its attachments, including the particularities of its social relationships, community ties, and historical context. In explaining what they mean by "community," communitarians typically refer to families, workplaces, religious organizations, tribes, nations, and the like.[2] They claim that these communities are partially, if not wholly, definitive of persons' perspectives and moral commitments, and that persons should willingly acknowledge their communal commitments in ethical and political discussions.

The communitarian ideal has found favor in the U.S. biomedical research enterprise. Although the National Institutes of Health (NIH) does not embrace a communitarian philosophy in its full complexity, NIH research initiatives aimed at women give expression to the central features of communitarianism. Articulating a commitment to study populations in terms of racial and ethnic characteristics, cultural norms, language, level of education, socioeconomic status, occupation, family configuration, and geographical location, these initiatives reflect the notion that women's identities, values, and life prospects are, to a great degree, constituted by the social context in which they are embedded.[3]

NIH researchers are charged with ensuring that efforts at recruitment and retention "conform with the needs and values of the research participants and their communities," underscoring a commitment to shared or communal values (both within communities and between communities and researchers) and to democratized decisionmaking.[4] In particular, they are urged to discuss the involvement of community members in such processes as establishing goals for recruitment and retention and evaluating the effectiveness of various strategies; achieving agreement on plans for the design, methodologies, implementation, and completion of research; and establishing and maintaining communication concerning the progress and findings of studies.[5] With these initiatives the NIH pledges to form "partnerships based on trust and mutual respect" with communities, acknowledging that "in the absence of common goals or shared recognition of the unique needs of the community, clinical studies cannot successfully coexist with a community."[6] Such provisions reflect a departure from the (illusory) notion that impartial experts are the only credible decisionmakers in research and that only they can adequately take account of the perspectives of others. "Subjectivities," in this case communal values, are to be incorporated in research projects, indeed, expressed by members of communities themselves.

Despite their welcome shift away from the reign of impartiality, I believe that when the ideals of communitarianism are *uncritically* embraced in research. They tend to undermine equality and inhibit women's ability to express their own experiences, to determine their own actions, and to lead their own version of a health life. Four objections to communitarianism are of particular relevance. First, communitarians tend to rely on models of community that do not necessarily enhance women's equality and self-determination. Second, communitarians have a tendency to "construct" the communities they study according to dominant social norms and to view subjects through distortive lenses, a tendency that undermines justice. Third, communitarians have a "desire [for] social wholeness," or "an urge to see persons in unity with one another in a shared whole,"[7] a tendency that functions to obscure the complexity of selves and social relations, and to exclude differences. Finally, even though it grants the significance of social situatedness, the conception of the self reflected in the NIH initiatives is impoverished, for it "situates" selves not for the purpose of supporting moral agency and enriching assessments of needs but for the (capitalistic?) purposes of promoting resource consumption. I turn now to discuss each of these challenges to communitarianism in detail.

Communitarianism Critiqued

Objection 1. In reference to communities that influence persons' identities and their moral commitments, readers will recall that most often communitarians refer to families, workplaces, churches, neighborhoods, social and civic organizations, tribes, and nations. These same models of community have been embraced by researchers. Elaborating on the goal of developing partnerships with communities, the NIH, for example, maintains that its aim is to "work with existing community structures." Outreach documents refer to health care institutions, community businesses and organizations, religious communities, social service agencies including public welfare offices, public housing offices, and neighborhood and tenant associations. Researchers, furthermore, are advised to identify "gatekeepers," "decisionmakers," "community leaders," and other "influential members" in such places for possible enlistment as recruitment agents.[8]

Although researchers invoking the insights of communitarians deserve praise for their recognition of the relevance of close human relations in people's lives, they are to be faulted for presenting as unproblematic "communities" that are typically very problematic for *women*. Families are often contexts for nurturing and self-development, but they may also serve to reinforce a coercive heterosexist culture and the sexual division of labor, and to provide a context for violence against women.[9] Workplaces are settings characterized more often than not by racism, sexism, and homophobia. Religious institutions rarely promote women to positions of formal leadership, despite the fact that the majority of their members are usually women.[10] What is more, their doctrines may make moral claims on women that contribute to their oppression.[11] Social service agencies and the legal system frequently stereotype and subject women to contestable interpretations of their needs.[12] Nations and tribes routinely exclude women from conceptions of communal good and from participation in governing bodies.[13] In particular, they generally fail to recognize women as leaders, with the exception of those few they view as exceptional on account of their high degree of education or preestablished political and financial ties, for example.[14] Even where such women are recognized as leaders, they can expect to face resistance and perhaps continued subordination through norms, moral rules, and laws.[15] When communities view them as less important, deserving of respect and equality, many women come to endorse their diminished status.[16]

Given the ways in which traditional models of community can and do oppress women, reliance on them and their "leaders" is a strategy that would seem to inhibit rather than enhance women's capacities to develop and exercise self-determination. If researchers rely uncritically on the notions of what is "good" for women that emerge from traditional communities—constituted according to patriarchal norms, racial and cultural biases, and ossified class structures—they will inevitably treat women unjustly either by denying them participation in research studies altogether or by embracing what are most likely impoverished and distorted assessments of women's health needs, just as impartialist approaches have done. For example, patriarchal communities with capitalist leanings might see reproduction among poor women of color as a hindrance to economic growth and so support contraceptive research projects on birth control methods that enhance compliance and inhibit choice (consider the debates surrounding Norplant and Depo-Provera).[17]

Objection 2.   When communitarian-minded researchers undertake efforts to involve community members in research planning, they often construct community boundaries themselves, grouping people together according to patterns they identify. As a result, they tend to impose certain identities on their research subjects. Worse, they impose these identities on the basis of racial, cultural, and other categorizations that have frequently been defined as deviant and inferior.[18] In other words, researchers influenced by communitarianism often construct communities in ways that can perpetuate injustice. They might, for instance, interpret the diseases of African Americans as owing to their "inferior" genes or "deviant" lifestyle choices instead of environmental factors such as lack of adequate health care insurance and education.[19]

Researchers relying on communitarian ideas have also manifested a tendency to view everyone in a community as essentially the same, thereby failing to capture the complex identities and social experiences of its very different members. In responding to HIV/AIDS in the United States, for example, categories such as the "gay community" or "community of color" have obscured the multiple relations and social networks that in fact compose identities.[20] Ultimately such constructions of community inhibit the development of effective strategies for disease prevention and treatment, including the design of research projects attentive to people's physical and psychological differences.

Objection 3.   Although problems occur when researchers construct and impose "community" identities on their research subjects, problems also occur when people construct themselves as a community. When used by persons counting themselves as members, the term "community" most often is meant to refer to those with whom one identifies, based on a shared history, culture, or set of beliefs and values. Commitment to an ideal of community may be associated, however, with valuing and enforcing homogeneity because membership typically entails an "oppositional differentiation" from other persons and groups. In other words, persons feel a sense of mutual identification only with some persons and not with others. Thus the ideal of community can express "desire for the fusion of subjects with one another which in practice operates to exclude those with whom the group does not identify."[21]

To take an example, although groups working around HIV/AIDS in the United States have invoked the concept of community "in order to create a sense of unity, where discrimination and assimilation have produced fragmentation" and to "thematize the power of collective action," some of these groups are still "guilty" of certain forms of exclusion.[22] In the "white gay community," for example, racism has precluded the inclusion of nonwhite gay men, whereas in "communities of color," the social stigma of homosexuality has made it difficult to embrace gay members of any skin color. Such exclusions made it especially difficult to develop research strategies that were meaningful and effective for all people.

Because of the considerations raised above, it is crucial to explore who is and who is not likely to be influential in designing research strategies. Again, consider research on AIDS in the United States. Invoking the language of "reproductive choice"—borrowed from feminists who claimed to represent all women—the pediatricians and public health officials who developed protocol AIDS Clinical Trials Group (ACTG) protocol 076 to decrease perinatal transmission of HIV/AIDS failed to see that the protocol might affect HIV-infected women of color differently than HIV-infected white women.[23] However well-intentioned these health care researchers were, they designed protocol 076 without consulting the women disproportionately affected by HIV/AIDS—particularly poor women of color with histories of substance abuse. Had they consulted these less-than-privileged women, chances are that protocol 076 would have been written differently.[24] Certainly, it would have been written so as to preclude forms of AIDS counseling and testing that inevitably target women whom the dominant society views as "drains" on public resources, poor candidates for motherhood, and irresponsible persons unable to control their urges, particularly their sexual desires.[25]

Objection 4. There is one final concern with strategies that acknowledge women's embeddedness in communities, namely, a view of women as consumers or receptacles of clinical research resources. This conception of women is evident in initiatives aimed principally at promoting successful recruitment of women in clinical studies, and gaining "maximized local acceptance of the program."[26] To the extent that proposals to involve women in designing research plans ultimately amount to efforts to promote and maintain enrollment, women are regarded as recipients of research resources and, eventually, as consumers of (markets for) health care products.

To summarize, the incorporation of communitarian ideals in health research for women cannot ultimately promote social justice for them, despite displaying appreciation for the social contexts in which women live and for the need to involve them in aspects of research planning. Although communitarian models of community may well be integral to women's lives, they often shape women's identities in ways that warrant critique. Beyond recognizing that selves are embedded in and constituted by communities, it is crucial to consider "*how* social selves are constituted, toward what ends, and with what costs and benefits for various individuals, groups, and relations."[27] Moreover, it is crucial to reckon with the relations of privilege within and among communities, and between communities and researchers, which distort determinations of women's needs.

Empowerment Models for Democratic Research in Developing Nations

In developing countries, as in the United States, researchers are struggling to identify democratic standards for decisionmaking. Although many of the empowerment models designed by researchers in developing countries are steps in the right direction, they stop short of securing the right kind of input from all the persons involved in and affected by research. In particular, they have some difficulty adequately attending to women's voices. Thus they too are ultimately unsuccessful in supporting women's social equality and capacities for self-determination.

Empowerment Approaches That Exclude Women in Planning

Recognizing the need for moral guidance in research projects that are international in scope, in 1992 the Council for International Organizations of Medical Sciences (CIOMS), in collaboration with the World Health Organization, published guidelines for the appropriate use of research subjects from "underdeveloped communities."[28] Among the rules for researchers' conduct is what seems to be a provision for democratizing decisionmaking. Because research projects in the developing world are often funded by government agencies, foundations, corporations, or associations based in or receiving support from powerful European and North American nations, places distant and in many respects different from where the research subjects reside, guideline 8 recognizes that persons in the developing world are socially and economically at risk of being exploited for research purposes. Thus the guideline states that investigators working in developing countries should try to ensure that "the research is responsive to the health needs and priorities of the community in which it is to be carried out . . . [and that] proposals for research have been reviewed and approved by an ethical review committee . . . familiar with the customs and traditions of the community."[29]

Regrettably, following the CIOMS guidelines does not ensure that justice will be realized. The same problems that plague communitarian initiatives in the United States can arise. Researchers may organize and approach communities according to troublesome conceptions of the identities of residents and ignore the complexity that characterizes people's actual social experiences. Moreover, to the extent that researchers are uncritical about the threats some communities' norms pose to women's lives, health, bodily integrity, freedom to move and assemble and to speak and participate in decisionmaking, they may perpetuate injustices.[30]

This last concern can be considered in light of a particular example. Housed within the Joint United Nations Programme on HIV/AIDS (UN-AIDS), an informal working group on prevention of mother-child transmission of HIV was responsible for coordinating a multinational and multiagency study of perinatal transmission of HIV/AIDS in developing countries, including Thailand, the Ivory Coast, and Uganda. The study was highly controversial, given the fact that a placebo group was measured against a modified regimen of zidovudine, or AZT, that fell below the standard of care in the United States—the major sponsoring country. In response to concerns that the study risked exploiting women from developing countries,[31] spokespersons from the nations and agencies involved claimed that decisions about the acceptability of the studies were made at the local level by local leaders and that they reflected the particular needs, circumstances, and values of the countries in which the research was to be conducted.[32] What remains unclear is the extent to which the women who participated in these trials were consulted. If asked about their particular needs, circumstances, and values, would the women targeted for study provide the same list their local leaders did? Would they assess benefit and risk in similar ways? Equipped with the benefit of hindsight, Western commentators suggested that HIV/AIDS researchers proceeded with their studies on the basis of some very flawed ideas about the needs of these research subjects.[33] To the degree that this also holds true from the standpoint of the women affected, the same concerns seen thus far arise: social equality for women and their capacities for self-determination are diminished, and research projects continue to reflect the interests of others, including in this case those who stand to profit from changes in standards of care for pregnant women with HIV/AIDS.

Empowerment Approaches That Include Women in Planning

Moving away from approaches that exclude women in planning, some researchers working on development projects with nongovernmental organizations (NGOs) have adopted what is known as an "empowerment" approach to research. This model is characterized by two features: analyses by women who reside in developing countries of the social and institutional relations, processes, and structures that create and sustain their oppression, and challenges to these analyses through the cultivation of participatory democratic processes. Project staff design and facilitate consciousness-raising workshops at which concepts like gender, race, class, and imperialism are discussed, and women's participation in setting goals and making plans for the community, including those related to research projects, is encouraged.[34]

Although respectful of this attempt at change, critics have found fault with this strategy. In their view, the expert knowledge of project funders and staff continues to be privileged, thus constructing the participants from developing countries as objects and perpetuating unequal relations of power. Even though participatory democracy is emphasized, it is still project staff who determine the categories for analysis, who the target groups are, and who will produce the knowledge that both comes to and emerges from discussions. Moreover, they continue to be in a position of economic power, receiving pay, benefits, and professional status for their work.[35]

Feminist Models for Democratic Research Worldwide

Situated within an increasingly complex matrix of social and institutional structures, including cultural norms and economic structures, research has great potential to violate women's dignity, to perpetuate their inequality, and to erode their capacity for choice. But research has great promise too, of course, due to its power to support women in achieving the ideals of social equality and self-determination—ideals that are universalizable because of a shared dignity among them. This promise can best be realized where there is attention to differences and particularity or, more precisely, to the complexity of women's identities.

Rather than rely on locations where women are compelled to conform to others' images of who they are and should be, taking social equality and self-determination seriously suggests a need to find or even support the creation of places where women can establish their own research norms. As women gain experience in reflecting on their identities, they may seek out, create, and discover new attachments, commitments, and communities of *choice*. These new places, perhaps best described as "alternative supporting communal frameworks" or "oppositional communities,"[36] may contribute just as much to the "constitution" of women's identities as their communities of *origin*.[37] Indeed, they may serve as ideal sites for the development of "strong moral definition," that is, the process of affirming *and critiquing* (emphasis added) various features of persons' identities so that they can further construct their moral persona, set courses for themselves, and make decisions in pursuit of these.[38] It is within these sorts of social spaces that women may come to understand themselves better, interpret the meaning of "woman," deliberate over the hindrances that economic deprivation, gender roles, and hierarchically arranged, expert-guided processes of decisionmaking may place on their potential for equality and choice, and, finally, formulate specific ideas about their capacities (many of which will hold for all women everywhere) and how to realize them in their particular settings, given differences in place, material conditions, and so on.[39] Ideally, then, decisions regarding research agendas, funding, and ethical review should emerge from sites where there is a commitment to challenging such dominant social and institutional structures, relations, and processes as gender, cultural norms, and economic structures. It will be crucial for such networks to participate in exchanges with other women locally or abroad and with researchers and their supporters. In these exchanges, relations of privilege and crosscutting social differences and similarities can be explored and *used* to set priorities that reflect diverse interpretations of research needs. In addition, researchers and their sponsors should go through processes of "self-interrogation" in order to "destabilize their given identities and to uncover their horizons of ignorance."[40] The proposal here reflects the view that there are smart knowers (including scientists and nonscientists) and imperfect knowledge systems, not one correct knowledge system to which only certain people have access.[41]

This approach to participatory decisionmaking in research is less vulnerable to the problems raised by other strategies. It reckons with the complexity of women's identities, taking seriously the role of community in women's lives and the importance of responding to women's actual needs and lived realities. When women are asked about needs, their expressed preferences may not necessarily be their own but those of a society that has shaped and imposed them on its members. Aware of the degree to which one's desires are not necessarily one's own, researchers will be able to maneuver the planning process away from the urge to see women as parts of some unified collective, and the tendency to define them and their research needs in terms of patriarchal, racist, and economist interests and frameworks. The crucial point is that spheres of choice, where women can realize their moral agency, must be recognized, or sometimes developed, so that women can consider and discuss their own ideas about what is "good" for them rather than living under others' interpretations.

This proposal recognizes the need for "strategic essentialism."[42] It assumes, contrary to deconstructionist or postmodernist views, that women do have particular standpoints on nature and social life and that they are valuable resources for social policy.[43] Moreover, although it is situated, it is nonrelativist. Based on the idea that women hold much in common in terms of what is required for flourishing, it puts forth a vision of justice that is applicable to all women. Yet it acknowledges that promoting this vision of justice requires attention to the specifics of particular contexts, to the concerns and the resources that reside there. Abstract values like social equality and self-determination—values that are not imperialist artifacts but are appealed to by women around the world—can be instantiated in particular contexts using the richness of local knowledge. Moreover, this view allows for the recognition of plural criteria of knowledge, recognizing that knowledge is not "culture free." But as I and others have shown, to give total deference to local norms would be to thwart women's abilities to flourish, to experience "the joy most people have in using their own bodies and minds."[44] International feminist politics is made possible by linking "cautiously circumscribed global conclusions" about ethical ideals with such "sensitive local mappings."[45]

In thinking further about the details of developing participatory decisionmaking structures, and especially ways of creating conditions of parity among participants (researchers, their sponsors, and the women who will be affected by research projects), it is important to consider more precise accounts of participatory decisionmaking processes. What do these really amount to, particularly when they involve diverse participants? Favored by many theorists is the model of deliberative democracy. As an alternative to an interest-based theory of democracy, in which persons pursue their own perceived interests primarily through voting, deliberative democracy usually refers to a discussion-based ideal aimed at realizing the common good.[46] Contemporary theorists of deliberative democracy—critics of the interest-based model—object to what they regard as its privatized, consumer-oriented political processes. Competing for the expression and satisfaction of their own private goods, individuals are not inclined to recognize others or their particular points of view. Ultimate outcomes are not determined through processes of reasoning but by the seemingly irrational desires of a majority of voters and/or by the influence of money and social power.

The deliberative conception of democracy, by contrast, understands politics as people coming together to deliberate rationally over social goals and public policies. According to this more inclusive, egalitarian model:

> Democratic processes are oriented around discussing [a] common good rather than competing for the promotion of the private good of each. Instead of reasoning from the point of view of the private utility maximizer [and of course, the ideal of impartiality] through public deliberation citizens transform their preferences according to public-minded ends, and reason together about the nature of those ends and the best means to realize them. In free and open dialogue others test and challenge these assertions and reasons. . . . The interlocutors properly discount bad reasons and speeches that are not well argued. . . . Putting forward and criticizing claims and arguments, participants in deliberations do not rest until the "force of the better argument" compels them all to accept a conclusion.[47]

Despite its appeal, this model is not without liabilities, some of which have been discussed above. Here the crucial point is that to the extent that critical argument is a "privileged" form of discussion, conceptions of deliberative democracy reflect a culturally biased understanding of deliberation. Although theorists claim to be "bracketing political and economic power," thereby making participants equal, they are in fact promoting ideals that are exclusionary, for

> the social power that can prevent people from being equal speakers derives not only from economic dependence or political domination but also from an internalized sense of the right one has to speak or not to speak, and from the devaluation of some people's style of speech [most notably women and cultural minorities] and the elevation of others' [typically white middle-class men or other privileged persons serving in the role of "expert"].[48]

These insights suggest the need to recognize and attend to structural inequalities in discussion. Although the most privileged speech is that which is dispassionate, assertive, and general in its argument, justice calls for eliminating biases against speech that incorporates expressions of emotion and bodily gestures, is "tentative, exploratory, or conciliatory," "halting and circuitous," or refers to particularities in making points and developing arguments.[49] Furthermore, greetings (e.g., smiles, handshakes, hugs), storytelling, and rhetoric should be recognized as forms of communication that can serve to strengthen political discussion. The virtues of these modes of expression are that they attend to the embodiment of participants and affirm their particularity, thus "providing ways of [communicating] across difference."[50] According to Iris Young, an ideal of *communicative* democracy best captures this respect for diverse "forms of communicative interaction where people aim to reach understanding."[51] This ideal of participatory, communicative democracy surpasses other models of democratization in its capacity to challenge the norms and structures that render the discernment of oppressed groups' views difficult.

Conclusion: Promoting Social Justice
for Women in Research

Diminishing esteem for the ideal of impartiality has presented us with a need to consider how best to incorporate the perspectives of the public, especially those who have faced oppression, in the funding, design, and review of health research. In this chapter we have explored different models of decisionmaking processes that aspire to be democratic. These explorations show the importance of illuminating the shifting personal or network allegiances lived by women. Further, they show the need for change in the social and institutional relations, processes, and structures that shape women's lives and are embedded in research. Acknowledging this and involving women as participants at all levels of decisionmaking is necessary if justice is to be realized for women in the context of research and, more broadly, health policy around the world. Offered here is one proposal, chosen for its capacity to promote justice, that is, to enhance rather than inhibit social equality and self-determination for women.

Notes

1. Liberalism, of course, is not a monolithic tradition. There are differences among liberal theorists when it comes to considering the role of community in moral development and moral life. The issue here is one of emphasis. For further discussion of this point, see Martha Nussbaum, "The Feminist Critique of Liberalism," in Nussbaum, *Sex and Social Justice* (New York: Oxford University Press, 1999), pp. 60–61.

2. See, for example, Alasdair MacIntyre, *After Virtue: A Study in Moral Theory* (Notre Dame, Ind.: University of Notre Dame Press, 1981), pp. 32, 204–205; Michael Sandel, *Liberalism and the Limits of Justice* (Cambridge: Cambridge University Press, 1982), p. 179.

3. National Institutes of Health, Office of Research on Women's Health, *Outreach Notebook for the NIH Guidelines Concerning the Inclusion of Women and Minorities as Subjects in Clinical Research* (Washington, D.C.: National Institutes of Health, 1994), pp. 7–10.

4. Ibid., pp. 14–15.

5. National Institutes of Health, *Outreach Notebook*, pp. 7, 12–19.

6. National Institutes of Health, Office of Research on Women's Health, *Recruitment and Retention of Women in Clinical Studies* (Washington, D.C.: National Institutes of Health, 1995), p. 20.

7. Young, *Justice and the Politics of Difference*, pp. 232, 229.

8. National Institutes of Health, *Recruitment and Retention*, pp. 12–13, 18, 20–21; National Institutes of Health, *Outreach Notebook*, pp. 10–11.

9. Barbara Ehrenreich, "On Feminism, Family, and Community," *Dissent* 30 (Winter 1983): 103–106; Heidi I. Hartmann, "The Family As the Locus of Gender, Class, and Political Struggle," in Sandra Harding, ed., *Feminism and Methodology* (Bloomington: Indiana University Press, 1987), pp. 109–134.

10. See, for example, Jacquelyn Grant, "Black Theology and the Black Woman," in Gayraud Wilmore and James Cone, eds., *Black Theology: A Documentary History, 1966–1979* (New York: Orbis, 1979), pp. 418–433. I am not suggesting that women do not play leadership roles in religious communities. See Kathryn Kish Sklar, "The 'Quickened Conscience': Women's Voluntarism and the State," *Report from the Institute for Philosophy and Public Policy* 18, no. 3 (Summer 1998) for evidence to the contrary. My point is that often they are not recognized as leaders.

11. See, for example, Susan Brooks Thistlethwaite, "Every Two Minutes: Battered Women and Feminist Interpretation," in Judith Plaskow and Carol Christ, eds., *Weaving the Visions: New Patterns in Feminist Spirituality* (San Francisco: HarperCollins, 1989), pp. 302–313.

12. Nancy Fraser, "Women, Welfare, and the Politics of Need Interpretation"; and Bernadine Dohrn, "Bad Mothers, Good Mothers, and the State: Children on the Margins," *Roundtable: A Journal of Interdisciplinary Legal Studies* 2, no. 1 (1995): 1–12.

13. Will Kymlicka, *Multicultural Citizenship: A Liberal Theory of Rights* (New York: Oxford University Press, 1995).

14. This was the case for gay white male AIDS treatment activists who were successful in attaining credibility in the eyes of scientists. See Steven Epstein, "The Construction of Lay Expertise: AIDS Activism and the Forging of Credibility in the Reform of Clinical Trials," *Science, Technology, and Human Values* 20, no. 4 (Autumn 1995): 408–437.

15. Mary Shanley and Carole Pateman, eds., *Feminist Interpretations and Political Theory* (Oxford: Polity, 1991).

16. For example, see Amartya Sen, "Gender and Cooperative Conflicts," in Irene Tinker, ed., *Persistent Inequalities* (New York: Oxford University Press, 1990).

17. See Peter L. Beilenson, Elizabeth Miola, and Mychelle Farmer, "Politics and Practice: Introducing Norplant into a School Based Health Center in Baltimore," *American Journal of Public Health* 85, no. 3 (1995): 309–311; Alix M. Freedman, "Why Teenage Girls Love 'the Shot'; Why Others Aren't So Sure," *Wall Street Journal*, October 14, 1998: p. A1. For an international perspective, see Phillida Bunkle, "Calling the Shots? The International Politics of Depo Provera," in Sandra Harding, ed., *The "Racial" Economy of Science: Toward a Democratic Future* (Bloomington: Indiana University Press, 1993).

18. See, for example, Stephen Jay Gould, "American Polygeny and Craniometry Before Darwin: Blacks and Indians As Separate, Inferior Species," in *"Racial" Economy*, pp. 84–115; Iris Marion Young, "The Scaling of Bodies and the Politics of Identity," in *Justice and the Politics of Difference*, pp. 122–155.

19. Nancy Krieger and Mary Bassett, "The Health of Black Folk: Disease, Class, and Ideology in Science," in *"Racial" Economy*, p. 161. As well, see Elena S.H. Yu, "Ethical and Legal Issues Relating to the Inclusion of Asian/Pacific Islanders in Clinical Studies," in Anna C. Mastroianni, Ruth Faden, and Daniel Federman, eds., *Women and Health Research: Ethical and Legal Issues of Including Women in Clinical Studies* (Washington, D.C.: National Academy Press, 1994), pp. 220–222.

20. See Cindy Patton, *Inventing AIDS* (New York: Routledge, 1990), as well as her more recent work, *Last Served: Gendering the HIV Pandemic* (Bristol, Penn.: Taylor & Francis, 1994), especially chapter 3, "Identity, Community, and 'Risk.'"

21. Young, *Justice and the Politics of Difference*, p. 227.

22. Patton, *Inventing AIDS*, p. 8.

23. Katherine Luzuriaga and John L. Sullivan, "Pathogenesis of Vertical HIV–1 Infection: Implications for Intervention and Management," *Pediatric Annals* 23, no. 3 (1994): 159–166; Arthur Amman, "Human Immunodeficiency Virus Infection/AIDS in Children: The Next Decade," *Pediatrics* 93, no. 6 (1994): 930–935.

24. Jeremy Manier, "AMA Supports HIV Tests for All Pregnant Women: Critics Fear Some Will Avoid Prenatal Care," _Chicago Tribune_, June 28, 1996; Karen Rothenberg and Stephen J. Paskey, "The Risk of Domestic Violence and Women with HIV Infection: Implications for Partner Notification, Public Policy, and Law," _American Journal of Public Health_ 85, no. 11 (1995): 1569–1576.

25. Young, _Justice and the Politics of Difference_, p. 59.

26. National Institutes of Health, _Recruitment and Retention_, p. 28; Ruth B. Merkatz, "Women in Clinical Trials: An Introduction," _Food and Drug Law Journal_ 48, no. 2 (1993): 164.

27. Penny A. Weiss, _Gendered Community: Rousseau, Sex, and Politics_ (New York: New York University Press, 1993), p. 130.

28. Council for International Organizations of Medical Sciences, _International Ethical Guidelines for Biomedical Research Involving Human Subjects_ (Geneva: CIOMS, 1993).

29. Ibid., p. 25.

30. For additional discussion, see Nussbaum, "Women and Cultural Universals" and "Religion and Women's Human Rights," in _Sex and Social Justice_, pp. 29–32, 81–102.

31. For example, see Lurie and Wolfe, "Unethical Trials."

32. Harold Varmus and David Satcher, "Ethical Complexities of Conducting Research in Developing Countries," _New England Journal of Medicine_ 337, no. 14 (1997): 1004. As well, see Danstan Bagenda and Phillipa Musoke-Mudidi, "We're Trying to Help Our Sickest People, Not Exploit Them," _Washington Post_, September 28, 1997; Salim S. Abdool Karim, "Placebo Trials in HIV Perinatal Transmission Trials: A South African's Viewpoint," _American Journal of Public Health_ 88, no. 4 (1998): 564–566.

33. See, for example, Carol Levine, "Placebos and HIV: Lessons Learned," _Hastings Center Report_ 28, no. 6 (1998): 43; Leonard H. Glantz et al., "Research in Developing Countries: Taking 'Benefit' Seriously," _Hastings Center Report_ 28, no. 6 (1998): 40.

34. Ann Ferguson, "Resisting the Veil of Privilege: Building Bridge Identities as an Ethico-Politics of Global Feminisms," _Hypatia_ 13, no. 3 (1998): 99–101.

35. Ibid., p. 101.

36. Marilyn Friedman, "Feminism and Modern Friendship: Dislocating the Community," in _What Are Friends For?_, p. 246.

37. Ann Ferguson, "Feminist Communities and Moral Revolution," in Penny A. Weiss and Marilyn Friedman, eds., _Feminism and Community_ (Philadelphia: Temple University Press, 1995), pp. 367–397.

38. Margaret Urban Walker, "Moral Particularity," _Metaphilosophy_ 18, no. 3–4 (1987): 108–109. As well, see Nussbaum, "Women and Cultural Universals," pp. 48–49; and Jane Mansbridge, "Feminism and Democratic Community," in _Feminism and Community_, pp. 341–365.

39. Nussbaum is keen on the idea that a universal account of human capabilities, tailored by attention to context, should serve as the focal point for international political action aimed at promoting justice for women. See "Women and Cultural Universals," pp. 39–50.

40. Ferguson, "Resisting the Veil," pp. 103–104.

41. See Harding, "Gender, Development," p. 160.

42. Gayatri Chakroavorty Spivak, *Outside in the Teaching Machine* (New York: Routledge, 1993).

43. Sandra Harding, "Women's Standpoints on Nature: What Makes Them Possible?" *Osiris* 12 (1997): 186–200.

44. Nussbaum, introduction to *Sex and Social Justice*, p. 11. For examples of the dangers of cultural relativism, see Frederique Apffel Marglin and Stephen A. Marglin, eds., *Dominating Knowledge: Development, Culture, and Resistance* (Oxford: Clarendon, 1990).

45. Lorraine Code, "How to Think Globally: Stretching the Limits of Imagination." *Hypatia* 13, no. 2 (Spring 1998): 76. For her part, Code is willing to embrace a particular form of epistemological relativism.

46. The discussion here is taken from Young, "Communication and the Other," pp. 121–135.

47. Ibid., p. 121.

48. Ibid., p. 122. As well, see Lucie E. White, "Subordination, Rhetorical Survival Skills, and Sunday Shoes: Notes on the Hearing of Mrs. G," in Katherine T. Bartlett and Roseanne Kennedy, eds., *Feminist Legal Theory: Readings in Law and Gender* (Boulder: Westview, 1991), pp. 404–429.

49. Young, "Communication and the Other," pp. 123–124.

50. Ibid., p. 129.

51. Ibid., p. 125.

20

What Can Survivors of Nazi Experiments Teach Us All?

A Feminist Approach to a Problem with Global Implications

CAROL QUINN

*The wrongs perpetrated were monstrous; those wrongs are over and done with. . . .
The most horrible crime we have experienced is made worse by adding to it a further
wrong, however minor; that is, refusing to use the data when it is known they could
be of clinical benefit.*[1]

—*philosopher Benjamin Freedman*

You are looking at the data, the living data, of Dr. Mengele.[2]

—*victim Susan Vigorito*

During the Holocaust, Nazi researchers exposed concentration camp inmates to nocuous diseases, lethal gas, pressurized environments, and poisoned seawater. Inmates were shot, burned, and frozen in the name of medical science.[3] Of late, much attention has been given to whether we should continue to use the data obtained from these experiments. Since World War II, Nazi medical data have been cited in at least forty-five medical and scientific journals. According to Arthur Caplan, "Nazi data and the claims of Nazi science in areas such as genetics, physiology, pathology, anthropology, and psychiatry have in the past been studied, cited, and absorbed into mainstream science with little comment."[4] Nazi data have been used in matters of national interest. The U.S. space program, for example, embraced and utilized Nazi data.[5] Nazi medical material has also been used as teaching aids at reputable universities worldwide. Until very recently, body parts and complete cadavers of victims were used for study at several German medical schools, including Tübingen and Heidelberg. In Britain, medical schools used an X-ray film of Nazi victims in motion. The doses of radiation used to produce the film were so great that the subjects would certainly have died from the effects of radiation. Cambridge University discontinued using the film in the late 1980s, only after new technology made it obsolete.[6] In the United States, controversy over whether to continue to use Nazi material broke out in the late 1980s, when the Environmental Protection Agency (EPA) included Nazi data in their draft report on the effects of phosgene gas. After much opposition from EPA staff, the agency excluded the Nazi data from their final report. Elsewhere in the United States, at about the same time, hypothermia expert Robert Pozos debated whether to use the Nazi hypothermia data. Earlier in the decade, Canadian scientist John Hayward used this data in his research, testing survival suits for trawlers in the Canadian Arctic; Pozos, however, was the first scientist to publicly question the data's use.[7] Although many consider much of the Nazi data worthless, some respected researchers judge the hypothermia data to be valuable.

Researchers at the Dachau concentration camp conducted the hypothermia studies to answer questions arising about how to treat downed pilots who were parachuting into the frigid waters of the North Sea. They wanted to develop hypothermia-protective suits that would enable the pilots to survive longer, and they wanted to establish the most effective rewarming methods once the pilots were retrieved. At that time, no data existed to determine how to protect and treat the downed pilots. German physiologists had established the most successful method to rewarm severely hypothermic animals. They first conducted these experiments on guinea pigs and then on large adult pigs. However, since neither animal has temperature-regulating abilities similar to those of humans, head researcher Sigmond Rascher got permission to conduct a series of immersion-hypothermia experiments on approximately 300 male concentration camp inmates. Researchers conducted the hypothermia experiments in a conscientious manner according to the scientific standards of the time, and they presented their findings at an October 1942 medical conference entitled Medical Questions in Marine and Winter Emergencies, attended by ninety-five of the most eminent physicians and scientists. In the experiments, some subjects were forced to dress in pilot suits while others were stripped naked. Some were anesthetized, others left conscious. Subjects were immersed in vats of water at temperatures ranging between thirty-six and fifty-three degrees Fahrenheit and left in the water for up to several hours and brought near death. As prisoners "foamed at the mouth, writhed in pain, emitted death rattles, and slumped into drowsy semi-consciousness,"[8] researchers measured their changes in blood, urine, cerebrospinal fluid, muscle reflexes, heart action (by electrocardiogram), and internal and external body temperatures. When subjects' body temperatures dropped below 79.7 degrees, researchers tried various rewarming methods, including rapid rewarming by hot bath (they threw some subjects into boiling water), and slower rewarming by "light box," heated sleeping bags, blankets, pharmaceuticals, diathermy of the heart, and body-to-body contact and sexual stimulation by naked women prisoners who were forced to warm them. Nearly one-third of the victims died from exposure.

The Nazi data controversy is part of the larger debate over whether it is ever ethical to use data obtained in unethical ways. Unethical experimentation certainly did not begin, nor has it ended, with the Nazis, and data from many of these experiments have been cited in medical and scientific literature. In 1966, Henry Beecher wrote a landmark paper for the *New England Journal of Medicine,* in which he describes twenty-two unethical experiments conducted in the United States since World War II.[9] Data from these experiments "still float through scientific literature"—the data have been neither banned nor purged.[10] Perhaps the most notorious examples of medical abuse in the United States are the Tuskegee syphilis study and the Willowbrook hepatitis study; the data from each of these experiments have been extensively cited.

In the Tuskegee study, hundreds of poor African American males, ostensibly being treated for "bad blood," were denied treatment for syphilis (even after penicillin became available in 1943) and deceived by physicians working for the U.S. Public Health Service. One-third of the research subjects died of syphilis or related complications; further, since the subjects were not treated, many transmitted the disease to others. The study was brought to an end in 1972, only after it was made public. The Willowbrook study was conducted from the mid-1950s to the mid-1970s. In this study, researchers, without their subjects' consent, infected residents of a Staten Island institution for the developmentally disabled with the hepatitis virus to study the course of this disease.

Unethical research in the United States did not stop after Willowbrook. In the late 1980s and early 1990s, the Centers for Disease Control (CDC) and Kaiser Permanente of California tested a dangerous high potency measles vaccine on poor black and Latino infants in Los Angeles, California. Researchers did not inform parents that the vaccine was experimental, nor did they tell them about its sometimes deadly effects. Similar experiments had been conducted in Mexico, Senegal, Haiti, Bangladesh, Zaire, and other impoverished places. Currently, studies sponsored by the U.S. government through the CDC and the National Institutes of Health are being conducted in Cote d'Ivoire, South Africa, Thailand, the Dominican Republic, and other developing countries, to try to find inexpensive ways to prevent the transmission of HIV from mother to infant. Until 1998, these studies included placebo groups, even though AZT has been proven to reduce transmission of HIV from mother to infant.[11] Such studies would not be tolerated in the United States because of their unethical nature. Indeed, in similar U.S. studies, researchers provide all subjects with AZT or similar drugs.

The question arises whether we should continue to use data obtained from these and other unethical experiments. The use of the Nazi data, however, has generated the most controversy. The central argument for using the Nazi data is its life-saving potential. Among the arguments against using the data include (1) the "tainted data" argument, according to which the evil of the Nazi atrocities has infused the data, and so in using the data we become morally tainted by this contact; (2) the "legitimizing the evil" argument, which states that by using the Nazi data we confer legitimacy on the Nazi doctors; and (3) the "deterrence" argument, which states that in refusing to use the data we deter future researchers from participating in similar experiments.

One essential part of the dialogue has been largely ignored, and even dismissed, namely, the victims' voice. For example, one victim, after speaking at a conference at which she was invited to discuss why she objects to scientists' using the data, was told by a member of the audience that she was an "emotional cripple," "ruled by emotions and not by the mind," and was therefore unqualified to participate in the debate.[12]

Most victims argue against using the Nazi data on the grounds that such use harms them. They claim that use of the data amounts to their "final indignity."[13] By using the data "we would dishonor [them] once more by feasting on their bodies."[14] And "to use the data without the consent of those who were violated is to violate the violated anew."[15] Other victims maintain that using the data will "affirm the value and dignity of men and women whom the Nazis treated like laboratory rats."[16] Importantly, the victims demand that they alone have the right to decide what should be done with the Nazi data. As Jay Katz points out, as it now stands, scientists are guaranteed, under the First Amendment, the right to use virtually any data, and so ultimately the decision falls on the conscience of each researcher.[17] But what about the victims' rights? Shouldn't their interests be protected? Protection under the First Amendment does not come at the expense of serious harm to others, and the victims claim that in using the data the scientists seriously harm them.

In what follows, I focus on the victims' claim that they (and not scientists or philosophers) have the right to control the data's use. I discuss arguments that the Nazi victims do (or could) make for this right. Throughout, I use feminist standpoint theory, which claims that knowledge is fully socially and historically located. Some locations, namely, those of the socially subjugated, "are better than others as starting points for knowledge projects."[18]

Validation vs. lifesaving [handwritten annotation]

Feminist Standpoint Theory

According to traditional, mainstream, scientific ways of knowing, knowledge is universal, transhistorical, and apolitical. Lorraine Code tells us that such epistemologies "presuppose a universal, homogenous, and essential human nature . . . that allows knowers to be substitutable for one another."[19] There are no privileged perspectives from which to engage in knowledge projects; indeed, there is no perspective at all. Knowers are socially and historically disembodied, even invisible.[20] But as Sandra Harding explains, despite the scientific community's claims to pure objectivity and universality, all knowledge bears "the fingerprints of the communities that produce them."[21] Further, Code tells us that these prints belong to a "small, privileged group of educated, usually prosperous, white men."[22]

This "dominant group" values rationality, objectivity, clarity, precision, the capacity to be verified or falsified, and so on,[23] and it discredits those who do not meet its standards. Vrinda Dalmiya and Linda Alcoff call this practice of discrediting those who do not meet the criteria for knowing "epistemic discrimination."[24] Members of the dominant group, whom Code calls the "masters of truth," determine what counts as knowledge and who counts as knowers by consigning to "epistemic limbo people who profess crazy, bizarre, or outlandish beliefs."[25] Of course, since the dominant group has the power, it decides what is crazy, bizarre, and outlandish.

Marginalized people's experiences, experiences of those cast into epistemic limbo, have been disvalued and ignored as legitimate sources of knowledge, yet feminist standpoint theorists claim that an epistemically better account is one that begins from the standpoint (the perspective) of subjugated lives. Harding explains that starting from the perspective of marginalized lives will generate "illuminating critical questions," problems, and research agendas that cannot arise from the perspective of the dominant group.[26] The dominant group's inability to critically "interrogate their advantaged social situation and the effects of such advantages on their beliefs" leaves them epistemically impoverished.[27] We see this in the Nazi data debate. The debate, when controlled by the dominant group, has been whether it is ethical to use the Nazi data; but in taking seriously the victims' voice, the debate shifts. The question now concerns who should make such decisions; whether the data should be used becomes secondary.

Feminist standpoint theory challenges some of the most fundamental epistemological assumptions of the scientific community. Adopting standpoint theory involves making a commitment to take marginalized people seriously. As Harding puts it, adopting standpoint theory is "fundamentally a moral and political act of commitment to understand the world from the perspective of the socially subjugated."[28] It is from such a perspective that I consider the following arguments.

Six Arguments

The "It's About Time
You Take Us Seriously" Argument

This argument is straightforward and powerful. The claim here is that it is especially important to legitimize the victims' voices, to help victims speak, especially since their history has taught them that it is dangerous to become visible, dangerous to be heard,[29] and since they undoubtedly feel ambivalent about speaking, knowing that their voices can be so easily drowned out by the scientific and philosophical communities. In the Nazi experiments, the victims' selves were robbed from them in the name of medical utility. After the war, in accordance with the German indemnification law, the victims had to prove their damages and justify their claims. But as Judith Milton Kestenberg explains, this "enforced remembering brought on a distinct feeling of renewed persecution, renewed interrogation, disbelief, and degradation,"[30] as "experts" questioned the veracity of the victims' claims. This is not unlike a rape trial, where the survivor often faces a legal system that is indifferent, and even hostile, to her. Psychiatrist Judith Herman tells us that "efforts to seek justice or redress often involve further traumatization, for the legal system is often frankly hostile to rape victims."[31] Discounting the victims' testimony in the Nazi data debate—calling them "emotional cripples"—perpetuates these injustices. It is about time we take them seriously. Importantly, we *owe* them that.

The "Expert" Argument

According to this argument, the victims alone are experts in this debate—in virtue of their having undergone perhaps the most heinous of traumatic experiences—and only experts should decide what should be done

with this data. Victim Susan Vigorito states, "It is not due to the scars of
Nazi torture that I cannot condone the use of Nazi data. Rather, those of
us who have lived and by chance survived the heinous tortures called experiments by the Nazis, have a clearer understanding of the ABSOLUTE
EVIL of the Nazi doctor."[32] The Nazi victims claim to have a "privileged
access" to the debate. This idea of "epistemic privilege," "cognitive advantage," and so on, has been suggested by Charles Mills, Dalmiya and
Alcoff, bell hooks, and Susan Babbitt, among others. According to Mills,
certain people (especially members of subordinated social groups) have
social experiences structured (or, perhaps better, constrained) such that
"epistemically enlightening experiences result from it."[33] Using Mills's
insight, we can say that the Nazi victims are in a "better cognitive position to form true beliefs" about the implications of using the data than
hegemonic groups like the scientists and philosophers in the debate.[34]
The victims alone know (affectively) that using the data harms them.
    Someone might argue that the victims' experiences have actually
harmed their ability to know. But this begs the question against their assertion that they are not emotional cripples. As Laurence Thomas teaches
us, we owe some people moral deference. "A fundamentally important
part of living morally is being able to respond in the morally appropriate
way to those who have been wronged."[35] Moral deference calls for a presumption in favor of victims' accounts of their experiences. Someone else
might object that the victims claim too much. That is, even if they are experts about being victims, they are not experts about the effects of the
data's use. The victims might respond that, in virtue of their being victims, they know what it takes for them to heal. To recover from trauma, a
victim must take back control over his or her life; the victims suggest that
this includes controlling the use of the data.
    One reason the victims' way of knowing has not been legitimized by
mainstream scientific and philosophical communities is that it is emotional and "experiential." Emotions and the body have traditionally been
thought to oppose rationality and are, for this reason, crippling. This, of
course, rules out "feminine" ways of knowing. Knowledge is ordered
and controlled. Victims are out of control. Victims, then, are "feminine."
In their paper "Are Old Wives' Tales Justified?" Dalmiya and Alcoff argue for what they call the epistemic legitimacy of "G-experiential knowledge," or gender-specific knowledge. They claim that midwives (Western
women who, before the nineteenth century, were usually older wives
past child-bearing years, valued in society because of their knowledge
and skill in helping women with pregnancy, childbirth, and lactation)[36]
have access to "perspectival facts" of childbirth not accessible to male obstetricians.[37] Experiential knowledge is "knowing from the inside," or
"knowing what it is like to be . . ." and thus is Nagelian in spirit. Thomas

Nagel, in his paper "What Is It Like to Be a Bat?" argues that there is a fact of the matter about what it is like to be a bat, and we (humans) cannot know this fact unless we ourselves become bats.[38] Similarly, the Nazi victims have what we might call "V-experiential knowledge" (victim-specific knowledge) not accessible to those who have not been in the camps. Far from being emotional cripples who have an impaired judgment in this debate, the victims know best concerning what we should do with the data.

This argument is convincing only if the Nazi victims can establish that they do indeed have a *privileged*, and not just a different, access to the debate. Intuition might help here. When women who have given birth tell those of us who have not about the pains, pleasures, and anxieties of childbirth, and claim to know about them better than we do, most of us take this to be true—after all, they have experienced childbirth. Similarly, when Nazi victims tell us that we harm them when we use the Nazi data (especially without their consent), we should take their words to be true. They, and not we, have experienced the agony, the blood, the death of the Holocaust, and so they alone know how our using the data harms them. I discuss the nature of their harm in the next argument.

The "Living Data" Argument

This argument states that the victims are the "living data" of the experiments. The victims probably do not mean this literally—as if they are identical with the data. Rather, by referring to themselves as "living data," the victims suggest that when we use the Nazi data (without their consent) we ipso facto use them. Victim Eva Kor states, with respect to using the Nazi data, "Today some doctors want to use the only thing left by these victims. They are like vultures waiting for the corpses to cool so they could devour every consumable part."[39] In the camps, the Nazis reduced their victims to mere objects—*Menschenmaterial*. In using the data without the victims' consent, we continue the Nazi project of treating victims as mere objects of medical research. Susan Brison argues that, in trauma, victims' selves are "annihilated." The victims lose control. To recover, a trauma victim must be able to regain that control. But this depends in large part on the cooperation of other people.[40] So although trauma dehumanizes the victim, a compassionate community can restore her humanity.

Someone might suggest that, since the Nazi victims' selves have been annihilated, they no longer have agency—as if agency were a membership card, and the victims' cards were seized from them at the time of the trauma. Since victims are no longer agents, we need not take them seriously; rather, *we* know what is in their best interest. From this it follows that we are the ones who should maintain control over the data's use. However, I suggest that "self-annihilated" does not mean "loss of agency" or "loss of subjectivity." Rather, it means "loss of dignity." Not only does the Nazi victim have subjectivity, she or he has a "privileged" subjectivity (supposing the "expert" argument is right). This allows us to talk about the victims' agency as being disabled, and yet we can still recognize that the victims can judge their own interests and the interests of the community. On this view, the victims' regaining their dignity requires their controlling the use of the data. Here dignity is connected with freedom and control. As Sol Roth notes, "The patient who is seriously ill and hospitalized often complains of having been robbed of dignity. This is due, not so much to the fact that he must undergo a series of procedures that he may find embarrassing, but to his helplessness and the recognition that he has lost . . . the power to exercise control over his life."[41] If we care about the restoration of the victims' dignity, and if that restoration can only be accomplished through our finally treating them as subjects (which means giving them control over the data's use), then we must give them that control.[42]

Another variation of this argument looks a lot like the "expert" argument given above. Vigorito argues that "only the survivors have the right to decide what should be done with the Nazi research. I have a *clearer sense* of the evil behind this data than you do. . . . This is the data. *It is my experience.*"[43] The Nazis made lampshades out of the dried skins of their victims. Few would deny that the victims whose skins were used to make these lampshades were harmed by this treatment. The victims would not want to be remembered as mere objects, but as subjects. We are rightly disgusted by such treatment, and we would view any person who displays the lampshade in his or her home as deeply morally defective. By the victims' account, the scientists who want to use the data are equally deficient. In each case—using the lampshade and using the data—we fail to acknowledge the victims' loss of dignity, and thus we implicitly condone the victims' being treated as objects.

From the victims' point of view, there is no difference between using the victims' dried skins for lampshades and using the data—both are intimately connected to the victims' experiences. Those who want to use the data focus on consequences, because they have never endured these thoroughly demoralizing experiences. From a consequentialist point of view, there is a significant difference between using the victims' skins for lampshades and using the Nazi data; there is no reason to have a lampshade made out of human skin except for aesthetic (?!), or perhaps political, reasons, but the other has great utility—saving lives. Consequentialists balance ethical considerations with the importance of the results. Consequentialists would thus regard the display of dried-skin lampshades as unethical but would view the use of the data, because of its (potentially) great utility, as ethically justified. But victims make no distinction between these two cases. This is because the data's historical association, and especially its association with the victims' experiences, is undeniable. If we take away the victims' experiences, there are no dried-skin lampshades; if we take away the victims' experiences, there are no data.

The lampshades represent the victims' experiences in the camps. Similarly, the data represent the victims' experiences in the camps. We can make this stronger. There is a sense in which the lampshades *are* a part of the victims' experiences. In one sense, the victims were part of the larger Nazi project that treated people like objects. In another, the victims probably knew people who died and whose skins were used for that end, and they probably saw tanned human skin piled high in the camps. Kor writes about remembering "the huge chimneys, the smell of burned flesh, the shots, the blood taking, the endless tests in Mengele's labs, the rats, lice, and dead bodies that were everywhere."[44] The data, too, *are* a part of the victims' experiences. One should have control over one's experiences, and even (it may be argued) the *telling* of one's experiences.[45] How we use the data is part of the telling of the victims' experiences. Kor powerfully states that, if she had control over the data's use, she would "shred [the data] and put them into a glass monument with the inscription underneath 'No human guinea pigs again.'"[46]

The "Moral Property" Argument

The structure of this argument looks something like this: the Nazi victims have a right to control the data's use because they somehow "own" the data. Perhaps, as Lynne McFall suggests, the data are the moral property (in an ownership sense) of the victims.[47] If you impoverish me by stealing my money, and you subsequently invest my money, I have a right not only to my money but to the investment earnings.[48] Analogously, the victims were used to produce something. The data came about as a result of the victims' pain, against the victims' will, and so the victims have a right to control their use. Perhaps this analogy will help: suppose a woman is beaten, raped, and left for dead outside of her apartment building, and suppose that a surveillance camera catches the assault on videotape. Most of us would agree that showing the tape on the evening news would be a moral outrage. Although the story would be newsworthy and the video credible, the victim should decide what details of her assault are made public. The victim does not "own" the videotape in the standard way in which we understand ownership. She did not purchase the tape. It was not given to her as a gift. The videotape and the camera do not belong to her at all. Her apartment's security company owns these things. And yet we feel that we should obtain her permission before showing the videotape. By contrast, showing a video of an animal attacking another animal would be morally permissible because the attack does not count as an exploitation of others; it does not violate a person's dignity.

Someone might worry that if the Nazi data are the moral property of the victims, then all data are the moral property of victims. Thus we cannot publish rape statistics, for example, without getting permission from rape victims. The reason this "slippery slope" type of objection will not work is that there is a morally relevant difference between rape victims and the Nazi victims. Rapes are not committed to generate statistics, and so the victims do not have their selves invested in the statistics; therefore, controlling these statistics will not help them heal. By contrast, the torturous experiments were conducted to generate the data, and since the victims' lives are invested in the data, controlling that data will help them heal.

The "Alienation" Argument

Another possible argument is based on Marx's conception of alienation. According to Marx, living a fully human life requires self-determination, a capacity every person within the community has. Self-determination is connected with freedom and control. When people engage in labor in a capitalist society, they become like animals—work horses or oxen. They are told what to do, and they work only for subsistence. Outside of work, people exercise their mental faculties. Work, then, alienates people from their full human potential. Similarly, people have certain capacities that are alienated through trauma—autonomy, sexual pleasure, trust, self-love, and so on. Giving victims control over the use of the data gives them back the power of self-determination.

All people have a right to self-determination. If the victims can accomplish this by controlling the use of the data, they must have that control. Marx claims that the end of alienation is possible only through revolution. What the Nazi victims demand is nothing short of a revolution in the Nazi data debate. One reason some argue for the data's continued use is that they assume the Nazi victims' suffering is over and done and that to use the Nazi data would in no way add to the suffering of these victims. In arriving at this conclusion, promoters of the data's use ignore or dismiss outright the victims' claims to the contrary. How does this bear on the alienation argument? When people engage in labor in a capitalist society, they are treated not as subjects but as objects. Similarly, the scientists who ignore the victims' claims of harm treat them as mere objects in not acknowledging their subjectivity. Saving lives becomes more important than any consideration of harm to the dignity of persons, and according to the victims, concern for the dignity of persons must take precedence over any other consideration, including saving lives. Saving lives should certainly not come at the cost of trampling over the dignity of others. — *But which is more valuable*

Someone might ask, after all of the victims have died, will it then be morally permissible to use the Nazi data? In response, once the victims are dead, control should be given to the victims' children or grandchildren. As Kestenberg explains, victims' children believe that they "have a mission to live in the past, and to change it so that their parents' humiliation, disgrace, and guilt can be converted into victory over the oppressors, and the threat of genocide undone with a restitution of life and worth."[49] Victims' children are thus very concerned with the restoration of their parents' dignity. If their parents (having died) were denied the control necessary to facilitate their healing, that control should be extended to their children. Some children might believe that, in using the data, the victims' dignity can be recaptured ("valuable data" equals "valuable lives")—even posthumously. If so, they should debate this matter (as we debate any other tough ethical question) with victims' families. The major point concerns who has the right to control the data's use. Scientists and philosophers have always assumed that they have this right (because they are better educated or more "rational," and so on), but this is a mistake.

The "If We Want a Better Society, Then . . ." Argument

According to this argument, a society that puts its members' dignity first—even at considerable cost—is a better society than one that does not. According to Dennis Klein, "Our object [as members of a moral community] is to preserve certain sacred values, and the value that stands above all is the sanctity of human beings."[50] On this view, any benefit gained from saving lives cannot possibly balance the weight of immorality and indignity of the Nazi experiments or the further harm that we inflict on its victims by using the data. In a moral community, the inviolability of a person's dignity should be the guiding principle in all pursuits, including science. Kor challenges the scientists "to do your scientific work, but please, never stop being a human being. The moment you do, you are becoming a scientist for the sake of science alone, and you are becoming the Mengele of today."[51]

Concluding Comments

Many people claim that my project is a "nonstarter" because the Nazi data are garbage. Why, then, do we need to worry about who has control over this data? On this view, the debate is over because the data are unreliable, being the product of sloppy methodology and poorly designed experiments. The research is shoddy, conducted by unqualified persons. The data are thus incomplete, inconsistent, and probably freely fabricated.[52] Robert Berger, for example, argues in this way in a paper that many claim has put an end to the debate by showing that the only Nazi data ever considered to be of any worth (the Dachau hypothermia data) are also worthless.[53] Berger claims that Dachau head researcher Rascher was completely unqualified. Although this is true, Rascher brought on two reputable scientists considered experts in hypothermia (Holzloehner and Finke) who took charge of the study, and their results were presented at a respected medical conference on the topic. Moreover, Katz and Pozos remark that the Dachau findings "either confirmed prior experimental data or produced new data that scientists in the West have considered valid and have cited in scientific journals in support of their own findings."[54]

Between 1933 and 1945, the German medical community published widely, and they did little to mask their source of data—much of the world knew of their experimental subjects.[55] According to Arthur Caplan,

> Much of the basis for the Nazi murder of Jews, Gypsies, and others lay in the work of internationally respected German scientists at a time when Germany was the most scientifically advanced country in the world. . . . Most of the world [now] believes that scientists and doctors who participated in horrifying experiments . . . were people "on the fringe," but I do not believe that the medical and scientific community was dragged kicking and screaming into the Holocaust.[56]

Half of German physicians belonged to the Nazi party "because Nazi ideas of 'racial hygiene' meshed with then-current scientific thought."[57] There is a strong desire among the medical profession today to "other" the Nazi doctors—to put a fence around them—so as not to have to face the ugly side of medicine. The Nazi experiments, however, were conducted by reputable, mainstream, university-affiliated scientists and physicians to obtain scientifically valuable data, and researchers often met their medical objectives.[58] As Caplan notes, many experts now believe that "scientists and doctors were enthusiastic supporters of euthanasia, 'race hygiene,' and racial superiority, and they may even have provided the foundation for Nazi ideology."[59]

People who claim that my project is a "nonstarter" conflate two different, but relevant, distinctions. The distinction is *not* between valid and invalid data (between "good" data and "garbage" data), but between used and unused data. The Nazi data have been (and are still being) used by respected researchers who do believe that they are valuable. Whether these researchers are correct or incorrect in their assessment of the data is irrelevant. The valid/invalid controversy avoids the more important (and more general) question, Is it ever ethical to use data obtained in unethical ways, and who should make such decisions? The Nazi experiments are certainly not the only example of unethical scientific research, although they are arguably the most heinous example.

What lessons should we take from the Nazi victims? First, they remind us that the disadvantaged and already exploited tend to be victims of unethical experiments. People of color, the poor, residents of impoverished postcolonial countries, and other marginalized people are already considered outcasts merely in virtue of who they are; using them in unethical experiments further undermines their sense of self and their ability to trust others. Data from unethical experiments are always gained at the expense of the victims' dignity, often with their pain, and sometimes with their lives. If the victims of such experiments have a right to control the data obtained from these experiments (as I argue they do), then we must honor that right. But this requires "personal change, a giving up of power, and an actual change in behavior and commitment."[60] To ignore the victims' right is to continue to treat them as objects and counts as a further harm. But when we give victims of unethical experiments control over the data's use, we show them that we take them seriously; we acknowledge their subjectivity. Further, we announce that they can make important ethical decisions. In so doing, we help them heal. Far from being a "dead" debate, the bioethics community has much to learn by listening to Nazi victims.

Notes

I want to thank Rosemarie Tong, Linda Alcoff, and Robert Fudge for helpful comments on earlier drafts of this chapter. I would also like to thank members of the 1998 FAB audience in Tsukuba City, Japan, whose comments inspired the writing of this paper. This paper is for my grandfather, Robert Quinn.

1. See Matthew Gwyther and Sean McConville, "Nazi Experiments: Can Good Come from Evil?" *London Observer*, November 19, 1989.

2. See Robert Leiter, untitled article, *Long Island Jewish World Newsletter*, July 4, 1989.

3. See Faye Sholiton, "The Moral Dilemmas of Swallowing Bad Medicine," *Cleveland Jewish News*, November 25, 1988.

4. Arthur Caplan, "The Meaning of the Holocaust for Bioethics," *Hastings Center Report* 19, no. 4 (1989): 3.

5. According to Robert Pozos, "The whole U.S. space program has inherited tainted data." See Faye Sholiton, "Scientific Community Wrestles with Using Tainted Data," *Cleveland Jewish News*, November 25, 1988.

6. Guyther and McConville, "Nazi Experiments," p. 5.

7. Barry Siegel, "Can Evil Beget Good? Nazi Data: A Dilemma for Science," *Los Angeles Times*, October 30, 1988, pt. 1, p. 1.

8. Ibid.

9. Henry K. Beecher, "Ethics and Clinical Research," *New England Journal of Medicine* 274 (1966): 1345-1360.

10. Siegel, "Can Evil Beget Good?"

11. See Sheryl Gay Stolberg, "Placebo Use Is Suspended in Overseas AIDS Trials," *New York Times*, February 19, 1998, p. 16A.

12. Leiter, *Long Island Jewish World Newsletter*.

13. See Isabel Wilkerson, "Nazi Scientists and Ethics Today," *New York Times*, May 21, 1989, sec. 1, pt. 1, p. 34.

14. See Jay Katz, quoted in *Long Island Jewish World Newsletter*, July 4, 1989.

15. Stephen Post, "The Echo of Nuremberg: Nazi Data and Ethics," *Journal of Medical Ethics* 17 (1991): 42.

16. Robert J. White, "Learning from a Failure of Western Culture," *Star Tribune*, May 25, 1988, p. 14A.

17. See Sholiton, "The Moral Dilemmas of Swallowing Bad Medicine."

18. Sandra Harding, "Rethinking Standpoint Epistemology: What is Strong Objectivity?" in Linda Alcoff and Elizabeth Potter, eds., *Feminist Epistemologies* (London: Routledge, 1993), p. 56.

19. Lorraine Code, *Rhetorical Spaces: Essays on Gendered Location* (New York: Routledge, 1995), p. 24.

20. Harding, "Rethinking Standpoint Epistemology," p. 63.

21. Ibid., p. 57.

22. Code, *Rhetorical Spaces*, p. 32.

23. See Elizabeth Grosz, "Bodies and Knowledges: Feminism and the Crisis of Reason," in *Feminist Epistemologies*, pp. 187-215.

24. Vrinda Dalmiya and Linda Alcoff, "Are Old Wives' Tales Justified?" in *Feminist Epistemologies*, p. 217.

25. Code, *Rhetorical Spaces*, p. 32.

26. Harding, "Rethinking Standpoint Epistemology," p. 56.

27. Ibid., p. 54.

28. Sandra Harding, "From Feminist Empiricism to Feminist Standpoint Epistemologies," in Lawrence Cahoone, ed., *From Modernism to Postmodernism: An Anthology,* (Cambridge: Blackwell, 1996), p. 624.

29. See Rachael Josefowitz Siegel, "I Don't Know Enough: Jewish Women's Learned Ignorance," in Rachael Siegel and Ellen Cole, eds., *Celebrating the Lives of Jewish Women* (New York: Harrington Park, 1997), p. 205.

30. Judith Milton Kestenberg, "Post-Nazi Era and German Indemnification Law," in Martin S. Bergmann and Milton E. Jucovy, eds., *Generations of the Holocaust* (Columbia: Columbia University Press, 1982), p. 60.

31. Judith Herman, *Trauma and Recovery: The Aftermath of Violence: From Domestic Abuse to Political Terror* (New York: Basic, 1997), p. 72.

32. Susan Vigorito, "Far from Emotional Cripples, We Survivors of the Holocaust Have Clearer Understanding," *Cleveland Jewish News*, May 26, 1989.

33. Charles Mills, *Blackness Visible* (Ithaca, N.Y.: Cornell University Press, 1998), p. 28.

34. Ibid., p. 35.

35. Laurence Thomas, "Moral Deference," *Philosophical Forum* 24 (1992–1993): 233.

36. Dalmiya and Alcoff, "Are Old Wives' Tales Justified?" pp. 221-222.

37. Ibid., p. 229.

38. Thomas Nagel, *Mortal Questions* (Cambridge: Cambridge University Press, 1979).

39. Eva Kor, "Nazi Experiments As Viewed by a Survivor of Mengele's Experiments," in Arthur Caplan, ed., *When Medicine Went Mad: Bioethics and the Holocaust* (Totowa, N.J.: Humana, 1992), pp. 3–8.

40. See Susan Brison, "Outliving Oneself," in Diana Tietjens Meyers, ed., *Feminists Rethink the Self* (Boulder: Westview, 1997).

41. Sol Roth, *The Jewish Idea of Culture* (Hoboken: KTAV, 1997), p. 70.

42. For a more thorough discussion, see Carol Quinn, "Taking Seriously Victims of Unethical Experiments: Susan Brison's Conception of the Self and Its Relevance to Bioethics," *Journal of Social Philosophy* (forthcoming, 2000).

43. Susan Vigorito, quoted in Leiter, *Long Island Jewish World*.

44. Kor, "Nazi Experiments," p. 4.

45. In his paper "The Naked Truth," Arthur Danto argues that one has a right to control one's representations of oneself. I suggest that, in controlling the telling of one's experiences, one controls how one is represented. Being denied that control is a violation of that right. See "The Naked Truth," in Jerrold Levinson, ed., *Aesthetics and Ethics* (Cambridge: Cambridge University Press, 1998).

46. Eva Kor, quoted in Gwyther and McConville, "Nazi Experiments."

47. Thanks to Lynne McFall for bringing this to my attention.

48. Thanks are owed to Robert Fudge here.

49. Kestenberg, "Post-Nazi Era," p. 101.

50. See Bjorn Sletto, "When Research Is Evil," *Minnesota Alumni Association Newsletter* (November-December 1988): 26.

51. Kor, "Nazi Experiments," p. 8.

52. For such a discussion, see Rabbi J. David Bleich, "Using Data Obtained Through Immoral Experimentation," in Fred Rosner, ed., *Medicine and Jewish Law* (New Jersey: Jason Aronson, 1993), 2:143.

53. Robert Berger, "Nazi Science: The Dachau Hypothermia Experiments," *New England Journal of Medicine* 332 (1990):1435–1440.

54. Jay Katz and Robert Pozos, "The Dachau Hypothermia Study: An Ethical and Scientific Commentary," in *When Medicine Went Mad*, pp. 135–140.

55. See Faye Sholiton, "Mandate for Murder in the Name of Medical Science," *Cleveland Jewish News Newsletter*, November 25, 1988.

56. Arthur Caplan, quoted in Jim Fuller, "Holocaust Casts Lasting Shadows on Science," *Star Tribune*, May 18, 1989.

57. Robert Proctor, quoted in Jim Fuller, "Scientists Say Holocaust Should Have Taught That Science Alone Falls Short," *Star Tribune*, May 19, 1989, p. 15A.

58. See Delores Lutz, "Holocaust Conference Debate Centers on Research Ethics, Use of Nazi Data," *Minnesota Daily*, May 18, 1989, p. 1.

59. Quoted in Mike Steele, "Conferees Will Study Holocaust and Bioethics," *Star Tribune*, May 17, 1989.

60. Susan Babbitt, "Feminism and Objective Interests: The Role of Transformation Experiences in Rational Deliberation," in *Feminist Epistemologies*, p. 256.

21

Organ Transplantation and Community Values: Concerns of a Feminist Grief Counselor

KATHLEEN S. KURTZ, C.S.W.

It is widely known that the need for human organs for transplantation greatly exceeds the supply available.[1] This fact seems to have automatically translated into the notion that we must increase the supply of organs. In this chapter I challenge this assumption by questioning the "consciousness" on which it is based.

I am a social worker practicing in bereavement counseling, and my interest in feminist approaches to bioethics is a relatively newfound one. Feminist theory and social justice theory complement my work and challenge me to seek deeper meanings in the complicated world of bioethics. They force me to picture issues globally when identifying problems and proposed solutions. As our planet becomes "smaller," our actions have ripples that extend farther than our own borders; thus, as a leader in the development and marketing of medical technology, including organ transplant technology, the United States must reflect on how its power affects the lives of not only its own citizens but also people everywhere.

In this discussion I attempt to draw on the synergy of my practice and theoretical interests to examine the ethical benefits and dangers we are facing with regard to organ transplantation. I believe that organ transplantation is a practice that begs us to stop and think about what we are doing and why. My approach to the issue of increasing the supply of organs is informed by one of the main tenets of feminist epistemology and bioethics, namely, that discussions about practices in bioethics must not be limited to "experts" or "academics." Rather, they must be expanded to include the ordinary persons or patients whom the field supposedly seeks to serve.[2]

In my work with dying patients and their family members, I have seen health care professionals impede the reasoning abilities and choosing capacities of this particularly vulnerable group of people. Specifically, for a patient living in hope of getting an organ, the option that might actually serve that patient's best interests—dying—is precisely the option that most health care professionals find difficult to mention, let alone thoroughly discuss. However, if health care professionals fail to give patients *all* the information they need or would like for autonomous decision-making,[3] we must, as feminists, be aware that patients are being deprived of the opportunity to decide for themselves whether they really want to live or to die. *My concern is that health care professionals are so committed to saving lives that the very real and necessary discussion of death as a viable option is routinely left out of the conversation concerning choice in organ transplantation.*

As a grief counselor, I am reminded every day that in our culture we don't like to talk about death *or anything having to do with our own mortality.* In fact, we totally avoid it. Unfortunately, we pay a great individual and social price for this aversion.[4] This discomfort destroys valuable opportunities for personal discussion with family and friends concerning one's wishes about death. In a society in which doing more, accomplishing more, and living as long as possible are valued goals, actions (even extreme ones) taken to avoid death are routinely praised. Those who may want to choose to die are confronted with the social stigma of such a decision—even if death is the choice most appropriate to their circumstances. They are told to "hang in there"—that an organ will at last be found for them. Understand that, of course, I am not advocating for death *as opposed to* organ transplantation. However, I am arguing that a discussion of dying be offered to a patient facing an organ transplantation and that we consider the possibility that our real problem may not be a limited supply of organs but a failure to question the increasing *demand* for more organs.

Introduction to Social Work Theory and Feminist Bioethical Theory

Like social work theorists, feminist bioethicists are convinced that all the systems and structures of health care, including its conceptual schema, shape medical decisionmaking. Therefore, feminist bioethicists insist that we examine the assumptions underlying traditional bioethics so that we can transform the health care system in ways that will permit those who work within it to serve their patients in a more responsible and responsive manner. With respect to concerns about organ transplantation, feminist bioethicists have focused on traditional bioethics assumptions about (1) agency, (2) power and dominance, and (3) criteria for identifying voices that should be heard and voices that should be silenced.

Traditional bioethics posits autonomy as an instrument of agency for individuals—the core idea being that individuals should be treated as separate, independent beings who are able to make their own rational decisions, except, of course, if there is reason to think that the person is not competent.[5] Feminist bioethics does not view this conception of autonomy as fully useful or correct in examining what agency really looks like in health care. In fact, *actual people are not independent.* They are fully interconnected beings not only with family and friends but also within a social context.[6] Persons have socially constructed identities based on their gender, race, ethnicity, or age that affect their "autonomy." We are not equally autonomous individuals; we exist in relation to other individuals, social groups, and the institutions that serve us. Therefore, while agency is a useful tool in *offering* a patient autonomy (or assuming a person has "autonomy"), it must be seen as an instrument that actually gives very different levels of power to particular individuals as well as collective groups.

Issues of power and dominance concern all feminists, including feminist bioethicists. This fact is relevant in regard to the delivery of health care. Among central feminist tenets is the belief that there is a greater danger of oppression where biases are so pervasive (or perceived to be inevitable) that they are invisible. Such a state of affairs almost always creates an atmosphere ripe with oppression. Therefore, feminist bioethicists aim to question the methodology and practices of institutions that have greater power in and of themselves than the individuals they serve. Health care is such an institution.

Finally, feminist consciousness seeks to teach us that even if we assume, as I do, that most health care professionals are benevolent individuals, they must be concerned with the voices they do not hear, the questions they or others leave unasked, and the assumptions that underlie the choices that *are not* offered to patients in specific situations.

Susan Sherwin says that traditional bioethics, as a discipline, reflects the power structures in our larger society by focusing attention almost exclusively on the dilemmas of physicians.[7] She reminds us that even when the patient is remembered and issues are examined from both sides of the physician-patient relationship, it is inaccurate to state that these two persons have equal autonomy. The fact is that in a hierarchical society, most patients have far less power than most physicians. As a result, many patients are, in the presence of physicians, virtually incapable of truly "autonomous" decisionmaking.

Assuming that the promotion of autonomous decisionmaking is the goal of traditional bioethics, the question then becomes how to achieve this goal in a society whose systems and structures impair the individual and collective agency of certain populations. Sherwin posits that feminist bioethics has rejected the "ontology of persons conceived as isolated, fully developed individuals."[8] Therefore, for feminist bioethicists, the concept of autonomy as traditionally conceived does not serve a person's agency. Instead, a relational conception of the self, in which others help strengthen the self, enables the individual to be self-determining. Social work theory also relies on a nonindividualistic ontology that says persons do not exist apart from their family systems and social circumstances. When these factors are taken into account, the choices that some persons are forced to make in life, as well as in their health care, greatly affect what we may call (or dismiss as) an "autonomous" decision.

Although many, if not most, health care professionals are caring, concerned individuals, there are systemic forces inside and outside the institutional medicine that limit a person's ability to act as a genuine moral agent in making medical decisions—especially if that person is a member of a socially oppressed group. This is not to say that such a person is *without agency*. However, it is to say that agency "looks" different for one who lives life as a member of a socially oppressed group rather than as a member of a powerful or privileged group.

One of the criticisms of feminist theory is that its well-intentioned goals look "nice on paper" and are well-meaning in intent but cannot be attained practically. In the health care arena, the feminist intent would be to create a system of egalitarian decisionmaking in which the patient receives *all* the information she needs to make the decision that best fits her circumstances. Achieving this end might require particular persons being present (or being excluded) during discussions, or having things explained in the patient's first language. This goal may seem unrealistic because we are easily convinced by health care professionals or ourselves that health care decisions are very complicated and thus we should simply "do what the doctor says." However, even if the technical intricacies of medicine cannot be explained to every patient, feminist bioethicists still insist that it is important to continually question who decides what information to offer and what to omit. Furthermore, it is not acceptable to allow an oppressive practice to continue simply because it is difficult to change it, for it is the work of bioethics to change whatever has to be changed irrespective of the difficulty of doing so. Feminism as a movement states that friction caused by passionate discussion of perceived problems and suggested solutions is a necessary, even welcomed, part of the process to reach change. Although it is acceptable for feminist bioethicists to begin such conversations at professional meetings, it is our responsibility to make sure that these discussions also occur among the persons they are intended to serve, particularly when they involve a medical technology that is labeled "life saving."

Who Is Deciding?

The cost of transplantation is one issue that many people feel uncomfortable discussing. In the 1960s, the federal government decided that no one should die from end-stage renal disease (ESRD). As a result, in 1972, Congress passed legislation to use Medicare funds to pay for dialysis and transplants for all patients suffering from kidney failure.[9] (The availability of these treatments is now tied to individual state decisions regarding how federally allocated Medicaid dollars are spent.) Congress justified allotting funds for kidney transplants as well as kidney dialysis on the basis that in many cases kidney dialysis was more costly than a kidney transplant. However, setting the stage for federal economic support for life-saving transplantation created a precedent that was difficult, if not impossible, to follow (if one refers to monetary concerns alone). Now that heart, lung, pancreatic, and liver transplants have caught up in efficacy to kidney transplants, people want the federal government to pay for *all* organ transplants. But the federal government is unwilling to pay for all the transplants its citizens need, pointing out that it cannot justify such steep expenditures as it did in the past. After all, there is no such treatment as "liver dialysis" with which to compare the cost and overall efficiency of a liver transplant, for example. Therefore, persons who need transplants other than kidney transplants must pay for them out-of-pocket or through insurance. But because only relatively affluent persons have the means to pay for costly transplants, only they can be said to autonomously choose whether or not to submit to such treatment. Feminist bioethicists point out that in a country which does not offer universal health care, it cannot be argued that patients without the means to pay for costly transplants freely decide not to have them.

In our Western, avoid-death-at-all-costs culture, the tension of the search and wait for an organ can take on monstrous proportions. In cultures that see death as part of the life cycle, the need to save lives may be looked at differently, with different values in the forefront. In developing countries, many people are strong believers in destiny, even if that destiny is death.[10] Expenditure of dollars on a better overall quality of life (food, clothing, shelter, education, basic health) might make more sense to persons sharing that belief. Even in the United States, a very affluent nation, it is reasonable to ask if governmental funding of organ transplantation is an appropriate use of (supposedly) scarce health care dollars and energy. This question is not easy to answer. For example, several years ago Oregon decided to redistribute its health care resources through a change in Medicaid benefits. The state eliminated paying for organ transplants in favor of using that money to address the public health issue of prenatal care for economically disadvantaged women. When a young boy died because his family could not raise the money for a necessary bone marrow transplant, there was a public outcry and Oregon restored Medicaid funding for transplants.[11] As a feminist bioethicist, I would ask whose concerns are prioritized here and whose are erased? The many faceless women and their fetuses who would benefit from prenatal care become less important than the one "real-life" boy who needs an organ to live.

In examining issues of social justice for allocation of scarce resources, most people do not like to think of medically necessary care being denied because of a person's inability to pay for it. The problem is that we cannot collectively agree what "medically necessary" health care is. In the last few decades, our society has struggled over the issue of unequal access to health care. These concerns probably reflect our collective guilt about failing to fulfill one of the founding principles of our nation, namely, the principle of "equal opportunity, justice for all." It is hard to espouse equal opportunity if we do not provide all of our citizens with certain basic needs, such as health care. Everyone needs it. The problem is how much, and what kinds of, health care are people *entitled* to? Even if one agrees that health care is deserved by all and should be decided by need, who decides what a "need" is? Does organ transplantation fall under "need"? The unpleasant truth is that health care costs have spun out of control and, absent clear public policy, physicians are put in the ethically tenuous position of having to make bedside rationing decisions about patient care. As the *structure* of delivering health care places more emphasis on cost savings than patients' best interests, physicians (as part of that structure) will be tempted to change their traditional behavior. This possibility raises questions as to whether physicians can maintain the best interests of their patients if they are also involved in the rationing of health care. By failing to publicly address the ethical dilemma of deciding how far to go in particular cases, how many procedures to employ, and at what cost, we place our physicians and patients in extremely difficult relationships.

Proposed Changes to the Current
U.S. Procurement System

The Uniform Anatomical Gift Act (UAGA) of 1968 was amended in 1987 *specifically in an effort to increase the supply of organs*. The amendment placed more importance on donor wishes, the ease with which one could donate,

the necessity for hospital and law enforcement personnel to seek documentation of a potential donor's wishes, and a "routine request" process of
asking patients entering a hospital about considering organ donation.
Health care professionals tell us, however, that in practice, the statute is not
enforced and the act has not increased the supply of organs or enhanced
the autonomous wishes of donors.[12] In practice, the authority/permission
to remove organs remains with the family. Their wishes, more than their
dying or already dead loved one's wishes, are more likely to be honored by
health care personnel. What's more, health care professionals continue to
find conversations about impending death difficult. As a result, many
health care professionals can't find what they regard as the "right" words
to make an organ donation request or to make it clearly and with conviction. This state of affairs is regrettable because long after their loved one
has died, many people say that they wish they had thought to donate their
loved one's organs. At the time, however, they were too emotionally dis-
traught to have this opportunity come to mind. Others say that because
they were asked to donate their loved one's organ in such a perfunctory
and cold manner, it seemed unthinkable for them to do so then, but now
they regret not having done so. If done appropriately, perhaps by bereavement counselors, families who are asked if they wish to donate the organs
of a loved one at the time of death might view the request as a blessing, a
decision they can make to ease their pain. Bereaved persons are often looking for a way to make sense of tragedy and death. Health care professionals miss the opportunity to offer this chance to the family if they allow their
own discomfort about death to prevent a candid, well-timed conversation
regarding organ donation.

The tension between our current individualistically autonomous system of deciding to donate and the public need for organs is not adequately addressed by the UAGA.[13] There is nothing in the UAGA that requires public education about organ donation or requires that
conscientious thought be given to this matter. If we move the level of discussion to an experiential level, is there a message there? Is the fact that
we rarely discuss beliefs and values about our bodies a sign that we do
not want to contribute to increasing the supply of organs because we do
not want to think of our bodies as being defiled at death? If so, who is deciding that this sort of belief can (and should) be "educated away"? Feminist bioethicists posit these questions because they feel it is essential to
hear all voices. They caution that the physician's worldview often prevails in discussions of highly technological medical treatments. Therefore, the plea to increase the number of organs could be viewed as a narrow medical goal, not a broad communal one, if full discussions have not
occurred in community forums. In other words, the assumption that increasing the supply of organs is right because it will save lives assumes

that the most important thing in all circumstances is to save lives. That is an understandable assumption on the part of health care professionals, but it may not be the natural priority for all patients.

In other cultures, including many European ones, individual autonomy in donating organs is not respected as a "positive right." Rather, it is respected as a "negative right," which is commonly referred to as "presumed consent." A person is presumed to want to be an organ donor at the time of death unless there is documentation verifying his or her *refusing* to be a donor.[14] This strategy makes organ donation something to which each person must give thought, putting the issue squarely in the public forum. In requiring that a person announce a *refusal*, rather than a *desire* to be an organ donor, autonomy is not disregarded; rather, the importance of people's need for organs is simply elevated to a conscious level. After reflecting on this need, individuals can then decide if, or how much, they want to contribute to this need. Although a "presumed consent" policy seems entirely laudable, feminist bioethicists have nonetheless expressed great concerns about the burden of choice being shifted in this manner. Because of the inherent hierarchy of our social structure, vulnerable groups such as the poor, illiterate, and uneducated may not have access to complete information about this kind of choice and therefore may not be able to fully understand it. Where would agency lie for these persons? Misunderstandings under such a system might result in unjustified organ removals, reflecting a policy so determined to increase the organ supply that it willingly erases agency for vulnerable populations.

Another suggestion in addressing organ shortage is whether, as a society, we ought not consider allowing the market to solve this problem by permitting organs to be bought and sold as commodities. Currently the UAGA and federal law prohibit the sale or purchase of organs. One of the basic arguments for this prohibition is that the poor might become vulnerable to financial incentives that would only benefit the rich. As feminist bioethicists remind us, issues of power and dependency greatly affect one's ability to "freely choose" particular solutions. If one's basic human needs are not being met, such as the need for food, clothing, or shelter, one might be tempted to sell some of one's bodily parts for cash. In such cases, fully informed and uncoerced consent is not possible.[15] Those who advocate for the option of "organ vending" must not be allowed to view it as a good way for poor people to solve their financial problems. Although traditional bioethicists might argue that the autonomous decision to sell an organ should be available to everyone, feminist bioethicists argue that autonomy/agency does not exist when a person is so impoverished that the only way for him or her to make money is by selling a body part.

Arguments against buying and selling organs also include the fact that to do so would radically alter an ethical paradigm our society operates on, namely, that there is "something different" about buying and selling things as opposed to body parts,[16] and that there is something wrong about poor people selling parts of themselves to rich people. Consider, for example, that countries such as Iraq, Egypt, and India are viewed and used as "organ markets" by wealthier countries.[17] Although the governments of Iraq, Egypt, and India officially prohibit the buying and selling of human organs, the practice continues[18] and, at least "on the books," we condemn this state of affairs.

Avoiding Death: Life at All Costs

In my work with families who are grieving, I am painfully aware of the lengths persons will go to avoid dealing with feelings they have about their own mortality. I would now like to reflect on that cultural reluctance in relation to the topic of organ transplantation. The ability to transplant organs from dead persons (cadavers) to living human beings in order to extend life is truly a medical miracle. Although not taking away from this, I am concerned that in the process of striving for the advancement of this science, we may have relinquished our responsibility to examine the values and assumptions that undergird our passion for extending life at all costs.

It is reasonable to assume that medical personnel need to continually focus on what they can do to prevent death and extend life. However, the rest of us are not bound by that occupational hazard—rather, we are the subject of it! Increasing public discussions regarding "the right to die" offer evidence that for many people, the endless perpetuation of life is not a worthwhile goal.

After spending over forty years as social scientists in the field of organ transplantation, Renee C. Fox and Judith Swazey announced their departure from the field. Their announcement caused quite a stir, for they specifically said that they now need to intentionally separate themselves

> from what we believe is an overly zealous medical and societal commitment to the endless perpetuation of life and to repairing and rebuilding people through organ replacement—and from the human suffering and the social, cultural, and spiritual harm we believe such unexamined excess can, and already has, brought in its wake.[19]

Fox and Swazey bring up an interesting point. They are taking a moral stance that "enough is enough" and that organ transplantation has become an example of a practice in medicine becoming widely accepted *be-*

cause it is possible, not because it is actually desirable. This point applies to a discussion of the use of transplantation in developing countries as well. Although horrendous living conditions contribute to widespread organ failure in persons living in developing countries, organ transplantation may not be the appropriate remedy for them. Successful transplantation requires extraordinary economic and social resources—resources that most struggling nations cannot afford to divert to what can only be perceived as medical "luxuries." Until people in developing nations have clean water, adequate nutrition, and basic immunizations and antibiotics, costly transplant programs had best remain within the borders of those nations that can sustain their costs without jeopardizing simple public health initiatives, for example. If feminist bioethicists expand their vision to include the problems of peoples in developing countries, they can initiate particularly honest discussions about if and when organ transplantation is both a desirable and a feasible goal.

Swazey talks of our vision of health care as a "mirage of health . . . complete and lasting freedom from disease."[20] She warns us that organ transplantation is but another way of fostering our sense that we are entitled to (and therefore should pursue) any means necessary to prolong life. It is uncomfortable to explore an alternative to this line of thinking because, as a culture, we are not taught to incorporate our own mortality into our personal vision of our lives.

We are a warmhearted and generous people, but most especially when a person in a tragic situation has a name and a face. There have been cases, usually involving children, in which a particular child's need for an organ has been brought to national light on news or talk shows. The whole country gets involved in the desperate plea for an organ. We never even question if it is the "right thing" to search desperately for an organ for such a child, yet some of these children have gone on to need multiple surgeries because of rejection of the primary transplant. They have spent months (or even years) hooked up to machines in sterile hospital environments, existing in this manner until another organ becomes available. As a feminist and social worker, I have concern for these children and their quality of life. Furthermore, I lament that we rarely give thought to the fact that one child has to die before another gets an organ. How that other child dies is an important question, yet it is one we do not fully address. Is it accident, crime, or lack of access to primary healthcare that is the reason some of these young donors die, thereby making organs available to the recipients who capture our hearts? As a matter of public policy (since much funding is through Medicaid), I worry about public funds being drained for one heartbreaking transplant case when we allow so many children to live below the poverty line without access to such basic necessities as food, clothing, health care, and a safe place to live.

In the case of transplantation, feminist bioethicists observe that the healthiest organs used in adult transplantation often come from young people who have died as a result of accident, murder, or suicide.[21] Many of these deaths would not have occurred had these young people been children of privilege. Nevertheless, society accepts this state of affairs as "a part of life," the way things are. Why, then, do not the people who receive organs view death as something they should have accepted as a natural inevitability? Why do they not accept death as an event to which they should simply submit?

Conclusions

Clearly, our culture assumes that we should increase the supply of organs simply because it also assumes that the best choice for everyone is extension of life. We must challenge this assumption and see it as grounded in our culture's enormous fear of death. We need to discuss death more openly, as the current euthanasia/physician-assisted suicide debate invites us to do. Organ transplantation may not be *the best solution for everyone*. In other words, *death* can be a person's best choice if, in his or her estimation, the quantity and/or quality of life an organ transplant purchases is simply not worth the attendant physical, psychological, material, and spiritual pain, suffering, hardships, and burdens.

Our medical capabilities do not come without a price. Collectively, we have to decide what price is acceptable to us. I am not arguing that organ transplantation is never a good option for a person, but I am insisting that organ transplantation is not always a good option. There are times when patients should be offered detailed explanations of what the cost of "living" might be, even if that leads them to choose nontreatment and subsequent death. This option is often not discussed with patients due to the discomfort of health care professionals, or it is glossed over in language that does not register the same meaning for the patient as the physician.[22]

The field of bioethics was born over thirty years ago because of the ethical dilemmas created by the growing ability of medicine, science, and technology to benefit people. It is my wish that we pause and take a breath, and look at these benefits as something that we *might* or *might not* want to choose. We do not have to accept the fruits of progress as something we must eat. It is up to us to decide, consciously, whether we wish to partake of these fruits or not. As for myself, I have decided to be an organ donor and often ask others to consider being donors as well. I tell you this so that you will clearly understand that I am not against organ transplantation per se. I am simply saying that my choice—or yours for that matter—is not the only one that should be recognized. In

order to guarantee thoughtful, conscientious responses to questions of
how far we should go with organ transplantation, we must encourage
all segments of the public to express their personal values and views
about this subject. As I see it, this is the charge of feminist bioethicists in
particular, for

> *We cannot live for ourselves alone.*
> *Our lives are connected by*
> *A thousand invisible threads.*
> *And along these sympathetic fibers,*
> *Our actions run as causes*
> *And return to us as results.*
> **—Herman Melville**

Notes

1. J. F. Blumstein, "The Use of Financial Incentives in Medical Care: The Case of
Commerce in Transplantable Organs," *Health Matrix: The Journal of Law and Medicine* 3, no. 1 (1993): 1–30.

2. Helen B. Holmes and Laura M. Purdy, eds., *Feminist Perspectives in Medical Ethics* (Bloomington: Indiana University Press, 1992), pp. 24–25.

3. Susan M. Wolf, ed., *Feminism and Bioethics: Beyond Reproduction* (New York: Oxford University Press, 1996), pp. 187–198.

4. T. A. Rando, *Grief, Dying, and Death: Clinical Intervention for the Caregiver* (Champagne, Ill.: Research Press, 1984), pp. 4–8.

5. Tom L. Beauchamp and James F. Childress, *Principles of Biomedical Ethics*, 4th ed. (New York: Oxford University Press, 1994), pp. 123–125.

6. Susan Sherwin, *No Longer Patient: Feminist Ethics and Healthcare* (Philadelphia: Temple University Press, 1992), pp. 51–54.

7. Ibid., pp. 3–4.

8. Holmes and Purdy, eds., *Feminist Perspectives*.

9. R. D. Blair and D. L. Kaserman, "The Economics and Ethics of Alternative Cadaveric Organ Procurement Policies," *Yale Journal on Regulation* 8, no. 403 (1991): 403–462.

10. M. Gaber, "Organ Transplantation in Developing Countries," *World Health Forum* 19, no. 2 (1998): 120–123.

11. B. R. Furrow et al., *Bioethics: Healthcare Law and Ethics*, 3d ed. (St. Paul: West, 1997), p. 362.

12. J. Prottas, *Altruism and the Public Policy of Organ Transplants: The Most Useful Gift* (San Francisco: Jossey-Bass, 1994).

13. Furrow et al., *Bioethics*, p. 364.

14. A. H. Berger, "Is 'Presumed Consent' the Best Policy for Increasing Voluntary Organ Donation?" *CQ Researcher*, August 11, 1995, pp. 721–727.

15. Sherwin, *No Longer Patient*.

16. Judith P. Swazey and Renee C. Fox, "Allocating Scarce Gifts of Life," *Trends in Healthcare, Law, and Ethics* 8, no. 4 (1993): 30.

17. A. S. Darr, "An Emerging Transplant Force—Developing Countries: Middle East and the Indian Subcontinent," *Transplantation Proceedings* 29 (1997): 1577–1579.

18. Gaber, "Organ Transplantation in Developing Countries," pp. 120-123.

19. Stuart J. Youngner, Renee C. Fox, and L. J. O'Connell, eds., *Organ Transplantation: Meanings and Realities* (Madison: University of Wisconsin Press, 1996), p. 252.

20. Swazey and Fox, "Allocating Scarce Gifts," p. 33.

21. Ibid., pp. 31–32.

22. R. Bogdan, M. A. Brown, and S. B. Foster, "Be Honest, but Not Cruel: Staff/Patient Communication on a Neonatal Unit," *Human Organization* 44, no. 1 (1982): 12.

22

Serving Nationalist Ideologies: Health Professionals and the Violation of Women's Rights: The Case of Apartheid South Africa

JEANELLE DE GRUCHY
LAUREL BALDWIN-RAGAVEN

Feminists have critiqued biomedicine as a form of patriarchy that controls female bodies, disregarding women's inherent rights to dignity and bodily integrity.[1] The health professions have also been criticized for their role in maintaining particular global power relations through their support of conservative money market agendas that often violate the human rights of those in the "developing" world. In particular countries, health professionals have participated in national agendas that ensure their hegemonic power, even when the rights of certain groups are violated. Concomitantly, governments have used "health-related activities as one of a number of tools to maintain control and power."[2]

For us—feminists, human rights activists, and medical doctors in South Africa—the case of health professionals during apartheid is illustrative. The great majority of South African health professionals and their institutions supported the apartheid state in its violation of the basic human rights of black people. In terms of reproductive health policies, South Africa both followed and rejected global trends. In this unique and stark context, the health sector participated in the racist and sexist construction of South African women as reproductive bodies and was complicit in the manipulation of their reproduction for political purposes. We discuss how the complementary relationship between bioethics and human rights was severely compromised by the South African health profession during apartheid, focusing specifically on reproductive agendas and policies to explore the complex interconnections between science and biomedicine, patriarchy, and racist nation building.[3] We end by presenting three examples of unethical practices by health professionals that led to violations of women's rights. Through these examples, we identify and discuss four explanations for health professional abuses. Despite the positive changes that have taken place in South Africa, we need to be aware that these patterns persist. Our concern now is to develop a culture of respect for human rights and professional accountability in the South African health sector. This involves challenging and ultimately changing the unethical behaviors that persist. In so doing, we will truly achieve respect for rights and informed choice on reproductive matters for women.[4]

A Sobering History of Professional Collusion

With the demise of apartheid, hastened by increasing opposition both within and without the country, the National Party was forced to the negotiating table in the early 1990s. A settlement was reached that released political prisoners, including the key figure Nelson Mandela, and unbanned antiapartheid organizations, which led to the first ever democratic elections in 1994. As part of the mandate of this "new" South Africa, a Truth and Reconciliation Commission (TRC) was established to document gross human rights violations, grant amnesty to perpetrators of politically motivated violence, and recommend the implementation of reparations for victims. The TRC has had a profound effect on the nation's psyche and consciousness, although its full implications are not yet evident. After more than two years of statement taking, investigation, and public hearings, the TRC delivered its final report to President Mandela in November 1998.[5]

From the start of the TRC hearings in May 1996, there was mounting evidence that health professionals were complicit in gross human rights abuses. This evidence led to a call for the TRC to institute special hearings on the health sector.[6] There was also increasing discussion within the health professions aimed at gaining an understanding of and dealing with abrogations of "professional ethics" and countering the suggestions that many health professionals, as individuals and organizations (many continuing to be major role players in the health sector), were suffering from a "selective amnesia" with regard to past human rights abuses or support for apartheid policy. These TRC health sector hearings, held over two days in June 1997, focused national and international attention on the healing professions' involvement with the repressive apartheid state.[7] Apartheid "permeated the entire health sector, distorting and corrupting health services and health professional training."[8]

The focal point of the hearings revisited the death in detention of Black Consciousness leader Steve Biko in 1977.[9] This case demonstrates how formal organizations of the profession condoned and covered up the behavior of the "Biko doctors," even after their conduct was shown to be unequivocally unethical. This situation epitomized the loss of honor by the medical profession through doctors' unwillingness to speak out against colleagues who put the interests of the state before the interests of their patients.[10]

The principles of health profession ethics and human rights have as their common aim the respectful and dignified treatment of people— both as individuals and collectively. Professional ethics are critical to the relationship between the profession and civil society, an "honoring" of an established social contract—a contract that depends on ethical practice and respect for human rights. At the societal level, health professionals have largely been given a free hand. In return for this right to self-regulation, society expects them to protect the rights of their patients and ensure that the highest standards of care and conduct are maintained. However, as evidenced by the treatment of Steve Biko, this trust can be open to abuse.

The South African statutory councils, organizations, and training institutions embraced the discourse of contemporary bioethics and created the perception that the health sector supported universalized norms for professional behavior, while at the same time ignoring the glaring disparities in the distribution of resources, population health indicators, provision of trained personnel, and eventually in the treatment of those in custodial care. Under apartheid the health sector constructed a situation in which behaving "ethically" with one's patients was separated from the imperative to engage with human rights tenets. "When confronted about its conduct, [the health sector] continually sought to defend its behaviour on traditional ethical grounds" so that "actions antithetical to human rights [were] justified within an ethical paradigm."[11] Disconnecting "ethics" from its common origins with human rights—for reasons of political expediency and self-interest—permitted the disingenuous adoption of all major international codes of ethics, including the Declaration of Tokyo, which condemns health professionals' participation in and complicity with torture. The split effectively rationalized violations of human rights as "political," well outside the purview of health profession ethics.[12]

The Biko case illustrates again that the complicity of health professionals in human rights violations was not the isolated activity of a few "bad apples." It was the inevitable result of an environment in which human rights abuses could be condoned by the medical establishment. It is the construction of this environment, as it pertains to reproduction, that we now address.

Population (and Women) Control

The development of contraceptive and reproductive technologies has been a major step in the movement to increase the control that women can exercise over their reproductive and sexual lives.[13] Although these technologies offer some women greater choice, they may not necessarily impact positively on all women's lives. Unfortunately, this technology can actually increase the ways in which women, particularly those in the "developing" world, are vulnerable to exploitation. This "potentially liberating technology"[14] has been abused for expressly political purposes in the population control project of apartheid South Africa.[15]

Population policies foreground the tension between the right of governments to intervene in their subjects' intimate lives and the protection of citizens' human rights. "Virtually all human rights can be infringed within population policies thus *all* basic human rights and fundamental freedoms ought to be applied in population policies as in other areas for which public authorities are responsible."[16] Population policies set demographic targets, whereas ideally family planning programs are meant to provide the means for women to exercise reproductive freedom. However, these distinctions can often become muddied as governments use women's bodies to achieve demographic goals.[17] Feminists have been active in challenging the distortion of family planning programs[18] and have successfully effected changes in the way in which governments develop population policies.[19]

In the apartheid state only whites were citizens with rights. They enjoyed a privileged status with entitlements, whereas black South Africans were systematically stripped of their rights and humanity. Black women were objectified as the bodies through which the black population grew. In reality, then, policies were made with scant regard for universal human rights, for black women's bodily integrity or autonomy did not count.

In her discussion of the role of women in "the biological reproduction of the nation,"[20] Nira Yuval-Davis describes three major discourses that "tend to dominate national policies of population control"—the eugenics and Malthusian discourses, and what she terms the "people as power" discourse.[21] In examining the deployment of these three discourses in South Africa, we first explore the eugenics movement and the use of scientific discourse, particularly "scientific racism," in legitimating apartheid theories and practices. Second, drawing on feminist critiques, we examine the apartheid state and its "double standard" use of both Malthusian and "people as power" discourses in its population policies.

Controlling Production: "Fit" Babies for a "Fit" Nation

> The State needs all the *good* children it can get. But it does not need the un-der-nourished, mal-adjusted brood of the overworked and underpaid slum dweller or the feebleminded, and so the woman eugenist would extend to them the knowledge of birth control. (Annie Porter, from a lecture presented at the inaugural public meeting of the Race Welfare Society [RWS], Johan-nesburg, August 14, 1930)[22]

Eugenics is concerned with improving the "quality" of "a people" through engineering the "fit" to reproduce and the "unfit" to be pre-vented from doing so. "Fitness" is defined through discourses such as "race," "national stock," class, and intelligence. The eugenics movement was influential during the late nineteenth and early twentieth centuries. Although discredited as an intellectual movement,[23] eugenics discourse, as a way of improving society and the fitness of humankind, continues today.[24]

In her study of the eugenics movement in Latin America, Nancy Stepan notes the privileging of a biologically determined nation, and the engagement of gender and "race" by nation-states to realize their politics of identity.[25] She writes:

> The desire to "imagine" the nation in biological terms, to "purify" the repro-duction of populations to fit hereditary norms, to regulate the flow of peo-ples across national boundaries, to define in novel terms who could belong to the nation and who could not—all these aspects of eugenics turned on is-sues of gender and race, and produced intrusive proposals or prescriptions for new state policies toward individuals. Through eugenics, in short, gen-der and race were tied to the politics of national identity.[26]

Despite science being "rarely examined as part of the project of nation-alism . . . it has been a powerful discourse regulating meaning."[27] Scien-tific racism provided the "scientific proof" of the superiority of the "white race." This was vital to the emerging nation-building quest of the Afrikaners, a mission that found its political realization when the Afrikaner-based National Party took power in 1948. The thinking that "race" was biologically determined, with essential heritable characteris-tics such as brain size, IQ, deviance, and fecundity, supported the National Party's classification of South Africans into four major "racial" groups. These groups formed the basis for the systematic brutality of apartheid.

Saul Dubow, in his book *Scientific Racism in Modern South Africa*, argues that "South African historical scholarship has tended to underestimate the extent or significance of intellectual racism in the context of white minority rule" and that "racial science helped to facilitate the realisation and ideological maintenance of white power and authority."[28] Scientific racism informed the country's medical research agenda, which has had "a powerful and damaging impact on perceptions of human diversity and the origins of disease."[29]

As already noted, this nation-building quest turned on not only issues of "race" but also of gender. Stepan emphasizes the centrality of the state's control of women's reproductive capabilities in any national project:

> Gender was important to eugenics because it was through sexual reproduction that the modification and transmission of the hereditary makeup of future generations occurred. Control of that reproduction, by direct or indirect means, therefore became an important aspect of all eugenics movements.[30]

The eugenics program, and that of Afrikaner nation building, required that the prohibition of sexual unions across "races" was critical for maintaining "racial purity," "since it was through sexual unions that boundaries between races were believed to be either maintained or transgressed."[31] It is not surprising therefore that key apartheid legislation included the Mixed Marriages and Immorality Acts, which defined permissible sexual relations and eligible marriage partners. Again, scientific justification was readily available with research such as that conducted by Fantham and Porter[32] from the 1920s, which "purported to prove that racial mixture led to physical abnormalities or 'disharmonies,' ranging from pulmonary complaints and deficient circulatory systems, to disproportionately sized organs and bodily parts."[33]

The eugenics movement in South Africa accommodated and promoted multiple agendas across a broad political spectrum, from "white" conservatives to social welfare reformers. Certain influential women of the early contraceptive movement, many of whom were doctors, also engaged in the eugenics discourse, which underscores the complex alliances that were formed.

In February 1945 Dr. Marie Stopes, president of the Mothers' Clinics (sponsored by the Society and Clinic for Constructive Birth Control and Racial Progress in London, England) sent a letter to Dr. Sallie Woodrow, a physician instrumental in establishing the Cape Town Mothers' Clinic.[34]

In the letter Dr. Stopes states passionately, "I have long felt that we had to
have birth control knowledge and materials available for everybody in
the whole world who has intelligence [to use] them, and then sterilisation
must be used for those who have not sufficient intelligence." Later, after
favorably reviewing the male sterilization procedure, Dr. Stopes opines, "I
should say that the best thing would be to popularize that [vasectomy] as
far as you can among the blacks who have got, say, two children, and also
among any blacks who ask for it, whether they have any children or not."
With regard to a "very simple method of the sponge and oil," which she
apparently advocated "for the problem in India," Dr. Stopes responds to
Dr. Woodrow that "from what you say of the black women I do not know
that one could rely on them using it, as simple as it is."[35]

This correspondence between two women doctors raises issues, pertinent today, with a particularly time-bound honesty.[36] The need to provide women with the safest, most reliable, and user-friendly contraceptives available was recognized and responded to by a medical doctor's
paternalistic concern. At the same time, informing her prescription is a
mixture of "scientific" justification, dubious ethics, eugenics motivation,
racist stereotypes, and colonial objectification. As we discuss later, these
elements are still found, although generally expressed more subtly,
among health professionals today.

The "Black" Population Explosion
and a Call for More "White" Babies

Just as eugenics saw control of reproduction as central to the improvement of humankind, so the idea of controlling women's reproduction for
greater social good informed neo-Malthusian thought, which identified
world "overpopulation" as the threat to social development and global
prosperity.

The World Population Conference in Bucharest in 1974 drew on neo-
Malthusian principles, as did South Africa's formal population policy
initiated in the same year. Whereas the Bucharest conference began to
approach issues of population growth through a "combination of economic growth and broad publicly funded family planning,"[37] the South
African policy "ignored [the] Conference's assertion that development
could not be effectively addressed in the apartheid context."[38] Instead,
the apartheid state's demographic policy was "the most blatant contemporary" example of a "double-standard approach," simply put, to
increase the white population and decrease the black.[39] From its inception, South African reproductive policy was "formulated with the intention of reinforcing . . . social relations of inequality under apartheid
and capitalism."[40]

Politicians[41] concerned at the declining numbers of "whites" used what Yuval-Davis terms the "people as power" discourse in which "the future of 'the nation' is seen to depend on its continuous growth."[42] They exhorted white women to reproduce and provided tax incentives for larger white families. They also actively recruited white immigrants.[43]

At the same time, as a result of policies through the century, the state had sufficient unskilled people for its labor purposes. With rising worker militancy, the state feared that the increase in the black population would lead to increasing numbers of poor and unemployed people, and the increasing potential for uprising. Speaking in 1972, the then prime minister, B. J. Vorster, said, "We would like to reduce them [the black population] . . . and we are doing our best to do so, but at all times we would not disrupt the South African economy."[44]

From 1974, "the government embarked on [the] mass provision of contraception, free of charge, through a vertical 'family planning' service based . . . on mobile clinics" in the rural areas, and on dedicated sites in nearly every urban center.[45] These services benefited from extensive resources and were available to all "racial" groups, but at segregated facilities.[46] By 1990, there were some 58,000 clinic locations.

Apartheid policy and capital cooperated extensively and in very practical ways to control the black working population. Over 60 percent of factories had on-site family-planning services. In a situation where women faced losing their jobs if they became pregnant, they had to use contraception to stay employed.[47] The contraceptive net was thrown wide; a pamphlet put out by the Department of Health and Welfare in the 1980s gave a clarion call to farmers' wives:[48]

> The wife that is a strong supporter of family planning instruction and clinical services on her farm, provides a unique service to her country and people. With her help, family planning will quickly reach every corner of the land—something that would not be otherwise possible. Begin today—your workers will appreciate it! [There are benefits for the farmer.] He will have a stable and productive workforce; he will have a motivated worker, with a planned family, with fewer problems to distract him from his work.[49]

Issues of reproduction globally could in fact be analogous to the double standard approach of the South African apartheid state. Women from wealthier nations are encouraged to reproduce, whereas those from poorer nations are discouraged. Although industrialized nations pioneer new technologies allowing women with capital to have children, there is little money for fertility programs in poor nations, despite high infertility rates. These industrialized nations do not apply population targets for their "own" populations, out of respect for human rights, while at the same time population targets "may be supported within their international population assistance" programs.[50] These nations spend vast amounts on family planning programs for the "developing" world—and link this money to other economic and social benefits.

"There Would Be Fewer Starving Kids": The Health Profession and Accountability

> If women are to be subjects and not objects in the medical encounter, this requires the highest ethical standards from health workers and it is clear that these are not always achieved.[51]

We maintain that health professionals, as clinicians, policymakers, and administrators, have particular ethical responsibilities toward all vulnerable groups, including women. Having examined some of the ways in which science and medicine contributed to the three discourses that informed the apartheid government's policy of population control, we now focus on the involvement of health professionals in unethical practices with regard to reproductive health care. More than farmers' wives and factory managers, health professionals were key to the successful implementation of apartheid's population policy.

As we have shown, the government's family planning program was synonymous with its population policy and clearly was not focused on improving the health status of women. The role of health professionals in a program designed primarily for population control in promoting "family planning" therefore raises challenging ethical questions. On whose behalf and for whose benefit were South African health professionals working?[52] Was it possible for health professionals to fully respect the autonomy of any "black" woman of childbearing age? Although we acknowledge that health professionals' complicity with the government's population policy is a complex issue, this in no way absolves the relationships cultivated between the state and the health professions to achieve population targets. Klugman articulates the problem clearly: "When providers of contraception are absolutely certain that stopping a woman from having another child will be a major contribution towards the national good, there is a serious ethical problem, especially when the majority of the nation have had no say in the formulation of the policy in the first place."[53]

To introduce our discussion of some of the ethical inconsistencies and challenges to the health sector, we have selected three examples in which health professionals actively suppressed (and might continue to suppress) professional ethics and human rights principles in providing for the reproductive health of women.

The Military Project to Develop an Antifertility Vaccine

The TRC heard evidence that "the most important project of the early stages of South Africa's secret biological warfare programme" was work done by scientists of the South African Defence Force (SADF) to develop an antifertility vaccine that "could have been used clandestinely on black people."[54] Dr. Wouter Basson, a cardiologist and former physician to President P. W. Botha, was head of the SADF's biological and chemical warfare program, which coordinated this project; Basson has thus far denied participating in experiments to control black female fertility.[55] Giving evidence before the TRC, Dr. Goosen, a veterinarian and pathologist, said that when he was recruited as managing director of the SADF front company which was to conduct the research, he was told that

> the growing black population, and of course "communism" were the overwhelming threats to white South Africa . . . [and] this anti-fertility project was approved by the SADF at the highest levels. . . . I joined the project for patriotic reasons. I thought we were involved in a war for our survival. [The surgeon-general had] not only ordered the project but said it was our most important task as there were "too many blacks." . . . we believed at the time, this was legitimate. If we developed an anti-fertility vaccine, we would have curbed the birth rate, there would be less starving kids. We believed a new government would also need it. It wouldn't have been like a contraceptive pill that has to be 100 percent effective. If we had done that and there were suddenly no babies coming out of Soweto . . . well, we couldn't do that, so we wanted a vaccine [to be only] 70 to 80 percent effective.[56]

Sterilization: Enthusiasm for a Cause

Parallel to its extensive promotion of reversible contraception, the apartheid state also embarked on a major program of female surgical sterilization. Here too the potential for abuse by health care workers was enormous. A pamphlet on sterilization that failed to mention the permanence of the procedure can, at best, be seen as purposely misleading.[57] A doctor who now works at the Medical Research Council recalls that as a medical officer, he observed surgical registrars (surgeons in training) sterilizing patients during appendectomies—without their knowledge, let alone consent. Furthermore, he recollects how surgeons regularly manipulated fallopian tubes with the intention of causing adhesions and subsequent infertility.[58] These practices were commonly known.

In 1987, the deputy director of family planning, Ms. Stockton, admitted in an interview with Barbara Klugman that "there is the problem of doctors in provincial hospitals doing sterilizations when they do a caesar; [and] district surgeons are [also] inclined to give Depo without the correct motivation."[59] As an explanation for the behavior of these health professionals, Ms. Stockton suggested that "it is partly a problem of enthusiasm for a cause . . . noting that the white population is well below replacement and that we're a minority group in the country."[60]

Depo-Provera: The "Fourth Stage" of Labor

By 1993, 70–80 percent of all black female clients in South Africa were using injectables, as compared to 10 percent of all white female clients.[61] This is in contrast to other family planning programs on the continent; specifically, there is hardly another program in Africa that supplies injectables for more than 20 percent of contraceptive usage.[62]

There are three medical stages to labor. In South Africa, the automatic administration of an injectable progestogen during childbirth has resulted in Depo's being known as "the fourth stage of labor." "Many women do not give informed consent for the injection, and women who try to refuse are often given a hard time."[63] This was certainly one of our experiences as medical students. "Every woman who I observed giving birth, was given the option only of the 'two month' or 'three month' [which refers to the administration period of the injectables]. I was present on one occasion when a woman requested the pill. The request was shared between the midwives and met with loud derision. The woman was summarily given an injection."[64]

These three instances describe some of the myriad unethical practices that occurred during apartheid. Some continue to occur. They lead us to examine four patterns of complicity: patterns which constructed the environment that allowed for these abuses.

Patterns of Complicity

Ideological Congruency

If we understand medicine itself as an institution of social control,[65] a dominant ideology that "is part of an extensive system of moral regulation of populations,"[66] we can see how easily medicine could have, and indeed did, serve the purposes of the apartheid state. The context for the examples cited above was apartheid. All of the role players were therefore classified according to "race," which in turn fundamentally determined their political positioning in society and in the medical hierarchy. The power of the health profession was vested predominantly in white male doctors, most of whom would have been been supporters of apartheid ideology. This ideological conviction informed their work as doctors and scientists as well as their relationships with other health professionals, the majority of whom were black female nurses.

The *South African Medical Journal (SAMJ)*, official mouthpiece of the Medical Association of South Africa (MASA), welcomed the government's 1974 population program, declaring that "South Africa is on the brink of a population explosion, especially with regard to its Black citizens." It furthermore branded this "population explosion . . . [as] the biggest problem in the history of humankind"[67] (our translation from the original Afrikaans).

This ideological conviction that *population growth* per se is the problem and "family planning" the answer persists among many South African health professionals. Responding to an editorial in the *SAMJ*, a doctor wrote:

> Your diehard intransigence in insisting that only socio-economic development will lead to a population decline is to be regretted. It is just not true. The best and most rapid aproach to population control is when a strong effective family planning campaign goes hand in hand with socio-economic development. *But . . . strong, effective family planning can work wonders even without collateral socio-economic development* (emphasis added).[68]

This privileging of contraception regulates women's reproduction and controls their social behavior instead of responding to their reproductive health needs. This informs our understanding of the extensive use of injectables in South Africa, a practice that remains unchanged: "If the driving force of [South Africa's family planning] programme was the fear of the white population about growing black numbers, then the widespread use of injectables may have developed as a tool of social engineering, and this pattern now established is difficult to break."[69]

Patriotic Science: A Neutral Vocation?

The ideological congruency between apartheid, patriarchy, and medicine facilitated the drive to control women's reproduction, determining the national contraceptive research agenda and condoning the covert participation of academic researchers in programs such as those conducted by the military. Bridgette Mabandla, South African deputy minister of Arts, Culture, Science and Technology, described the TRC hearings on biochemical warfare as "mind-boggling accounts of the lurid and somewhat astonishing activities of scientists in service of apartheid. These highlight the capabilities of science and technology in an era symbolized by torture, genocide and moral subversion of society."[70]

A veneer of professionalism covered the close partnership between "science" and a repressive state, allowing for these "astonishing activities." A reporter in the *British Medical Journal* commenting on the hearings noted that "because doctors were running the programme it was generally assumed that the programme was ethical and above board."[71]

This presumption that doctors and medical scientists would behave ethically reflects the hegemony of scientific positivism specifically, and of rationalism more generally. It furthermore exposes the myth of scientific objectivity and impartiality. In a recent Listserv discussion of Basson and his unit's work, the research itself could be separated from its context and thus seen as inherently neutral, albeit with a potential for abuse. One respondent commented:

> Any effective and safe method of family planning would surely be welcome if used responsibly. The key issue for me would be to demonstrate scientifically that the vaccine will be effective, safe and can be used responsibly by the health workers and policy makers. It could be a better alternative to tubal ligation.[72]

We would argue, however, that science is never objective or impartial.[73] In this instance, locating the antifertility vaccination experiments in apartheid military laboratories and not subjecting them to the same regulatory mechanisms as other research, protecting the secrecy of this project in the interest of "national security," and allegedly recruiting university-based academics from the nearby Pretoria University to work there covertly render this "science" quite pernicious.

An analysis by the World Health Organization, moreover, shows that contraceptive research never takes place without political determinants. Rather, contraceptive research internationally has

- focused on population growth, too often ignored women's health, and sometimes resulted in coercive approaches
- produced methods more reflective of scientists' interests than women's preferences
- ignored the risks posed by provision and use of systemic and clinic-based methods in inadequate, inaccessible, or inappropriate health services[74]

The antifertility vaccine research conducted by the SADF clearly did all three.

A Profession of "Othering"

Widely acknowledged as part of becoming a health professional is learning appropriate "professional boundaries." Too often, however, constructing barriers between "professional" and "patient" results in a process of "othering" that negates human dignity and respect. In other words, this socialization process ends up off-centering respect and devaluing caring. As we have illustrated, in apartheid South Africa, with its constructed social and political divisions, professional "othering," itself problematic, too often worsened to become "objectification."

Women were objectified by the population control policies of the apartheid state and often by those implementing its programs. By objectifying women, health professionals withheld their respect, across "race" and hierarchy. Respect of personhood, however, is a prerequisite to any other ethical principle, such as autonomy, nonmaleficence, beneficence, equity, and justice. We have already seen how South African health professionals routinely injected Depo-Provera or sterilized women, often without obtaining informed consent. Yet there has been little acknowledgment that these activities constituted human rights violations or even breaches of professional ethics.

Ethical dilemmas in South Africa during apartheid were effectively camouflaged. Although problematic for some, the overriding group consciousness relegated the Other to the status of nonpersonhood, or certainly less than full personhood. Although it was never explicitly articulated in the professional literature, an unspoken belief existed that ethical norms were only applicable to full persons; nonpersons, or lesser persons, could be dealt with in an attenuated and "appropriately" altered manner. It never seems to have occurred to anyone that these standards of ethics, to which all South African health professionals "adhered," could and should be applied universally. After all, in one way or another, and to greater or lesser degrees, every "black" person was already legally assigned an inferior status of personhood.[75]

Reproductive Choice: A Surgeon's Decision?

The fact that so many South African women, on balance, chose to use contraception suggests that in their estimation these services met real needs. Women still retained some degree of agency, albeit in desperate situations. However, when contraception or sterilization was undertaken either violently or covertly, it was extremely difficult, if not impossible, for women to question decisions and assert their rights. In such situations, women's limited agency in contraceptive choice was clearly negated.

Dr. Esther Sapire posits that many health professionals perceived their involvement in family planning programs as part of their duty in the "fight against poverty" or even in promoting socioeconomic rights.[76] A distorted understanding of poverty, however, produces a paternalistic "ethics,"[77] setting up health professionals as qualified to make decisions on behalf of women. The health professional believes that he or she is in a better position than the "ignorant" consumer to choose a contraceptive method. This reveals the construction of "black" women as incompetent in making their own decisions with regard to their health.

Gains and Vulnerabilities: Postapartheid South Africa

Running parallel to the TRC process has been the drafting and adoption of South Africa's new constitution and bill of rights (1996). Feminists and activists embarked on well-organized and effective action to ensure that the constitution reflects the interests of women and promotes gender equality. Our bill of rights now contains clauses that safeguard and promote women's rights as human rights, with explicit reference to reproductive rights and violence against women.[78] The constitution also creates structures[79] to facilitate the drive to gender equality. Legislation has been enacted operationalizing the state's commitment to ensuring that constitutional rights are not infringed. The passing of the Choice on Termination of Pregnancy Act (1997) has further strengthened the reproductive freedom of women in South Africa. Launched in July 1999, the white paper on population policy is a milestone, marking

> a critical shift from a population programme designed to lower women's fertility, to a policy supporting better planning and monitoring of development programmes generally, and pushing government to focus on priorities for intersectoral action so that the country's resources can be most optimally used. It is probably the first population policy in the world which is not demographically driven and offers a new interpretation of the paradigm-shift ascribed to the International Conference on Population and Development (ICPD) held in Cairo in 1994.[80]

Internationally, South Africa has committed itself to human rights for women by ratifying in 1995 the Convention on the Elimination of All forms of Discrimation Against Women (CEDAW)—the only country to ratify CEDAW without qualification. Although these are important gains, their impact may be compromised because of the lack of transformation in the sectors responsible for their realization. There have been articles in the local press recently commenting on the deep entrenchment of patriarchal, sexist thinking in South Africa. There have also been disturbing reports in regard to women's reproductive health, such as research conducted by the Medical Research Council showing that "violence of various forms is a feature of care at the [Midwife Obstetric Unit]."[81] Frank physical assault, including battering, verbal abuse, and lack of privacy were commonplace. Also, there have been many problems with the funding and implementation of the Choice on Termination of Pregnancy Act. Women still die from illegal abortions, some of them having been turned away from hospitals where they sought terminations.[82] The legacy of apartheid in the health sector, as well as the racist and sexist constructions of women by the health profession, have the potential therefore to sabotage important legislative and policy developments.

How can human rights now be guaranteed in a setting that has historically abrogated the rights of black women? Given the history of their collusion with apartheid patriarchy, how can South African health professionals be expected to begin adopting women-centered practice styles and redress power imbalances that derived from apartheid health legislation and reproductive policy? What transformation is required in the health sector for nascent reproductive rights to realize comprehensive health care for women?

Although we welcome South Africa's important legislative and policy changes, we hold that it is only through understanding how and why health professionals colluded with apartheid policies, as well as developing interventions to change the unethical behaviors that persist, will we truly achieve respect for rights such as privacy, confidentiality, and informed choice on reproductive matters. The role players involved in the health sector—individual health professionals, professional organizations, the statutory councils, state services, training institutions, and organizations in civil society and the private sector—all need to undertake particular activities and engage in far-reaching interventions which affirm their commitment to social transformation. As examples, we suggest beginning with self-study, research, and reflection on their positioning vis-à-vis apartheid population policy. Education and training institutions have a further responsibility to acknowledge their role in socializing professionals into certain worldviews, norms, and values that devalue human dignity and caring. The South African health professional orginizations and statutory councils must explicitly prioritize human rights and institute disciplinary action against those who conducted dubious contraceptive research or violated women's autonomy. Health professionals "have to consider their responsibility not only to respect human rights in developing policies, programs and practices, but to contribute actively from their position as health workers to improving societal realization of rights."[83] There is much work to be done in order to develop a culture of respect for human rights and professional accountability in the health sector.

Notes

The Health and Human Rights Project: Professional Accountability in South Africa (HHRP) is a joint initiative of the Department of Community Health, University of Cape Town, and the Trauma Centre for Survivors of Violence and Torture. The authors, both medical doctors, are research fellows with the HHRP in Cape Town, South Africa.

1. See, for example, Edward S. Williams, *Where Have All the Children Gone?* (Johannesburg, South Africa: Ernest Stanton, 1980); H. Graham and A. Oakley, "Competing Ideologies of Reproduction: Medical and Maternal Perspectives on Pregnancy," in H. Roberts, ed., *Women, Health, and Reproduction* (London: Routledge & Kegan Paul, 1981); J. Ussher, *The Psychology of the Female Body* (London: Routledge, 1989); and J. Altekruse and S. Rosser, "Feminism and Medicine: Cooptation or Cooperation?" in C. Kramarae and D. Spender, eds., *The Knowledge Explosion: Generations of Feminist Scholarship* (Great Britain: Harvester Wheatsheaf, 1993), pp. 27–40.

2. Anthony Zwi, "The Political Abuse of Medicine and the Challenge of Opposing It," *Social Science and Medicine* 25, no. 6: 649.

3. The "racial" terminology used in this paper employs categories legislated by the apartheid state. We submit that "race" is a social construct that serves particular political purposes; in no way do we suggest that "races" exist as essential groupings.

4. Although for the purposes of this paper we have employed the homogenizing signifier "women," we acknowledge the diversity of "women," whose heterogeneity includes age, marital status, race, sexual orientation, professional status, and class.

5. TRC [Truth and Reconciliation Commission], *Truth and Reconciliation Commission of South Africa Report* (Cape Town: TRC, 1998).

6. This call to examine the accountability of health professionals also resulted in the establishment of the HHRP, which helped to facilitate the TRC health sector hearings as well as document and analyze the involvement of health professionals in human rights violations during apartheid.

7. The hearings were internationally historic for being the first time that a truth commission has held a hearing dedicated specifically to the activities of a nation's health sector. B. Hayner, "Fifteen Truth Commissions—1974 to 1994: A Comparative Study," *Human Rights Quarterly* 16 (1995): 597–675.

8. Jeanelle de Gruchy et al., "The Difficult Road to Truth and Reconciliation— The Health Sector Takes Its First Steps," *South African Medical Journal* 88 (August 1998): 976.

9. Steve Bantu Biko was a leader of the Black Consciousness movement who died in detention following torture in 1977. The doctors involved in his care were

found to be grossly negligent and unethical in their conduct. It took concerted effort over a number of years by certain outraged doctors, including two Supreme Court challenges, to force the South African Medical and Dental Council to take disciplinary action.

10. Laurel Baldwin-Ragaven et al., "Restoring the Honour of Our Profession," *South African Medical Journal*, August 1998, 969–970.

11. Leonard Rubenstein and Leslie London, "The UDHR and the Limits of Medical Ethics: The Case of South Africa," *Health and Human Rights* 73, no. 2 (1998): 160–161.

12. Laurel Baldwin-Ragaven, Jeanelle de Gruchy, and Leslie London, eds., "Submission Date June 1999, on Target," *Commission, Omission, and Resistance: Health Professionals, Human Rights, and Ethics in South Africa* (Cape Town: UCT Press, 1999).

13. Issues of women's health, especially reproductive health, have been concerns at the forefront of the feminist struggle since the 1970s. Judith Clark and Ellen Annandale, "What Is Gender? Feminist Theory and the Sociology of Human Reproduction," *Sociology of Health and Illness* 18, no. 1 (1996), write that the struggle over women's health was "virtually synonymous with the emergence of second wave feminism." Feminists challenged the lack of women's visibility and voice with demands that women take control over their own bodies, epitomized by the slogan "Our Bodies Ourselves."

14. Zwi, "Political Abuse of Medicine," p. 650.

15. See, for example, Barbara B. Brown, "Facing the 'Black Peril': The Politics of Population Control in South Africa," *Journal of Southern African Studies*, April 3, 1987, pp. 256–273; Zwi, "Political Abuse of Medicine"; Barbara Klugman, "Balancing Means and Ends—Population Policy in South Africa," *Reproductive Health Matters*, May 1, 1993, pp. 44–57; Barbara Klugman, "The Politics of Contraception in South Africa," *Women's Studies International Forum* 13, no. 3 (1990): 261–271; Helen Rees, "Contraception: More Complex Than Just Method?" *Agenda* 27 (1995): 27–36.

16. Katarina Tomasevski, *Human Rights in Population Policies: A Study for SIDA* (Lund: Swedish International Development Authority [SIDA], 1994), p. 5.

17. Cognizant that family planning programs can be abused by states for demographic ends, leading to tension between human rights and government policies, the 1974 World Population Plan of Action laid down three requirements for population policies: "(1) absolute respect for the fundamental rights of the human being, (2) respect for dignity of the family, and (3) prohibition of coercive measures" (Tomasevski, *Human Rights*, p. 21).

18. Feminists from the "developing" world have particularly "challenged the economic and demographic theories used to justify population policies that are harmful to women." Sonia Correa, *Population and Reproductive Rights: Feminist Perspectives from the South* (London: Zed, 1994), p. 4.

19. The ICPD in Cairo (1994) was a landmark global forum that heralded a paradigm shift in the approach to sexuality and reproduction. The change was from seeing reproduction as an approach to population control to seeing women as human beings in their own right, with human rights; promoting women's health and well-being; promoting reproductive health care, including family planning;

and promoting women's sexual health without coercion. The Fourth World Conference on Women at Beijing (1995) reaffirmed the direction of Cairo but emphasized women's health as not just about reproductive and sexual health, extending the focus to life cycle health issues, from infancy to old age.

20. Nira Yuval-Davis, *Gender and Nation* (London: Sage, 1997), p. 29.

21. Ibid.

22. Stephanie Klausen, *The Race Welfare Society: Eugenics and Birth Control in Johannesburg, 1930 to 1944* (Centre for Southern African Studies, University of Sussex, 1998), p. 1.

23. Saul Dubow, *Scientific Racism in Modern South Africa* (Cambridge: Cambridge University Press, 1995), p. 1, notes that "a curious form of collective amnesia has, until quite recently, obscured the centrality of intellectual racism in Western thought during the early part of the twentieth century." In reaction to the horror of the scale of the eugenic plan of Nazi Germany, which included the forced sterilization of hundreds of thousands of people, intellectuals in Europe and America were quick to disassociate from their previously championed cause.

24. A letter to *Asijiki*, the newsletter of a South African NGO, suggests possible solutions to "the problem of street children and vagrants." Among these is "some form of compulsory or incentive driven sterilisation [which] should be introduced for street adult parents with two children" (E. V. Rapiti, letter to the editor, *Asijki*, March 1998). A letter to *Time* magazine written by a Mr. Smith from Cape Town trumpets: "Should we not restrict breeding where there are genetic problems? . . . Few people have the guts to stand up and say humans should be forced to restrict their breeding" (Andrew B. Smith, letter to the editor, *Time*, November 3, 1977 1997).

25. Nancy Stepan, *The Hour of Eugenics* (New York: Cornell University Press, 1991), p. 105.

26. Ibid.

27. Ibid., p. 106.

28. Saul Dubow, *Scientific Racism*, pp. 284, 86.

29. G. Ellison et al., "Desegregating Health Statistics and Health Research in South Africa," *South African Medical Journal* 86 (1996): 1257–1267.

30. Stepan, *Hour of Eugenics*, p. 103.

31. Ibid., p. 104.

32. Dr. Annie Porter and her husband, Dr. Fantham, were scientists. They were both members of the RWS.

33. Dubow, *Scientific Racism*, p. 184.

34. Letter from M. Stopes to E. P. Woodrow, February 8, 1945, PPASA Archives, Cape Town. Dr. Woodrow was an eminent leader in South African reproductive health. She died in 1997 at the age of ninety-six.

35. Ibid.

36. Stepan, *Hour of Eugenics*, pp. 108–109. Stepan discusses how women like Stopes and Woodrow "accepted unthinkingly the more reprehensible racial and class biases of eugenics, thereby reflecting their own privileged status as members of the middle class." That women, early "feminists" and social reformers,

found career opportunities in the eugenics movement also characterizes the complex relations between race, gender, class, and eugenics.

37. Correa, *Population and Reproductive Rights*, p. 1.

38. Klugman, "Balancing Means and Ends," p. 44.

39. Correa, *Population and Reproductive Rights*, p. 42.

40. Klugman, "The Politics of Contraception," p. 263.

41. That is, white politicians in the whites-only government.

42. Nira Yuval-Davis, *Gender and Nation*, p. 29.

43. Fred Sai, Helen Rees, and Steve McGarry, *Reproductive Health and Family Planning Consultancy: National Review and Recommendations, Final Report* (Johannesburg: Commission of the European Communities: Special Program for South Africa, 1993); Correa, *Population and Reproductive Rights*; Brown, "Facing the 'Black Peril,'" pp. 256–273.

44. HHRP, *The Final Submission of the HHRP to the Truth and Reconciliation Commission* (Cape Town: Health and Human Rights Project, 1997).

45. Klugman, "Balancing Means and Ends," p. 44.

46. Pamphlets on contraception were provided in all of the African languages, something not done in any other area of health service delivery. Zwi, "Political Abuse of Medicine."

47. In 1988, women interviewed from a factory in Natal related how, when looking for jobs, they were told that they would be injected every three months to stop them from "breeding a lot." They were told that childbirth should not interfere with production. The women said they felt defenseless and had to agree to the injections because they needed jobs. Rees, *Women and Reproductive Rights*, p. 211.

48. Typically, the demographics of farming in South Africa would be a white farmer and family, assisted by black farm laborers who traditionally live on the farm, even for many generations.

49. Department of Health and Welfare, *How the Farmer's Wife Can Promote Family Planning* (South Africa: Department of Health and Welfare, 1980). In Afrikaans.

50. Tomasevski, *Human Rights*, p. 9.

51. Lesley Doyal, "Gender, Justice, and Medical Ethics," in S. Benatar, ed., *Human Needs, Human Rights, Gender, and Medical Bioethics* (Cape Town: University of Cape Town, 1996), pp. 57–73.

52. A white doctor wrote a book called *Where Have All the Children Gone?* in which he spoke of the effectiveness of the medical profession in determining behavior. The book claimed that the profession was being duped by the government to implement family planning and that this had led to a decline in the white birthrate. However, blacks had not gone along with the program, and their rate was increasing. Edward Williams, *Where Have All the Children Gone?* (Johannesburg, South Africa: Ernest Stanton, 1980).

53. Klugman, "Politics of Contraception," p. 264.

54. Peta Thornycroft and Sam Sole, *Sunday Independent*, April 20, 1998, pp. 1–2. SADF used chimps in project to curb black fertility.

55. Basson has thus far denied his participation in experiments to control black female fertility.

56. Thornycroft and Sole, *Sunday Independent*, pp. 1–2.

57. Zwi, "Political Abuse of Medicine," p. 651.

58. Doctor at MRC, personal communication with Jeanelle de Gruchy, Cape Town, July 22, 1998.

59. Klugman, "Politics of Contraception," p. 265.

60. Ibid.

61. Sai, Rees, and McGarry, *Reproductive Health*, p. 16.

62. Ibid.

63. Helen Rees, "Women and Reproductive Rights," in S. Bazilli, ed., *Putting Women on the Agenda* (Johannesburg: Raven Press, 1991), p. 210.

64. Jeanelle de Gruchy, personal statement.

65. Michel Foucault, *The Birth of the Clinic* (London: Tavistock, 1973).

66. Bryan Turner, *Medical Power and Social Knowledge* (London: Sage, 1987), p. 13.

67. A. S. Alberts, "Die Medies Implikasies van de Versnellende Bevolkinsaan-was" [The medical implications of the population explosion], *South African Medical Journal*, September 27, 1975, pp. 1690–1694.

68. V. P. Villiers, "Bringing Down the Birth Rate," *South African Medical Journal* 84, no. 12 (1994): 870–871.

69. Sai, Rees, and McGarry, *Reproductive Health*, p. 16.

70. Brigitte Mabandla, "Sucking Out the Poison of Apartheid Science," *Sunday Independent*, June 21, 1998.

71. Pat Sidley, "Doctors Involved in South Africa's Biological Warfare Programme," *British Medical Journal*, June 20, 1998, p. 1852. Additionally, we note that no action has as yet been instituted against these doctors by the South African Health Professions' Council.

72. Otto, a participant in a Listserv discussion of Dr. Bassun's work on deveoping a fertility-regulating vaccine, made this comment.

73. Among its supporters, the anti-HCG vaccine is perceived as a promising new contraceptive technology in the global marketplace. South African research into antifertility vaccinations as methods of nonsurgical female sterilization would have been of "value" locally and internationally. Basson's diary of a visit to the United States in 1981 was brought to the TRC. It said that he was welcomed warmly by scientists and others who were more concerned with the communist threat than the increasingly unpopular racial policies of his government. . . . [U.S.] Air Force officials encouraged him to develop joint "medical projects" with the United States while other top military and defense officials extolled the virtues of chemical weapons. "He feels that chemical warfare is an ideal strategic weapon because infrastructure is preserved together with facilities and only living people are killed," Basson wrote of a conversation with Maj. Gen. William S. Augerson, who was deputy assistant secretary of defense for health resources and programs. He has since retired from the military.

This potential connection with the international scientific community is reminiscent of other situations in post–World War II history that have successfully shielded dubious research efforts, such as the cover-up of the Nazi research agenda post-Nuremberg, with the granting of asylum and new identities to those engaged in chemical warfare.

74. Helen Rees, "Contraception: More Complex Than Just a Method?" p. 31.

75. HHRP, 1997.

76. Personal interview with Dr. Esther Sapire, former chair and later president of the Planned Parenthood Association of South Africa, as well the head of the Family Planning Unit at Groote Schuur Hospital over a twenty-year period, from 1976 to 1996. HHRP August 1998.

77. De Gruchy et al., "Difficult Road to Truth and Reconciliation," pp. 975–979.

78. For example, the new South African constitution (1996) covers equality before the law; nondiscrimination on numerous grounds, including race, gender, sex, pregnancy, marital status, and sexual orientation; the right to life and human dignity; (12)(1) "the rights to freedom and security of the person, which includes the right—(c) to be free from all forms of violence from either public or private sources"; (12)(2) "the rights to bodily and psychological integrity, which includes the right—(a) to make decisions concerning reproduction (b) to security in and control over their body; and (c) not to be subjected to medical or scientific experiments without their informed consent"; (27)(1) "the rights to have access to (a) health care services, including reproductive health care."

79. Office of the Status of Women in the Vice-President's Office, the Commission on Gender Equality, the Parliamentary Joint Committee on Improvement of Quality of Life and Status of Women.

80. Barbara Klugman, bklugman@wn.apc.org. 1998. Re: Basson's fertility-regulating vaccine. 199808270935.LAA28778@wn.apc.org. Repro-L, August 27, 1998.

81. Rachel Jewkes, Zodumo Mvo, and Naeema Abrahams, "Violence Against Patients in a Cape Town Obstetric Unit," *Urbanisation and Health Newsletter (MRC)* 34 (September 1997): 25–30.

82. Mzilikazi Wa Afrika, "Schoolgirl Dies After Illegal Abortion," *Sunday Times,* September 6, 1998.

83. J. Mann et al., "Health and Human Rights," *Health and Human Rights* 1 (1994): 6–23.

Epilogue

NANCY M. WILLIAMS

What did I learn about feminist bioethics while participating in the production of this anthology? As one of the team members who brought forth this project, I discovered the many challenges that feminist bioethicists face when confronted with the task of assimilating diverse, and oftentimes conflicting, crosscultural perspectives. Primarily, I found the overriding challenge to be the reconciliation between global feminist diversity and feminist political solidarity. Can feminists from different cultural backgrounds unite in political solidarity without any one of them needing to forsake her unique "voice"? Can we "globalize" feminist bioethics without a dominant culture coming forward to assume the role of ultimate moral arbiter?

In my estimation, the international effort that this anthology represents has provided some possible answers to these pressing questions. Twenty-one authors, each articulating her or his cultural and/or theoretical perspective, demonstrated one of the common goals that all feminists share, namely, the creation of an environment in which individuals can speak freely about their own needs, interests, and rights as they perceive them so that they can join together in their resistance to any system, structure, or ideology that serves to oppress people. Only by speaking to each other honestly about the disparities in health care they perceive—indeed live—can feminists find the will and power to work together throughout the world on behalf of women and the men and children to whom they are related.

As I communicated with the authors of *Globalizing Feminist Bioethics*, I came to witness the dismantling of one of the walls that has separated feminists in the past, namely, the wall between feminists who stress personal (sexual and reproductive) issues and those who stress social (economic and political) issues. *Globalizing Feminist Bioethics* proclaims the end of this limiting dichotomy. The personal is indeed the political. In choosing (or being forced to "choose") one chooses (or is forced to choose) for others. In addition, as I worked on this anthology, I came to understand that feminist theory needs to guide men's and women's practices proportionally. Women's reproductive freedom depends, for example, on men's reproductive responsibility and vice versa. Men must be caregivers as well as carereceivers. Women must be lawmakers as well as lawabiders. The public world belongs to women no less than to men, and the private world's quality, particularly its safety, depends on men's efforts no less than women's.

The more I reflect on this volume, the more I am aware of the passion that pulses through it. I suppose I should define more precisely what I mean by passion. Obviously, passion can mean sexual desire and love, but in this context it means a strong devotion to some activity or concept. Devotion to values such as liberty, justice, equality, freedom, security, and comfort are a form of passion, in my estimation. Each one of the articles in this anthology speaks of its author's commitments and values, of her or his desire to help globalize feminist bioethics. Had I not *felt* the importance of this project, I might have found the logistics of putting it together overwhelming. Language barriers, computer glitches, and e-mail failures routinely tried my patience; but never did it occur to me or the editors of this book to give up their efforts. On the contrary, they motivated all of us to try harder.

On a final note, *Globalizing Feminist Bioethics* offers significant opportunities for conceptualizing and practicing a global feminist bioethics. Women and men everywhere are coming together in the shared hope of helping each other recognize and resolve the problems that result in some people's pressing health care needs not being met in a just and compassionate manner. While writing this epilogue, I came across lines from Rosemarie Tong's reflections on feminist bioethics.

> There is no such thing as feminist armchair bioethics. Feminist approaches to bioethics require actual discourse. . . . We need to remember what our goal is, namely, to make the world of health care one that structures and organizes itself so as to serve men and women (as well as all races and classes) equally.[1]

I believe the production of *Globalizing Feminist Bioethics* moves us closer to the goal that Tong envisions.

If feminist theory can persuade people (women and men) to think and behave differently than they have in the past, then (in the words of Richard Rorty) it deserves the title of "revolutionary" philosophy. I am very proud to have played a role in what I regard as very revolutionary philosophy. Indeed, one would be hard-pressed to find another collection of essays that goes as far as this one does in the direction of globalizing bioethics. This project presents new ways of thinking about existing health care ideologies and institutions. It has enhanced my understanding of feminism and how it can inspire hope for all people, but particularly women worldwide. Moreover, this anthology has further politicized me, inviting me to fight against the routine injustices that distort the quality, cost, and availability of health care goods and services in my own nation, the United States, and elsewhere. Finally, *Globalizing Feminist Bioethics* has further freed my philosophical imagination, enabling me to vision what truly healthy people might look, be, and act like. Readers of *Globalizing Feminist Bioethics* have their work cut out for them, for the message of this volume is that contemplation without action is idle speculation and that practice without theory is random motion.

Notes

1. Rosemarie Tong, *Feminist Approaches to Bioethics: Theoretical Reflections and Practical Applications* (Boulder: Westview, 1997), p. 245.

About the Editors and Contributors

William M. Alexander is Emeritus Professor of World Food Politics at California Polytechnic State University. Since retiring in 1988, Dr. Alexander has worked to solve the mystery of the Kerala phenomenon—high well-being measures in the Indian state of Kerala, which accords women high status, within the low well-being measures of all India. In this work, he has served as consultant for the Institute for Food Development Policy and as principal investigator for Earthwatch Expeditions.

Gwen W. Anderson, one of this book's coeditors, has a Ph.D. in nursing and is a postdoctoral fellow at Stanford University's Center for Bioemedical Ethics and is a research associate and faculty member at the Shriver Center for Mental Retardation. From 1998 to 1999, she was the principal investigator at the National Institutes of Health's Human Genome Research Institute. Recent publications have covered such topics as genetic services, nursing and genetics, and genetics and ethics. With P. Field and P. Mack, she contributed "Uncertain Motherhood: When All Is Not Well In the Childbearing Years" to *The Experience of Motherhood* (1994). She is an advisory board member of the Feminist Approaches to Bioethics Network.

Laurel Baldwin-Ragaven is a lecturer at the Department of Primary Health Care and Family Medicine at the University of Cape Town in Cape Town, South Africa. She is also a member of the health sciences faculty at the Groote Schuur Hospital in Cape Town, South Africa. She is the Feminist Approaches to Bioethics Network country representative for South Africa.

Mary A. Bendfeld is working toward the completion of a master's in philosophy at Dalhousie University in Halifax, Canada. She has done research with the Provincial Health Ethics Network and with the John Dosseter Bioethics Centre at the University of Alberta, Edmonton. She was the recipient of the Olga Hunchak Memorial Bursary and the Louise McKinney Scholarship as an undergraduate student at the University of Alberta, Edmonton. She has been nominated for the Izaak Walter Killam Fellowship by the Department of Philosophy at Dalhousie University.

Vangie Bergum has a Ph.D. in philosophy. She is a professor of nursing at the University of Alberta, Edmonton, and the interim codirector of the John Dossetor Health Ethics Center. Her publications include *Relational Ethics: The Full Meaning of Respect*, "Relational Ethics: What Is It?" in *In Touch: Provincial Health Ethics Network Newsletter*, and "Awakening the Moral Self: The Meaning of Quickening" in the *Bioethics Bulletin*. She has also presented on the topics of ethics, relational ethics, and health care ethics at workshops and conferences. From 1997 to 1999 she chaired the Conference Planning Committee of the Canadian Bioethics Society and the International Association of Bioethics conference in October 1999.

Fernanda Carneiro has a master's and a Ph.D. in production engineering from the Knowledge, Power, and Ethics Program of the Federal University of Rio de Janeiro. She has been a parliamentary adviser on reproductive rights. Currently she is a consultant in research ethics for the Oswaldo Cruz Foundation, works for the Fernandes Figueira Hospital in Rio, and coordinates the Ethics Committee in Pesquisa. She is coauthor of *Human Genetics Resources: Access Limits*.

Leonardo D. de Castro, Ph.D., is professor and chair of the Department of Philosophy at the University of the Philippines. He is the recipient of a National Book Award given by the Manila Critics Circle and a University of the Philippines Diliman Chancellor's Award for a book on bioethics and technology written in Filipino.

Jeanelle de Gruchy is a medical doctor with a master of arts degree in women's studies. She has worked clinically both in South Africa and the United Kingdom and is currently training to be a specialist in public health. She has been involved in health and human rights work, particularly through her work as a research fellow (1997–1999) with the Health and Human Rights Project (HHRP), a South African nongovernmental organization. The HHRP documented the involvement of health professionals in human rights abuses during apartheid and made a submission to South Africa's Truth and Reconciliation Commission (TRC) in 1997. Jeanelle was a coeditor of the book that was based on this submission, *An Ambulance of the Wrong Colour: Health Professionals, Human Rights, and Ethics in South Africa* (1999). She has published numerous articles in peer-reviewed journals, including the *Lancet*, *South African Medical Journal*, and *Feminism and Psychology*. She is a Feminist Approaches to Bioethics Network advisory board member.

Debora Diniz is an anthropologist. She is a lecturer of bioethics and feminist ethics and is a member of the health science faculty at the University of Brasilia, Brazil. She is a member of the board of directors of Anis, the Institute of Bioethics, Human Rights, and Gender. She is the Feminist Approaches to Bioethics Network country representative for Brazil.

Anne Donchin is a professor of philosophy at Indiana University. She was one of the cofounders and original co-coordinators of the Feminist Approaches to Bioethics Network. Currently, she is the organization's treasurer. With Laura Purdy, she edited the book *Embodying Bioethics* (1999). She has published extensively on the topics of autonomy and reproductive technology and is widely regarded as one of the major figures in feminist bioethics.

Roberto dos Santos Bartholo Jr. has a master of science degree in mathematical models applied to production engineering from the Federal University of Rio de Janeiro, as well as a doctorate in economic and social sciences from the University of Erlangen-Nurnberg in Germany. He is a professor at the Federal University of Rio de Janeiro, where he created the laboratory for technology and social development. His recent publications include *Sustainable Amazon*, with Marcel Bursztyn, and "The United States' Influence in the Making of the Contemporary Amazon Heartland" in David Slater and Peter Taylor's *Challenging the American Century: Consensus and Coercion in the Projection of American Power* (Blackwell).

Lisa A. Eckenwiler has a Ph.D. in philosophy and is a professor of philosophy at Old Dominion University in Norfolk, Virginia. Her areas of specialization include moral philosophy and biomedical ethics. Her publications include "Justice and Access to Therapies for AIDS," "Pursing Reform in Clinical Research: Lessons from Women's Experience," and *Institutional Policy in Pediatric Practice: Documenting Canadian Experience*, with Francoise Baylis and Louise Kunicki (1994). She is a member of the Feminist Approaches to Bioethics Network.

Helen B. Holmes has a Ph.D. in genetics and currently coordinates the Center for Genetics, Ethics, and Women in Amherst, Massachusetts. She was one of the cofounders and original co-coordinators of the Feminist Approaches to Bioethics Network. Among the many programs she has organized was a workshop funded by the Ethics Branch of the National Center for Human Genome Research. Her research on reproductive technologies has taken her to the Netherlands and New Zealand (as a Fulbright scholar). With Laura Purdy, she edited *Feminist Perspectives in Medical Ethics*.

Loretta M. Kopelman has a Ph.D. in philosophy and is a professor of medical humanities at East Carolina University's school of medicine. She has held panel positions at the National Endowment for the Humanities (NEH) and the National Institutes of Health (NIH) since 1982 and has been a member of the board of directors and the editorial board of the *Journal of Medicine and Philosophy* since 1986. She was the founding president of the American Society for Bioethics and Humanities from 1997 to 1998. She is editor of the forthcoming *Decisions at the End of Life and Physician-Assisted Suicide* and *Building Bioethics: Conversations with Clouser and Friends on Medical Ethics* (Kluwer Academic Publishers).

Kathleen S. Kurtz is working toward the completion of her Ph.D. in social sciences from Syracuse University, where she also earned a master's degree in social work. Kathleen has taught courses in conjunction with Syracuse Law School, the School of Social Work, the Center for Policy Research, and the Women's Studies Program. She is currently an adjunct professor of human services at Cazenovia College. Recent publications include a contribution to the *Encyclopedia of Feminist Theory* and a review of *Killing the Black Body* for the Feminist Approaches to Bioethics *Newsletter*.

Wang Jin-ling is a professor at the Zhejiang Academy of Social Sciences in Hangzhou, China. Her main research interests are in gender studies, especially in women's health, prostitution, and the development of rural women. Her publications include *The Man in Chinese Society* (1993), *Growing Up in Family: From Childhood to Adulthood* (1994), and *Analysis of Prostitutes in Mainland China* (1998). *Analysis of Prostitutes* is considered the first work researching prostitutes' issues in mainland China from a feminist perspective.

Florencia Luna received a master of arts degree from the University of Columbia and a Ph.D. in philosophy from the University of Buenos Aires. She teaches bioethics at FLASCO (Latin American University of Social Sciences) and at the University of Buenos Aires (UBA). She has been a board member of the International Association of Bioethics (IAB) since 1999. She is also the Feminist Approaches to Bioethics Network country representative for Argentina. She is a temporary adviser to the World Health Organization and CIOMS. She is directing a research program on bioethics at FLASCO and is editing *Perspectivas Bioeticas*, the first Argentinian journal wholly devoted to bioethics. She has coauthored the books *Decisiones De Vida y Muerte* and *Bioetica*.

Mary B. Mahowald is a professor in the College, the Department of Obstetrics and Gynecology, the MacLean Center for Clinical Medical Ethics, and the Committee on Genetics at the University of Chicago. A philosopher by training, Dr. Mahowald taught in the philosophy departments at Villanova University and Indiana University before moving to a medical school/hospital setting in 1982. Since then, she has published numerous articles in health care as well as in philosophical journals. She has had grants or fellowships from the National Institutes of Health, the Department of Energy and the National Endowment for the Humanities (NEH). Her most recent books include *Women and Children in Health Care: An Unequal Majority* (1996); *Disability, Difference, Discrimination: Perspectives on Justice in Bioethics and Public Policy* (1998). With Anita Silvers and David Wasserman, she coauthored the third edition of her *Philosophy of Woman: Classical to Current Concepts* (1994) and *Genes, Women, Equality* (2000).

Naoko T. Miyaji received her M.D. and Ph.D. from Kyoto Prefectural University of Medicine. She was a visiting fellow in the Department of Social Medicine at Harvard Medical School in 1989 and in the Human Rights Program at Harvard Law School from 1990 to 1992. She is currently an assistant professor at the Department of Hygiene at Kinki University School of Medicine. Her academic interests are in cultural psychiatry, medical anthropology, feminism, bioethics, and public health. She also organizes an NGO—AMDA at the International Medical Information Center Kansai—that provides aid to foreign patients. She is the Feminist Approaches to Bioethics Network country representative for Japan.

Rita B. Monsen has her doctor of science degree in nursing and is a nursing education consultant. She was formerly an adjunct graduate faculty member at the University of Central Arkansas and at the College of Nursing at the University of Arkansas for Medical Sciences. Rita has also held positions as a genetic counselor with the Spina Bifida Clinic at Arkansas Children's Hospital and was the genetics division coordinator at the University of Southern California Medical Center. Her work has been published in the *Journal of Pediatric Nursing, Nursing Forum,* and *Omega: The Journal of Death and Dying.* She is an executive board member of the International Society of Nurses in Genetics, was a representative for the American Nurses Association, and was interim cochair of the National Coalition for Health Professional Education in Genetics.

Julien S. Murphy is professor of philosophy and associate dean of the College of Arts and Sciences at the University of Southern Maine. She is the author of the *Constructed Body: AIDS, Reproductive Technology, and Ethics* (1995). She is the editor of *Feminist Interpretations of Jean-Paul Sartre* (1999).

Jing-Bao Nie, M.D., Ph.D., is a lecturer in the Bioethics Centre at the University of Otago, Dunedin, New Zealand. Dr. Nie has published numerous Chinese and English works on the history and philosophy of Chinese medicine, comparative medicine, medical sociology, and bioethics. He is finishing a book titled *Voices Behind the Silence: Mainland Chinese Views and Experiences of Abortion.*

Carol Quinn is a doctoral candidate in the philosophy department at Syracuse University. She teaches courses in feminist philosophy and ethics. She has published papers and given talks on the topic of ethics and the Holocaust. Her other research interests include social philosophy, bioethics, and the philosophy of trauma.

Mary V. Rorty has a doctorate degree in philosophy and a master's degree in clinical ethics. She has written on topics in ancient philosophy, feminism, and bioethics. She was director of advanced studies at the University of Virginia Center for Biomedical Ethics for five years and is currently associated with the Stanford University Center of Biomedical Ethics. She is one of the authors of *Organizational Ethics in Health Care* (1999). She is a Feminist Approaches to Bioethics Network advisory board member.

Alejandra A. Rotania is an Argentine Brazilian with a master's degree in social sciences and a Ph.D. in production engineering from the Federal University of Rio de Janeiro. She is on the board of directors of Ser Mulher, the Center for the Study of Urban and Rural Women. Her publications in Portuguese include her dissertation, "New Reproductive Technologies and Genetics, Ethics, and Feminism: The Celebration of the Fear." She is the Feminist Approaches to Bioethics Network country representative for Brazil.

Aida Santos, one of this book's coeditors, is the project director of the Philippine Network Against Trafficking in Women and is a faciliator-trainer at the Institute for Women's Studies. She previously was the executive director of women's education. She has served as a consultant to such organizations as the National Commission on the Role of Filipino Women and the World Health Organization's office in Manila. Her publications include *Woman-to-Woman* (1994) and *Women Empowering Women* (1993). She is a Feminist Approaches to Bioethics Network advisory board member and is the country representative for the Philippines.

Susan Sherwin has a Ph.D. in philosophy and is a professor of philosophy at Dalhousie University in Halifax, Nova Scotia. She was the principal investigator for the SSHRC Strategic Research Network Grant for Feminist Health Care Ethics from 1993 to 1998 and principal research fellow for the Rockefeller Foundation's International Study and Conference Center in Italy in 1999. Her publications include *The Politics of Women's Health: Exploring Agency and Autonomy* (1998), *No Longer Patient: Feminist Ethics and Health Care* (1992), and *Health Care Ethics in Canada* (Harcourt Brace, 1995). She is an advisory board member of the Feminist Approaches to Bioethics Network and of the International Association of Bioethics.

Nadine Taub received her B.A. from Swarthmore College and her LL.B. from Yale. She has a diploma in graduate legal studies from Stockholm University. She has been on the Rutgers faculty since 1974, where she is now a professor of law and S.I. Newhouse Scholar. She authored *The Law of Sex Discrimination* and writes widely on issues of equality theory, reproductive freedom, and women and work. Her litigation victories include one of the first cases to establish the right to sue for sexual harassment and the case that required the State of New Jersey to pay for abortions as part of its Medicaid program. Other publications include *Reproductive Laws for the 1990s*, with Sherrill Cohen (1988),

Rosemarie Tong, one of this book's editors, is Distinguished Professor in Health Care Ethics in the Department of Philosophy at the University of North Carolina at Charlotte. An award-winning teacher and prolific writer and lecturer, she is the author of *Women, Sex, and the Law* (1984), *Feminine and Feminist Ethics*

(1993), *Feminist Approaches to Bioethics: Theoretical Reflections and Practical Applications* (1997), and *Feminist Thought: A More Comprehensive Introduction* (1998). Tong currently serves as co-coordinator of the International Network on Feminist Approaches to Bioethics Network.

Ana Cristina González Vélez is a medical doctor who has done postgraduate research on social aspects of sexual and reproductive health. She is a researcher for the private organization SISMA-MUJER. She is also a member of the Latin American and Caribbean Women's Health Network (LACWHN) and the National Organization for Women in Colombia, as well as FAB's country representative for Colombia. Currently she represents LACWHN on the steering committee of the International Conference for Health Research for Development.

Jurema Werneck is a physician who has worked in community health in the slums of Rio de Janeiro. She is a master's degree candidate in production engineering in the Knowledge, Power, and Ethics Program of the Federal University of Rio de Janeiro. Currently she is general coordinator of CRIOLA, a black women's nongovernmental organization. She has written about mass sterilization and from 1990 to 1992 coordinated the National Campaign Against Mass Sterilization.

Nancy M. Williams is currently an instructor at the University of North Carolina at Charlotte, where she teaches philosophy and feminist theory. She earned a master's degree in philosophy from the University of South Florida in 1997. In 2001, she will continue her studies as a Ph.D. candidate at the University of Georgia. She has published articles on feminist ethics and has presented several papers on feminist theory at various universities.

Index

Abdalla, Ruquiya H. D., 223, 225, 226, 227
Ableism, 28
  and sex selection, 170, 176(n12)
Aboriginal people, organ transplantation among, 23
Abortion, 89
  in China, 151, 157–159, 159–163
  economic stake in, 94(n50)
  in Japan, 85–89, 94(n54), 149(n19)
  in Japan, personal accounts of, 151–157
  and male responsibility for contraception, 136–137
  rate per year, 94(n50)
  and reproductive technologies, 96, 98
  and sex selection, 173
  and spouse's consent, 149(n19)
  in United States, 162
  See also Pregnancy termination; Sex-selective abortion
Absolutism, 28
  and sex selection, 174–175
  and women's oppression, 29
Abstract reasoning
  and metaphors, 15
Accountability
  and health care professionals, 320–322, 328(n6)
ACTG. See AIDS Clinical Trials Group
Adoption, 124–125, 133(n29)
  and infertility, 122–123
  vs. conception, assisted, 128–130
Aesthetics
  and metaphors, 15

Africa
  female genital mutilation in, 71(n21)
African Americans
  and sickle cell screening, 39
  and unethical medical research, 284
Africa (north)
  female genital circumcision in, 223
AIDS
  and men's sexual behavior, 147
  research, 261–263
  See also HIV/AIDS
AIDS Clinical Trials Group (ACTG), 257, 271
Alcoff, Linda, 286, 288
"Alienation" argument, 292–293
AMA. See American Medical Association
American Medical Association (AMA)
  and female genital circumcision, 220, 234
Animals
  and cloning, 200
Antifertility vaccine
  in South Africa (apartheid), 321, 324, 332(n73)
Antifoundationalism
  and bioethical reasoning, 28
Anti-HCG vaccine, 332(n73)
Antinomy, 120
Antisperm vaccination, 149(n21)
Apartheid
  health care professionals during, 312–315
  reproductive health policies during, 312–315

and scientific racism, 315–317
See also South Africa (apartheid)
Arabia (southern)
female genital circumcision in, 223
Arapesh
adoption among, 124
Argentina
and International Criminal Court,
256
research on women in, 259–260
Aristotelianism, 70(n19)
Artificial reproduction, 123
Artificial insemination
and reproductive technologies, 97
Artificial insemination-husband,
132(n24)
Artificial wombs, 132(n24)
Asexual Reproduction (Sang), 202
Asia
adoption in, 133(n29)
well-being statistical data,
185(table)
Atomism, 43
Attentional dynamics, 81–82
Attitude of realism, 86
Augerson, William S., 332(n73)
Authentic insider
and third world development, 30,
31
Autonomy, 115–116
and black women, 131(n2)
and female genital circumcision,
169
and fetal monitors, 104
meaning of, 167, 175(n3)
relational, 110
and reproductive technologies,
97–99, 110–111, 120
respect for, and cultural difference,
166–169
respect for, and cultural values,
165–166
and right to choose, 130
and traditional bioethics, 65–66,
301–303
and ultrasound technology, 104
See also Women's autonomy

Avoid-death-at-all-costs culture, 303
AZT drug trials, 254, 262, 273
on HIV-infected women, 254
and unethical practices, 285
in United States, 257–258

Babbitt, Susan, 288
Bangladesh, 191
unethical medical research in, 285
Basson, Wouter, 321, 324, 331(n55),
332(n73)
Bauman, Zygmunt, 92(n14)
Bayles, Michael, 178(n30)
BDPA. *See* Beijing Declaration and
Platform for Action
Beauchamp, Tom, 62–63, 67, 68(n1)
Beauty
and female genital circumcision,
226–227
Beecher, Henry, 284
Behavior roles
and moral behavior, 63
Beiguelman, Bernardo, 123
Beijing Declaration and Platform for
Action (BDPA), 135, 148(n5),
149(n17)
Belgium
infanticide in, 209(n1)
Beneficence, 115, 116
and *kagandahang loob*, 55
and traditional bioethics, 65–66
Berger, Robert, 294
Bergum, Vangie, 76
Berlinguer, Giovanni, 127
Biko, Steve, 314–315, 328–329(n9)
Biko doctors, 314
Biodiversity
and cloning, 200
Bioethical reasoning
and relativism, 28
Bioethics
in Brazil, 67, 69(n6)
in Canada, 67
future of, 127
and health care, 70(n17)
in Latin America, 134(n43)
and metaphors, 15

Flew, Anthony, 221
Floyd-Davis, Robbie, 83
Ford Foundation, 1
Form of the personal, 75, 80–81,
    89–90, 91(n5)
Foundations model
    moral theories as, 14–15, 17–19, 20,
    25
Fourth World Conference on Women
    (Beijing), 330(n19)
Fox, Renee, C., 307
Frameworks model
    moral theories as, 15, 19–23
France
    and female genital circumcision,
    220
    Intracytoplasmic sperm injection
    by micromanipulation in,
    133(n26)
Freedom, 32, 167, 175(n4)
    and cloning, 198, 203–204, 205
    and population control, 315
    and women's difference, 29
Free will, 53–55
Friendship
    and feminist practical dialogue, 33

Gametes, uniting, 132(n24)
Ganda, 52
Gandhi, Mahatma, 187
Garcia Lorca, Federico, 122
Garrafa, Volnei, 127
Gay men
    and cloning, 206–207
GDI. *See* Gender-Related
    Development Index
GEM. *See* Gender Empowerment
    Measure
Gender
    and eugenics, 317
    and justice, 167–168
    and sex selection, 174
Gender differences, 180–181
Gender-differentiated ethics, theory
    of, 63–64
Gender Empowerment Measure
    (GEM), 147

Gender equality
    and well-being, 186, 188, 196
Gender identity
    and moral behavior, 63
Gender inequality
    in China, 163
Gender liberation, 35
Gender-Related Development Index
    (GDI), 147
Gender roles
    and health care decisions, 165
Gene-linked diseases
    and cloning, 208–209
Genes
    and well-being, 198
Genetic counseling
    in Brazil, 214, 218(n4)
    and dialogue, 212, 214
    and freely given consent, 214,
    218(n4)
    and I-Thou/I-It, 213
    personal account of, 214–217
Genetic diagnosis
    of fetus, 149(n20)
Genetic factors
    for breast cancer, 212, 214–217
Genetic health care services
    need for, 38–40
    and nursing, 37, 38, 40–48
    See also Health care
Geneticists
    female, and sex selection, 178(n35)
Genetic research, 123–124
Genetics
    and models of practice, 43–46
Genital cancer
    and reproductive technologies,
    102–103
Genital mutilation. *See* Female
    Genital Circumcision; Female
    genital mutilation
German Democratic Republic
    adoption in, 124–125
German medical community, 294
German medical schools
    and Nazi medical data, 283
Gilligan, Carol, 63–64, 162

female infanticide in, 190–191
and female-to-male ratio, 188–190,
189(figure), 190(figure), 191
girl child neglect in, 191
and health care discrimination,
179–180
organ vending in, 307
sex selection in, 172, 173, 174
sustainability in, 183–184
well-being in, 183–184
well-being statistical data,
185(table), 185–186
See also Kerala, India
*Indian Economic and Social
Opportunities*, 185
Individual freedom
and state intervention, 145,
150(n24)
Individualism, 14
and cloning, 199
Infanticide
in Belgium, 209(n1)
female, in India, 190
Infant mortality
and female literacy, relationship
between, 186–187, 187(figure)
and health care discrimination, 191
in India, 185(table), 185–186
in poor countries, 105–106
Infertility
and adoption, 122–123
and reproductive technologies,
106–107
research, and feminists, 207–208
Infibulation, 220, 221, 222, 224, 228
See also Female genital
circumcision; Female genital
mutilation
Information, categorization of,
93(n30)
Intellectual racism, 317, 330(n23)
Intentions to act, 80–81
Interdisciplinary genetic model of
practice
and health care delivery, 44–45
International Association of Bioethics,
72(n33)

International Conference on
Harmonisation (ICH), 249,
252
International Conference on
Population and Development
(ICPD), 135, 326, 329(n19)
International Criminal Court, 256,
264(n3)
International Federation of
Gynecology and Obstetrics
and female genital circumcision,
220
International Reproductive Rights
Research Action Group
(IRRRAG), 34
Intracytoplasmic sperm injection by
micromanipulation (ICSI),
133(n26)
Intravaginal ejaculation, 148(n13)
In vitro fertilization (IVF), 107–110,
123, 132(n24), 133(n26), 201
personal account of, 118–120
and reproductive technologies,
96–97
in Seoul, 207
Iraq
organ vending in, 307
Irreversibility of action, 92(n29)
IRRRAG. *See* International
Reproductive Rights Research
Action Group
Islam
and female genital circumcision,
220
Israel
sex selection in, 178(n31)
I-Thou relationship, 120, 132(n12),
213, 218(n2)
"It's About Time You Take Us
Seriously" argument, 287
IUDs, 98
IVF. *See* In vitro fertilization
Ivory Coast
HIV/AIDS in, 273

Jadeja Rajput, 190, 192
Jaggar, Allison, 32–34

Moral theories, 12, 13
 as foundations model, 14–15,
  17–19, 20, 25
 as frameworks model, 15, 19–23
 as lenses model, 15, 23–25
 and metaphors, 14–16
 See also Moral beliefs
Morgan, Robin, 32
Mortality, female
 and fatal daughter syndrome,
  195–196
Mothers' Clinics, 317–318
Multicultural feminism
 and health care, 31–32
Multidisciplinary genetic model of
  practice
 and health care delivery, 44
Mundugumor
 adoption among, 124
Muslims, 192
 and female genital circumcision,
  220, 224
Mutuality of restrictions, 58

Nagel, Thomas, 288–289
Nagmamagandang loob, 51
Nairobi
 female genital circumcision in, 219
Nambudiri Brahmins, 194, 195
Nankurrai, Priscilla, 219
Narayan, Uma, 29–30, 31
National Institutes of Health (NIH),
  267–268
 and unethical medical research,
  285
Nationalism
 and scientific racism, 316–317
National Sample Survey, 185
Nayars, 194–195
Nazi Germany
 eugenic plan of, 330(n23)
Nazi medical data, 282–295, 332(n73)
 and feminist standpoint theory,
  286–293
Neglect, child. *See* Child neglect
Negotiating Reproductive Rights
 (Petchesky and Judd), 34

Neonatal intensive care units, 97
Neonatal surgery, 97
New England Journal of Medicine, 257,
  284
New Guinea
 adoption in, 124
New reproductive technologies
  (NRTs), 123–125, 132(n24)
 perversion in use of, 132(n24)
 in Third World countries, 130
 See also Reproductive technologies
New York City
 female genital circumcision in, 220
NGOs. *See* Nongovernmental
  organizations
Nietzche, Friedrich, 70(n11)
Nigeria, 34
NIH. *See* National Institutes of Health
Noddings, Ned, 54
No Exit (Sartre), 198
Noncontraceptive sex, 148(n13)
 education about, 149(n18)
 forced, 140, 148(n14)
 legal formulations for, 137–139
 and paternity, proof of, 142,
  143–144
 and women's vulnerability,
  140–141
 and written consent, 144
Nondualist cultures
 and pregnancy, experience of, 74–75
Nonfeminist moral relativism, 65
Nonfeminists
 and feminists, friendship between,
  33
Nongovernmental organizations
  (NGOs)
 and empowerment approaches to
  research, 273
Nonmaleficence
 and traditional bioethics, 65–66
"Normal" baby
 and cultural imaginary, 92(n26)
 and visualization technologies, 80,
  92(n26)
North America
 contraception in, 98

See also Technology
Technology, 27
  and scarcity, 199
  See also Technological worldview
Thailand
  HIV/AIDS in, 263, 273
  unethical medical research in, 285
Thalidomide, 102, 209(n1), 249, 253
Theories, moral. *See* Moral theories
Third World countries, 32
  adoption in, 124
  new reproductive technologies in,
    130
  reproductive technologies in,
    134(n44)
Third world development
  and cultural diversity, 30–31
Thomas, Laurence, 288
Throughput
  and efficiency, 183
  and knowledge, 182–183
  and sustainability, 182–183
  and zero population growth, 183
Tissue banking, 132(n24)
Togo
  female genital circumcision in, 221
Tong, Rosemarie, 64, 69(n7), 69(n8)
Torture
  and health care professionals, 313
Traditional bioethics, 67–68
  and autonomy, 301–303
  principles of, 65–66
Traditional societies
  and genetic health care services,
    38–39
Transcultural/ahistorical ethics,
  71(n32)
Transcultural medical practice
  in Brazil, 67
Transdisciplinary genetic model of
    practice
  and health care delivery, 44, 45–46
TRC. *See* Truth and Reconciliation
    Commission
Truth and Reconciliation Commission
  (TRC), 313–314, 321, 323–324,
    328(n6), 328(n7), 332(n73)

Tuskegee syphilis study, 284

UAGA. *See* Uniform Anatomical Gift
  Act
Uganda
  HIV/AIDS in, 263, 273
Ultrasound technology, 77–78, 83, 90,
    100, 101–104
  and autonomy, 104
  in Japan, 94(n48)
  and sex selection, 171, 177(n19)
  in United States, 177(n19)
UNAIDS. *See* Joint United Nationals
  Programme on HIV/AIDS
Understanding, 93(n35)
  and knowledge, 82, 93(n34)
UNICEF
  and female genital circumcision,
    220, 227
Uniform Anatomical Gift Act
  (UAGA), 304, 305
Uniqueness
  and cloning, 201–202
United Kingdom
  cloning in, 206
  and female genital circumcision,
    220
United Nations
  and female genital circumcision,
    220
United Nations Development
  Program, 147, 180
United Nations Security Council, 256
United States
  abortion in, 75, 98, 162
  adoption in, 133(n29)
  AZT drug trials in, 257=258
  bioethics in, 67
  civil rights in, 28
  democratic research in, 267–272
  drug trial regulation in, 249–252
  and female genital circumcision,
    220
  and International Criminal Court,
    256
  and male responsibility for
    contraception, 137

CPSIA information can be obtained
at www.ICGtesting.com
Printed in the USA
FFHW021349241218
49986346-54680FF